THE BLOOD BRAIN BARRIER

THE BLOOD BRAIN BARRIER

TOMAS R. HELIO
EDITOR

Nova Science Publishers, Inc.
New York

For permission to use material from this book please contact us:
Telephone 631-231-7269; Fax 631-231-8175
Web Site: http://www.novapublishers.com

LIBRARY OF CONGRESS CATALOGING-IN-PUBLICATION DATA

The blood brain barrier / Tomas R. Helio, editor.
p. ; cm.
Includes bibliographical references and index.
ISBN 978-1-60456-894-3 (hardcover)
1. Blood-brain barrier. I. Helio, Tomas R.
[DNLM: 1. Blood-Brain Barrier. WL 200 B6545 2008]
QP375.5B5269 2008
573.8'621--dc22 2008024681

Published by Nova Science Publishers, Inc. ✦ New York

CONTENTS

PREFACE

The blood-brain barrier (BBB) is a membranic structure that acts primarily to protect the brain from chemicals in the blood, while still allowing essential metabolic function. It is composed of endothelial cells, which are packed very tightly in brain capillaries. This higher density restricts passage of substances from the bloodstream much more than endothelial cells in capillaries elsewhere in the body. Astrocyte cell projections called astrocytic feet (also known as "glia limitans") surround the endothelial cells of the BBB, providing biochemical support to those cells. The BBB is distinct from the similar blood-cerebrospinal fluid barrier, a function of the choroidal cells of the choroid plexus, and from the Blood-retinal barrier, which can be considered a part of the whole (the retina of the eye is an extension to the central nervous system and as such, can be considered part of the BBB).

Chapter 1 - Homeostatic regulation of the central nervous system (CNS) micro-environment and its immune-privileged status are maintained by the blood brain barrier (BBB). The capillaries in the CNS, formed by a continuous layer of endothelial cells with tight junctions between them, are the main structural component of the BBB. Other cells contributing to the regulation of the BBB function are the astrocytes, pericytes and perivascular microglia. Disruption of the BBB is a key feature of many conditions such as stroke, multiple sclerosis, Alzheimer's disease and head injury. Increased leakiness of the BBB in these disorders results from enhanced pinocytic activity of the endothelial cells and derangement of the tight junction proteins. Swelling of astrocytic end feet associated with the capillaries, activation of microglia and pericyte loss are associated with dysfunction of the BBB which results in cerebral edema. Many factors such as enhanced production of vascular endothelial growth factor, nitric oxide, degradation of extracellular matrix, free radicals and inflammatory cytokines may mediate the BBB breakdown. Although future research is needed to look into possible therapeutic strategies to improve the functioning of BBB in CNS disorders, experimental studies so far have reported beneficial effect of melatonin, curcumin, simvastatin, minocycline and some other drugs in ameliorating the increased BBB permeability in various neurological disorders.

Chapter 2 - Multiple Sclerosis (MS) is an inflammatory demyelinating disease of the Central Nervous System (CNS), characterized by multifocal perivascular infiltrates made up predominantly of lymphocytes and macrophages, in which lymphocyte recruitment into the brain across the blood-brain barrier (BBB) is critical to disease pathogenesis. Recent investigations have identified crucial components involved in leukocyte migration, providing new insights into mechanisms modulating these neuroinflammatory reactions, as well as novel targets for potential therapeutic strategies aimed at altering CNS inflammatory cell influx. Benefits of interferon β (IFN-β) and methylprednisolone treatment for example, have been associated with adhesion molecule (AM) pathway regulation. Likewise, monoclonal antibodies (mAb) against α_4 integrin have been shown to reduce clinical and MRI activity in experimental autoimmune encephalomyelitis (EAE), decreasing transmigration of lymphocytes to areas of inflammation, and reducing leukocyte activation and proliferation. Similarly, humanized mAb against α_4 integrin (natalizumab) has recently been successfully tested in MS patients. Interference in chemokine-chemokine receptor interactions may represent yet another new molecular target for novel MS therapies, such as IFN-β and statins. Beneficial effects of IFN-β in MS are mediated through T cell metalloproteinase (MMP) production suppression and increased transcription of inhibitory factors such as tissue inhibitor of metalloproteinase (TIMP). Recently minocycline for example, a tetracycline analogue, has demonstrated EAE severity attenuation through inhibition of MMP-2 and MMP-9 activity.

The presence of the BBB significantly limits therapeutic efficacy of anti-inflammatory molecules or neurotrophic factors administered systemically to patients affected by immune-mediated inflammatory diseases of the CNS like MS. Among some of the novel approaches attempting to overcome this barrier, current research has focused on the study of endogenous peptides that naturally cross it (e.g. insulin, and transferrin) through receptor-mediated endocytosis; the specific receptors involved in this process tend to preserve their transportation properties when linked to potential therapeutic agents, presenting an interesting new platform facilitating drug access into the CNS. Another alternative is the encapsulation of molecules into liposomes, which can then be directed to enter the brain. Under this approach, drugs, neurotrophic peptides, antisense oligonucleotides or genes would be incorporated into the centre of a liposome, and its surface then coated with polyethylene glycol (PEG) to prolong half-life. Current knowledge of cell-trafficking across BBB endothelium and into the CNS has increased significantly in recent years, promising further advances in the rational design of new therapeutic alternatives for the treatment of inflammatory neurological conditions such as MS.

Chapter 3 - Cerebrovascular disease with inadequate blood supply to brain and ischemic stroke is largely a disease of later life and results in death or permanent disability in around 2/3rds of cases. An early event in stroke is damage to the brain microvasculature and disruption of the blood-brain barrier (BBB) which in itself can lead to neuronal damage since the BBB normally maintains homeostasis of the delicate brain environment. Current treatments for stroke focus on re-establishment of cerebral blood flow and on neuro-protection, however there is concern that blood reperfusion contributes to further BBB disruption with subsequent edema and the increased possibility of hemorrhage. There is increasing interest in the mechanisms underlying BBB disruption, both to further understanding of the pathogenesis of cerebral ischemia and to identify new therapeutic targets aiding vascular (and thus neuronal) integrity. The cause of BBB disruption is multi-factorial and may involve matrix metalloproteinases, reactive oxygen species, nitric oxide and inflammatory cytokines. A complicating factor is that, although stroke is more common in older population, many of the pre-clinical studies have used young adult animal models which do not adequately account for underlying age-related deficits in cerebral microvessels. This may contribute to the reasons why promising therapies at a pre-clinical stage later fail at clinical trial. Aging itself is associated with a host of changes in both BBB and brain, such as increased BBB permeability, reduced cerebral blood flow and neuronal atrophy and loss. These changes alone may not necessarily result in clinical symptoms, however they would render the old brain vulnerable to ischemic insult. Recent studies on stroke using aged animals indicate larger infarct volume, greater BBB permeability, more neuronal loss, less functional recovery and higher mortality compared to the young. Future pre-clinical research on stroke would benefit from attention to both BBB disruption and age-related tissue vulnerability to help development of targeted therapies of relevance to the clinical setting.

Chapter 4 - Blood brain barrier (BBB) is a dynamic regulated system which is responsible for selective filtering of substances to and from the brain. This action has important significance in various pathophysiological processes of the central nervous system, including anoxia and stroke. Different animal model studies have demonstrated early disruption of the BBB ischemic cascade onset. Matrix metalloproteinase (MMP), serum proteinase (SP) and free radicals were found to have key roles in the breakdown of the BBB during stroke. It has been shown that MMP and SP have an affect on the early ischemic process of the extracellular matrix around the cerebral vessels and neurons. The reactive oxygen activated the signaling pathways influencing specific enzymes which lead to an ongoing disruption of the BBB during ischemia and anoxia. It has also been shown that VEGI and the proinflammatory cytokines, especially IL1β, TNFα, MCPI and E-selectin are actively involved in the post stroke BBB disruption. Probably neutrophil recruitment, damage of the tight junction system and adherens junction and loss of vital proteins - occludin and zonula occludens and vinculum - act also on this process. Molecular changes in the BBB during ischemia have been researched by application of the genomic and proteomic techniques.

The role of BBB disruption during stroke was less intensely evaluated in humans in vivo. Two main methods, MRI with contrast agent gadolinium-diethylene-triamine-pentaactic acid (Gd-DTPA) and DTPA single protein CT (SPECT), are used for demonstration of the BBB during stroke in patients. The cardinal role of BBB disruption in humans during stroke has been hypothesized, but not proven. Its role has also been discussed involving small lacunar infarctions, ischemic damage of the white matter and diabetes mellitus patients. Little information is known about the etiology and clinical applications for BBB in the subchronic and chronic stages after stroke. The review will discuss these issues.

Chapter 5 - There is emerging evidence that the blood brain barrier (BBB) is dysfunctional in neurodegenerative diseases such as Parkinson's disease (PD). Studies from our laboratory and others reveal that areas of BBB dysfunction occur in regions of the brain undergoing neuroinflammation including the substantia nigra and striatum. Thus, the authors have shown that several different tracers enter brain parenchyma in conjunction with microglia activation, cytokine release and up-regulation of integrins only expressed by angiogenic vessels [1] The authors have proposed that this BBB dysfunction contributes to disease progression by facilitating the entry of peripheral immune mediators producing a secondary immune response [2]. Such dysfunction would also facilitate the entry of dopamine (DA) neurotoxins into areas of active degeneration further contributing to disease progression. Such dysfunction similarly raises the possibility that the time-honored approach to delivering therapeutic treatments across an intact barrier by overcoming P-glycoprotein, utilizing existing transport mechanisms, or requiring high lipid solubility may be misguided. If the authors' hypothesis is correct, they should be able to deliver neuroprotective agents that normally do not cross the BBB, directly to an area of active degeneration thereby providing targeted therapy. Since this treatment could be delivered at low circulating doses because of BBB dysfunction, it is likely that central side effects that might otherwise complicate treatment could be avoided.

Chapter 6 - The blood brain barrier (BBB) is a highly selective barrier of brain microvascular endothelial cells that shields the brain from toxic substances in the blood, supplies brain tissues with nutrients, and filters harmful compounds from the brain back to the bloodstream [1]. Transport across the BBB is strictly limited through both physical (tight junctions) and metabolic barriers (enzymes, diverse transport systems). BBB breakdown or alterations in transport systems play an important role in the pathogenesis of many CNS diseases (HIV-1 encephalitis, Alzheimer's disease, ischemia, tumors, multiple sclerosis, and Parkinson's disease).

Chapter 7 - Since the meninges, cerebrospinal fluid (CSF), and the blood-brain barrier (BBB) effectively shield the central nervous system from other tissues, it was once believed that the brain was an "immunologically privileged" organ. Over the last two decades, however, various resident cells have been shown to mount a full immune response during CNS trauma, infection and disease, and thus the long-standing view that the brain was exempt from processes observed in the periphery has been re-examined and revised. How astroglial cells affect the induction and maintenance of the BBB under physiological and pathological conditions remains an area that requires much attention. More specifically, the potential involvement of astrocytes in neurodegenerative conditions and in neurorestorative attempts appears to be important, but more intense experimentation is required to elucidate the precise role of these cells. For example, astrocytes are clearly implicated in the initiation, maintenance, and suppression of immune responses, and appear to propagate both CNS damage and repair, depending on the milieu of the micro-environment. Various factors produced and released by astroglia can also influence the properties of the BBB (e.g., sustaining tight junctions), however, these same factors may contribute to a compromised BBB when dysregulated. Therefore, the objective of this chapter is to review recent evidence of connections between, and bi-directional signaling among, astrocytes and other resident brain cells, as well as examining the part played by astrocyte-derived factors in modulating the integrity of the BBB in health and during CNS disease.

Chapter 8 - The barrier between blood and CSF contributes to homeostasis of the CNS and protects it from potentially harmful substances present in the blood.

Lipoproteins present in the CSF are clearly distinct from their plasma counterparts. Human CSF lipoproteins contain mainly Apo AI and Apo E, the former deriving mostly from plasma after crossing the blood–cerebrospinal fluid barrier, the latter being also produced by CNS. Apo AI and E containing lipoproteins in the brain are key players in transport and delivery of lipids, cholesterol homeostasis, and are also involved in CNS remodeling mechanisms. On the other hand, the isoform apo E4 represents the most important genetic risk factor for sporadic and familial late-onset Alzheimer's disease and is involved in brain injury and neurodegenerative diseases.

Apo B containing lipoproteins are not produced by CNS and the characterization of normal human CSF lipoproteins did not allowed the isolation of low density lipoproteins. Lipoprotein(a) is a low density lipoprotein-like particle with the unique protein apo(a), which is characterized by a dimensional polymorphism. Lipoprotein(a) is a well known risk factor for athero-thrombosis. The pathological role of Lipoprotein(a) is strictly associated with its plasma concentrations and the size of apo(a) isoforms, with inverse relation. The pathophysiology of Lipoprotein(a) in cardio and cerebrovascular system is widely studied. Recently, we demonstrated that, in neuroinflammatory and neurodegenerative disorders, Lipoprotein(a) can cross a dysfunctional blood-CSF barrier and be found in the CSF.

This chapter focuses on the physiological presence of the lipoproteins in CNS, on the pathological aspects deriving from their isoforms, and in particular on the anomalous presence in CSF of Lipoprotein(a).

In: The Blood-Brain Barrier
Editor: Tomas R. Helio

ISBN 978-1-60456-894-3

Chapter 1

BLOOD-BRAIN BARRIER IN HEALTH AND NEUROPATHOLOGICAL CONDITIONS

C. Kaur* and E.A. Ling

Department of Anatomy, Yong Loo Lin School of Medicine, National University of Singapore, Singapore 117597.

ABSTRACT

Homeostatic regulation of the central nervous system (CNS) microenvironment and its immune-privileged status are maintained by the blood-brain barrier (BBB). The capillaries in the CNS, formed by a continuous layer of endothelial cells with tight junctions between them, are the main structural component of the BBB. Other cells contributing to the regulation of the BBB function are the astrocytes, pericytes and perivascular microglia. Disruption of the BBB is a key feature of many conditions such as stroke, multiple sclerosis, Alzheimer's disease and head injury. Increased leakiness of the BBB in these disorders results from enhanced pinocytic activity of the endothelial cells and derangement of the tight junction proteins. Swelling of astrocytic end feet associated with the capillaries, activation of microglia and pericyte loss are associated with dysfunction of the BBB which results in cerebral edema. Many factors such as enhanced production of vascular endothelial growth factor, nitric oxide, degradation of extracellular matrix, free radicals and inflammatory cytokines may mediate the BBB breakdown. Although future research is needed to look into possible therapeutic strategies to improve the functioning of BBB in CNS disorders, experimental studies so far have reported beneficial effect of melatonin, curcumin, simvastatin, minocycline and some other drugs in ameliorating the increased BBB permeability in various neurological disorders.

* Correspondence concerning this article should be addressed to: C. Kaur, Department of Anatomy, Yong Loo Lin School of Medicine, Blk MD10, 4 Medical Drive, National University of Singapore, Singapore 117597. E-mail : antkaurc@nus.edu.sg; Fax: 65-67787643; Phone: 65-65163209.

Introduction

The concept of a blood- brain barrier (BBB) was formulated by Ehrlich (1885) more than 120 years ago and later supported by Goldman (1913). This concept was based on observations that blood-borne substances did not leak into the brain. Following the first descriptions, a variety of methods such as electron microscopy and freeze fracture studies were used to get insight into the structure of BBB. With the advent of many molecular methods over recent years, the components of BBB such as the tight junction (TJ) proteins, transporters and receptors have been unfolded.

The BBB plays an important role in the homeostatic regulation of the brain microenvironment (Abbott, 2002) and maintains the immune-privileged status of the brain by restricting the entry of T lymphocytes. The integrity of BBB is breached in several neurological disorders, including multiple sclerosis, stroke, Alzheimer's disease (AD), brain trauma and tumors (Shivers et al, 1984) as well as in old age. Brain capillaries are continuous capillaries characterized by the presence of TJ between the endothelial cells. Intercelleular junctional complex between cerebral microvessel endothelial cells, absence of fenestrations and paucity of pinocytic vesicles are unique characteristcs of BBB (Thiel and Audus, 2001). The intercellular junctional complex consists of 2 types of junctions: TJ (zona occludens) and adherens junctions. Although the endothelial cells form the proper barrier, their interaction with the surrounding cells is important for maintenance of this function (Hamm et al, 2004). The endothelial cells of the capillaries are surrounded by a basal lamina outside which there are: (1) processes of the astrocytes called astrocytic end -feet and, (2) perivascular microglia (Figure 1). Pericytes, located between the endothelial cells and the basal lamina, are the third cell type related to the capillaries.

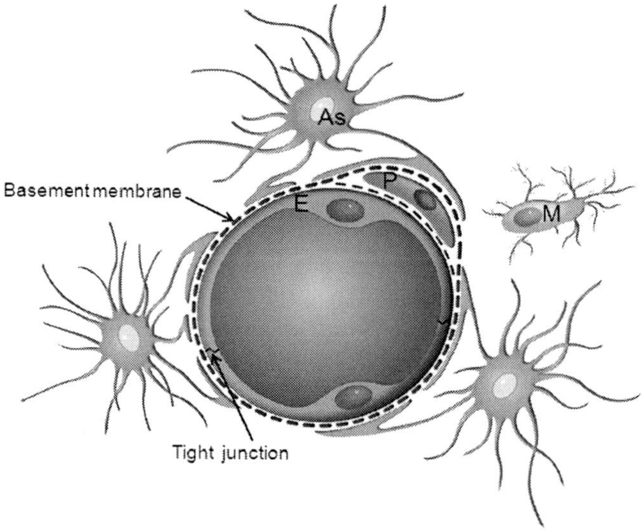

Figure 1. A Diagram showing components of the blood brain barrier: E, endothelial cells of the capillary resting on the basement membrane and with tight junctions (arrow) between them; As, astrocyte; P, pericyte; M, microglia.

Certain areas of the brain e.g. the circumventricular organs, hypothalamus and the median eminence lack this barrier as the capillaries in these areas are fenestrated and the tight junctions are lacking.

ENDOTHELIAL CELLS

Many functions are attributed to the endothelial cells including barrier, transport of nutrients, receptor-mediated signaling, leukocyte trafficking, and osmoregulation. Different mechanisms of transport across the BBB have been described: carrier-mediated transport, ion transport, active efflux transport, receptor-mediated transport, and caveolae-mediated transport. Ion transporters on the endothelial cells control ion flux across the BBB under normal conditions whereas transport of other molecules occurs by endocytosis or via specific transporters (Brown and Davis, 2002).

The endothelial cells contain membrane bound vesicles known as endothelial vesicles or plasmalemmal vesicles/caveolae at their luminal surface (Connell and Mercer, 1974; Stewart et al., 1985, 1987; Coomber et al., 1988; Simionescu et al., 1974). Transcellular permeability is controlled by caveolae which regulate endocytosis and transcytosis at the BBB (Parton and Richards, 2003) which may be receptor mediated or fluid phase requiring ATP (Simionescu, 1988; Simionescu et al., 2002; Schnitzer et al., 1995). A large number of mitochondria, required for active transport of nutrients to the brain (Persidsky et al., 2006), are present in the endothelial cells (Oldendorf et al., 1977). They may also be related to maintenance of ion differentials between blood plasma and brain extracellular fluid (Oldendorf et al., 1977). A cytoskeleton composed of microfilamants, intermediate filaments and microtubules is present in the endothelial cells (Nag et al., 1978; Nag, 1995). The maintenance of the BBB has been reported to depend on integrity of the microfilaments as actin disrupting agents such as cytochalasin B have shown to increase the permeability of BBB (Nag, 1995) and disrupt the structure of tight junctions (Bentzel et al., 1976).

Glucose, used as a primary fuel by the brain to generate energy, enters the brain by facilitated diffusion across the BBB. The endothelial cells contain a large intracellular pool of glucose transporter-1 (Glut-1) (Cornford et al., 1994; Stewart et al., 1994) which is the main transporter utilized for glucose transport (Qutub and Hunt, 2005). Receptors for transferrin, insulin, albumin and low density lipoprotein (LDL) present on the caveolar membrane are involved in receptor–mediated transport of transferrin (Jefferies et al., 1984), LDL (Meresse et al., 1989), leptin (Zlokovic et al., 2000), immunoglobulin G (IgG) (Deane et al., 2005), insulin and insulin-like growth factor (Pardridge, 2005). Endothelial cells possess a highly active Na-K-Cl cotransport system that is of major importance in endothelial cell volume regulation (O'Donnell, 1993; Sun et al., 1995). The endothelial cells also express a number of enzymes on the plasma membranes, including aminopeptidases, endopeptidases, cholinesterase, γ-glutamyl transpeptidase and others which provide a metabolic barrier by modifying endogenous and exogenous molecules crossing the BBB (Pardridge, 2005).

The dysfunction of the BBB in neurological disorders has been reported to result from disruption of ion homeostasis and transporter function (Jakobsen et al., 1987; Pan et al, 1996; Banks et al., 1997; Abbruscato and Davis, 1999; Kalaria, 1999). AD, epilepsy, ischemia, diabetes and many other central nervous system (CNS) disorders are associated with changes in glucose transport across the BBB (Gerhart et al., 1991; Saija et al., 1992; Lee and Bondy, 1993; Simpson et al., 1994; Boyle et al., 1995; Mooradian et al., 1997; Janigro, 1999). In vitro studies have also shown impairment of the BBB-associated Glut-1 in isolated brain microvessels and in cortical membrane fractions obtained from subjects with AD (Kalaria and Harik, 1989). Drastic changes in cerebral microvessels such as thickening of the vascular basement membrane, thinning of the endothelium and loss of endothelial mitochondria are found in AD patients (Kalaria, 1996) and advancing age (Stewart et al., 1987).

Studies investigating the effects of hypoxia-ischemia on the integrity of the BBB have reported that in the early post-ischemic period, tracers such as horseradish peroxidase (HRP) administered intravenously were transported by pinocytosis through endothelial cells in the brain (Petito, 1979). HRP was found to diffusely leak into the brain through the necrotic walls of vessels in the late post-ischemic period (Petito, 1979). Enhanced pinocytotic vesicle formation that may be induced after transient focal ischemia has been reported as a major mechanism of BBB opening (Cipolla et al., 2004) and several factors including nitric oxide production, release of neurotransmitters, inflammatory mediators and hemodynamic alterations may be responsible for this alteration. Other studies have reported that small molecules such as sodium fluorescein and ionic lanthanum may pass through the interendothelial cleft into the extracellular space in acute ischemic stage (Nakagawa et al, 1990).

Tight Junctions

Endothelial TJ are specialized contact zones critical for maintaining brain homeostasis by restricting diffusion of molecules from the lumen to the tissue parenchyma (Farquhar and Palade, 1963; van Meer and Simons, 1986). They are located at the apical region of the junctional complex between the endothelial cells (Ballabh et al., 2004) and are formed by fusion of the outer layer of plasma membranes of adjacent cells. The adherens junctions are composed of trasmembrane glycoproteins of the cadhedrin superfamily (Petty and Lo, 2002) and serve to hold neighbouring cells together (cell-cell adhesion).

The TJ are composed of a combination of transmembrane and cytoplasmic proteins linked to an actin-based cytoskeleton which allows these junctions to form a tight seal (Nag, 2003). The molecular components of TJ include transmembrane proteins like occludin (Furuse et al., 1993) and claudins (Furuse et al., 1998) which form the tight junction. Occludin was the first identified component of the TJ (Furuse et al., 1993) and is related to increased electrical resistance across the barrier and decreased paracellular permeability (Hirase et al., 1997). Claudins form the primary seal of the TJ (Furuse et al., 1999) and are believed to be the major transmembrane proteins at the TJ. Although the claudin superfamily consists of 24 members, claudin-1 and claudin-5 have been shown to be expressed primarily in the endothelial cells of mammalian capillaries especially in the endothelium of the brain capillaries (Morita et al, 1999; Liebner et al, 2000a,b; Lippoldt et al, 2000) and their increased expression is correlated with enhanced barrier properties of the BBB. Junctional adhesion molecule (JAM) such as JAM-1 is another transmembrane protein localized at the

TJ and is involved in the regulation of junctional integrity and permeability (Martin-Padura et al, 1998; Naik and Eckfeld, 2003). Zona occludens (ZO) proteins are members of the membrane-associated guanylate kinase family consisting of ZO-1 -2 and -3 expressed at the TJ (Haskins et al, 1998; Stevenson et al, 1986; Balda and Anderson, 1993; Jesaitis and Goodenough, 1994). The ZO-1,-2,-3 and cingulin are accessory cytoplasmic proteins associated with the TJ (Stevenson et al., 1986; Jesaitis and Goodenough, 1994; Balda et al., 1993; Haskins et al., 1998; Citi et al., 1989) that are necessary for structural support. Absence of ZO-1 immunoreactivity in blood vessels of the subcortical white matter in HIV-1 encephalitis (Dallasta et al., 1999) indicated a significant TJ disruption which led to the entry of HIV-1 infected monocytes in the CNS.

The adherens junctions are located near the basolateral side of endothelial cells. They hold the neighbouring cells together by forming a continuous belt (Petty and Lo, 2002). They are composed of transmembrane glycoproteins of cadherin superfamily. Cadherins are linked intracellulary to another group of proteins, α-, β- and γ-catenins (Gumbiner, 1996), and are not specific to the cerebral endothelium as they have been found in non-neural tissues also (Lampugnani and Dejana, 1997).

Dysfunction of BBB is a hallmark of various neurological disorders. Disruption of TJ has been reported in multiple sclerosis (Plumb et al., 2002; Kirk et al., 2003; Minagar and Alexander, 2003), stroke (Brown and Davis, 2002) and other neurological disorders. Occludin dephosphorylation preceding changes in BBB permeability has been reported to occur in experimental autoimmune encephalomyelitis, a model of multiple sclerosis (Morgan et al., 2007). In hypoxic-ischemic conditions, alteration in expression of claudin-3, ZO-1, ZO-2 (Mark and Davis, 2002; Witt et al., 2003) and claudin-5 (Koto et al., 2007) correlating with increased permeability has been reported.

Basement Membrane and Extracellular Matrix

The perivascular space around the brain microvessels is restricted by the basement membrane surrounding the endothelial cells which plays a major part in maintaining the microvascular integrity (Hamann et al., 1995). The basement membrane of cerebral endothelium has been described to consist of collagens, laminin, fibronectin, entactin, thrombospondin, heparan sulfate proteoglycans such as agrin, and chondroitin sulfate proteoglycans and versican (Abrahamson, 1986; Yurchenko and Schittny, 1990; Vorbrodt et al, 1988, 2003; Barber and Lieth, 1997; Gladson, 1999; Savettieri et al, 2000). Both the endothelial cells and the astrocytes generate the components of the basement membrane (Wang and Shuaib, 2007). Cellular differentiation and the barrier properties of cerebral microvascular endothelial cells are reported to depend on basement membrane components such as type IV collagen, fibronectin, and laminin (Tilling et al., 2002). These components are thought to be involved in transport of molecules through the BBB besides providing support to the the brain microvessels (Dermietzel and Krause, 1991). Matrix metalloproteinases (MMPs) are proteinases involved in many neuroinflammatory and ischemic conditions of the CNS as well as in acute brain injury. They are known to degrade components of the extracellular matrix and basal lamina and contribute to the breakdown of the BBB (Mandal et al., 2003; Gasche et al., 2006) resulting in increased permeability (Lukes et al., 1999). More than 20 members of MMP family have been identified so far. MMP-2 and MMP-9 expression has been reported to be increased in the brain following ischemic insults (Planas et al., 2001). It has also been demostrated that the constituents of the basement membrane are destroyed in neuropathological conditions such as ischemia (Hamann et al, 2002), AD (Zipser et al., 2007) and multiple sclerosis (van Horssen et al., 2006) resulting in migration of inflammatory cells in the CNS (Man et al., 2007).

Glial Cells and BBB

Endothelial cells of the brain capillaries need constant input from the neuroglia to maintain their BBB related properties (Prat et al., 2001). Astrocytes, microglia (Prat et al., 2001) and pericytes (Allt and Lawrenson, 2001; Lai and Kuo, 2005) are important cells that contribute to the proper functioning of the BBB.

Pericytes

Pericytes are perivascular cells in close association with the endothelial cells. They are enveloped in a basement membrane which is continuous with the basal lamina of the capillary endothelial cells. The portion of the basal lamina interposed between the pericytes and endothelial cells has been described to be significantly thinner than elsewhere (Frank et al, 1990). Besides their close proximity to endothelial cells, pericytes have direct contact with these cells through gap junctions, adhesion plaques and peg-and-socket junctions (Rucker et al, 2000). *In vitro* and *in vivo* studies have reported that the gap junctions between the two cell types allow passage of small molecules (Sims, 1986, 1991; Larson et al., 1987; Diaz-Flores et al, 1991; Shepro and Morel, 1993). Adhesion plaques anchor the pericytes to endothelial cells (Diaz-Flores et al, 1991; Sims, 1986, 1991) and peg-and-socket contacts are points where evaginations from the pericytes invaginate the endothelial cells and vice versa (Ho, 1985; Sims , 1986, 1991; Simionescu et al., 1988) and anchor the cells.

Each pericyte extends several long cytoplasmic processes over the endothelial cells (Allt and Lawrenson 2001) covering them partially. These processes have been reported to penetrate the basal lamina and contact the endothelial cells or contact them through gap junctions (Allt and Lawrenson 2001; Diaz-Flores et al, 1991; Fujimoto, 1995; Sims, 1986). The coverage of endothelial cells by pericytes appears to be functionally determined and interaction between them is important for the maturation and maintenance of the vascular system (Balabanov and Dore-Duffy, 1998; Allt and Lawrenson 2001).

Different functions have been attributed to the pericytes. They are thought to be contractile elements as they possess a cytoskeleton similar to muscle cells (Herman and D'Amore, 1985; Skalli et al., 1989) and play a part in cerebral blood flow regulation. Evidence for this function comes from the findings of many studies which have demonstrated that contractile response of pericytes is altered by vasoactive substances such as nitric oxide (NO) and endothelin-1 (Chakravarthy and Gardner, 1999; Rucker et al., 2000). The presence of endothelin receptors on the pericytes has also been documented (Chakravarthy et al., 1992; Dehouck et al., 1997; Lee et al., 1989; Yamagishi et al., 1993). A macrophagic function for the pericytes has also been proposed (Castejón et al., 2005) evidence for which comes from the recent studies of Kaur et al., (2006) in which pericytes in the cerebellum of hypoxic rats were found to phagocytose horseradish peroxidase that was extravasated from the capillaries (Figure 2).

Pericytes have also been reported to express macrophage markers such as complement type 3 receptors and ED1 antigens (Graeber et al., 1990; Hickey et al., 1992), major histocompatibility complex class I (MHC I) and II (MHC II) antigens (Streit et al., 1989; Kida et al., 1993), and hence may be involved in phagocytic and antigen presenting functions.

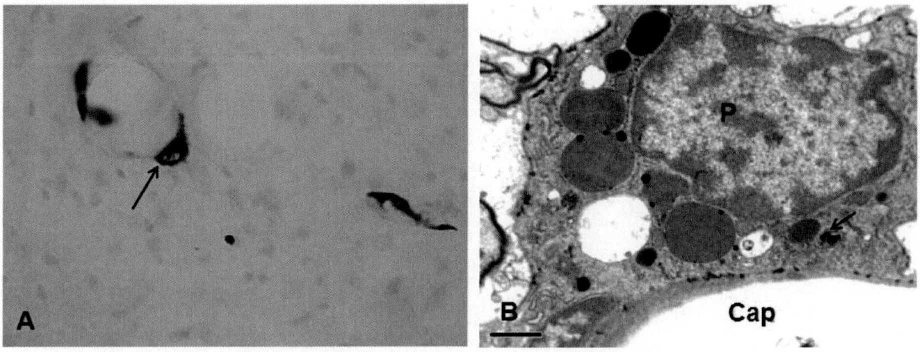

Figure 2. A pericyte (arrow) laden with HRP in the cerebellum of a hypoxic rat is seen in A. B is an electron micrograph of a pericyte (P) close to a capillary (Cap) in the cerebellum of a hypoxic rat. Arrow in B indicates HRP reaction product.

Pericytes may also play an important role in regulating T cell infiltration into the CNS (Verbeek et al., 1995) as they express adhesion molecules such as intercellular cell adhesion molecule-1 (ICAM-1) and vascular cell adhesion molecule-1(VCAM-1). Pericytes also release growth factors such as basic fibroblast growth factor (Folkman, and D'Amore, 1996; Beck and D'Amore, 1997) which promotes endothelial cell proliferation and differentiation. They have been also reported to release vascular endothelial growth factor (VEGF) (Takagi et al, 1996; Kim et al, 1998) which is strong mitogen for the endothelial cells (Nomura et al, 1995; Benjamin et al, 1998).

In vivo and in vitro studies have reported that various hormones and neuromodulators such as angiotensin II and vasopressin affect the pericytes (Ferrari-Di et al., 1996; Matsugi et al., 1997). Lack of pericytes has been reported to correlate with endothelial hyperplasia, increased capillary diameter and changes in junctional proteins suggesting increased transendothelial permeability (Hellstrom et al., 2001) resulting in edema (Bergers and Song 2005). Increased BBB permeability observed in hypoxic conditions and brain injuries has been associated with a migration of pericytes away from brain microvessels (Gonul et al, 2002, Dore-Duffy et al, 2000).

Astrocytes

Astrocytes play an important role in the development, maintenance as well as breakdown of the BBB. Regulation of brain water and electrolyte homeostasis under normal and pathological conditions is mediated by astrocytes through their direct or indirect interactions with endothelial cells (Abbott et al., 2006). Astrocyte processes, known as astrocyte-end-feet, ensheath the abluminal surface of brain capillaries (Janzer and Raff, 1987). About 99% of the brain surface of the capillary basement membrane is invested by astrocyte-end-feet (Partridge, 1999) which form a network of fine lamellae closely apposed to the outer surface of the endothelium (Kacem et al., 1998). Astrocytes are considered to induce both the barrier and permeability properties of the cerebral endothelium (Risau, 1991) and a direct contact between the endothelial cells and astrocytes has been reported to be necessary for generating an optimal barrier (Tao-Cheng et al., 1987; Rubin et al., 1991). Cultured astrocytes implanted into areas with normally leaky vessels were shown to induce tightening of the endothelium (Janzer and Raff, 1997). Astrocyte-derived humoral factors have been suggested to be responsible for maturation of the endothelial cells at the BBB (Neuhaus et al., 1991) and to contribute to tight junction formation (Arthur et al., 1987; Wolburg et al., 1994). One of the mechanisms by which astrocytes enhance the barrier properties is increasing the ZO-1 protein expression at the TJ (Gardner et al., 1997). Studies have shown that when astrocytes were removed from an in vitro BBB model where brain endothelial cells were in co-culture with astrocytes, increased permeability of the endothelial cells to horseradish peroxidase was observed (Hamm et al., 2004). In contrast to the *in vitro* experiments, *in vivo* studies have provided conflicting results with some of them indicating that the BBB integrity is not compromised in the brain when extensive loss of astrocytes occurs (Krum et al., 1997) whereas others have reported that focal loss of astrocytes resulted in microvascular damage (Willis et al, 2004). However, the BBB could self-repair despite the apparent absence of direct astrocytic-endothelial contact (Willis et al., 2004).

Astrocytes express glial fibrillary acidic protein (GFAP) and release several vasoactive substances including ATP (Guthrie et al., 1999; Queiroz et al., 1999), adenosine, (Zhang et al, 2003), NO (Murphy et al., 1993) and VEGF (Kaur et al., 2006). They are also known to express the water transporting protein, aquaporin 4 (AQ4) (Figure. 3). The astrocyte-end -feet also express noradrenergic receptors (Mulligan and MacVicar, 2004; Paspalas and Papadopoulos, 1996), PLA_2 (Sun et al., 2005), nitric oxide synthase (NOS) (Calka and Wolf, 2003), hemichannels (Nagy et al., 1999; Simard et al., 2003), AQ4 (Nicchia et al., 2000), Ca^{2+} activated K^+ channels (Price et al., 2002) and purinergic receptors (Simard et al., 2003). They have been also shown to express inflammatory molecules such as interleukin-1beta (IL-1β), interleukin-6 (IL-6) and MMP-12 (Wasserman et al., 2007).

BBB leakage is known to trigger the activation of astrocytes (Dietrich et al., 1994; Hirano et al., 1994). Up regulation of GFAP is a hallmark of reactive astrocytes. Knock-out mice lacking GFAP were found to develop dilated blood vessels in the brain and the spinal cord (Pekny et al., 1999).

It has been shown recently that GFAP is upregulated in the astrocytes in hypoxic brain (Kaur et al., 2006). GFAP is thought to be important in modulating astrocyte motility and shape by providing structural stability to astrocytic processes (Eng et al., 2000). Besides an increase in GFAP expression, swelling of astrocyte end feet around the capillaries (Figure. 4) occurs in response to hypoxia-ischemia (Panickar and Norenberg, 2005; Kaur et al., 2006). Disruption of ionic homeostasis and reduction in intracellular Na+ as well as high levels of K+, glutamate, free radicals and energy failure during ischemia-hypoxia are some of the factors responsible for astrocyte swelling (Panickar and Norenberg, 2005). AQ4 has also been reported to contribute to swelling of these cells (Papadapolus et al., 2002, 2004 a, b, 2005). An increase in AQ4 mRNA and protein expression in hypoxic rats was reported in the cerebellum (Kaur et al., 2006). Specific localization of AQ4 expression on astrocytes supports the notion that these cells are involved in the transport of water from the blood vessels to the brain parenchyma, hence, may contribute to edema formation in hypoxic conditions.

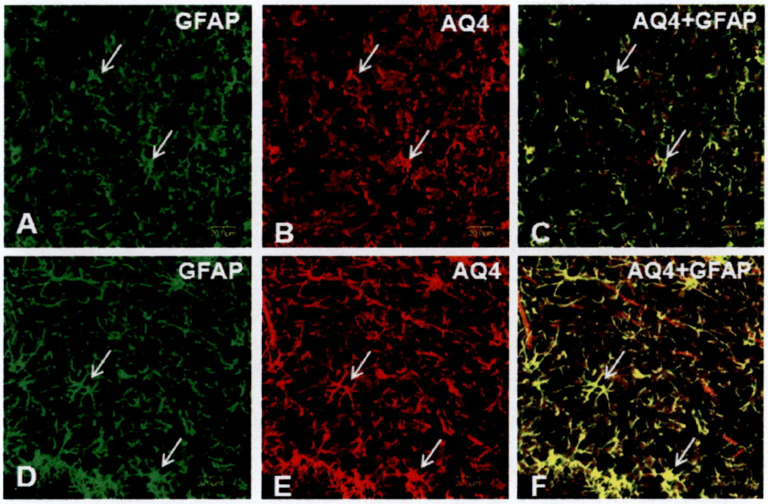

Figure 3. Astrocytes (arrows) in the cerebellum of a normal rat express GFAP (A, green) and AQ4 (B, red). C shows colocalization of GFAP and AQ4. The expression of GFAP and AQ4 is increased in the astrocytes (arrows in D, E and F) in hypoxic injury to the cerebellum.

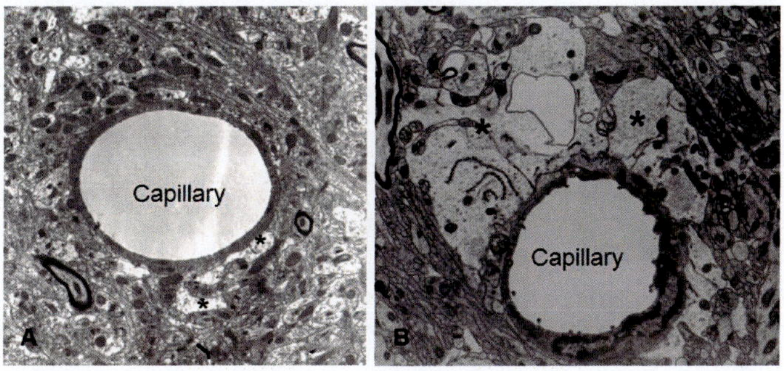

Figure 4. A capillary in the cerebral cortex of a normal rat is surrounded by astrocyte end feet (*) in A. The astrocyte end feet (*) in association with the capillary in B are markedly swollen following a hypoxic insult to the brain.

Up regulation of endogenous VEGF on astrocytes in ischemia is believed to interact with receptors for VEGF on the ischemic vessels and contribute to the disruption of BBB and leakage (Zhang et al, 2000, 2002). VEGF binds and activates two tyrosine kinase receptors, VEGFR1 (Flt-1) and VEGFR2 (KDR/Flk-1) which regulate physiological as well as pathological angiogenesis (Shibuya, 2006). Inhibition of VEGF reduces the BBB permeability (Zhang et al, 2000).

Microglia

Microglial cells are present ubiquitously throughout the brain parenchyma (Figure.5) with some of them being closely associated with the blood vessels (Grossmann et al, 2002). These juxtavascular microglia make direct contact with the vascular basal lamina (Gehrmann et al, 1995). Microglia have been reported to be involved in the functioning of BBB as they mediate the uptake of macromolecules such as low density lipoprotein, horseradish peroxidase and ferritin injected either into the blood or into the cerebral ventricles (Mato et al, 1996).

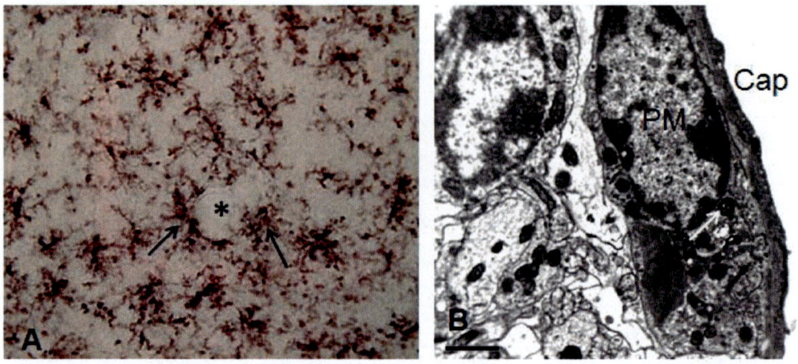

Figure 5. Microglial cells (arrws) stained with OX-42 antibody, a specific microglia marker, surrounding a blood vessel (*) in the cerebral cortex and a perivascular microglial cell (PM) in close association with a capillary (Cap) in the cerebellum of a hypoxic rat can be seen in A and B, respectively. The cell in B shows horseradish peroxidase reaction product (arrow).

Microglia are the immune effector cells in the CNS having phagocytic and antigen presenting capability (Dheen et al, 2007). They share phenotypic markers of monocyte–macrophage lineage and express complement type 3 receptors and MHC I antigens in the normal CNS and MHC II antigens under pathological conditions. Under normal conditions, they are in a quiescent state and exhibit many ramifications but are activated in brain injuries, infection, ischemia, and neurodegenerative disorders (Thomas, 1992; Morioka et al, 1993; McGeer and McGeer, 1995; Davies et al, 1998; Gonzalez-Scarano and Baltuch, 1999). Upon activation, microglia pass through a series of morphological and molecular changes that support neuroprotective and/or cytotoxic roles (Kaur and Ling 1992; Bruce-Keller, 1999). Their neuroprotective action upon activation is evidenced by phagocytosis of degenerating elements such as axons or dying cells and removal of substances leaking through a disrupted BBB such as exogenously administered horseradish peroxidase (Figure 5) in injuries of the brain (Kaur and Ling, 1992; Kaur et al, 2006). Activated microglia release a variety of inflammatory factors (Han et al, 2002), NO (Ha et al, 2008) and growth factors that can damage the components of BBB (Yenari et al, 2006). Cytokines/chemokines participate in modulation of inflammation and immune responses. IL-1β (Koprich et al, 2008), IL-6 (Heyen et al, 2000), tumour necrosis factor-α (TNF-α) (Benveniste, 1997; Persidsky et al, 2000) and interferon-γ (IFN-γ) (Kawanokuchi et al, 2006; Wang and Suzuki, 2007) are among many of the inflammatory cytokines produced by the microglia. These cytokines and toxic factors such as NO released by microglia (Chao et al, 1992) promote neurodegeneration and may also activate astrocytes which further affect the integrity of the BBB. Several studies have shown TNF-α mediates endothelial TJ disruption (Gloor et al, 2001; Poritz et al, 2004; Wang et al, 2005). *In vitro* studies have shown that IFN-γ and TNF-α can induce fragmentation of ZO-1 (Blum et al, 1997; Youakim and Ahdieh, 1999) leading to an increase in paracellular permeability via disorganization of the TJ.

Blood-Brain Barrier in Neurodegenerative Disorders

BBB disruption is an early phenomenon in many conditions such as multiple sclerosis (van Horssen et al, 2007a,b), AD (Bowman et al, 2007; Zlokovic 2002, 2005, 2008) and Parkinson's disease (Kortekaas et al. 2005). Opening of TJ, capillary basement membrane disintegration , swelling of astrocyte end feet and activation of perivascular microglial cells are featutures of BBB disruption (Figure. 6) Several factors such as increased production of VEGF, NO, inflammatory cytokines and reactive oxygen species may be responsible for a breakdown of BBB.

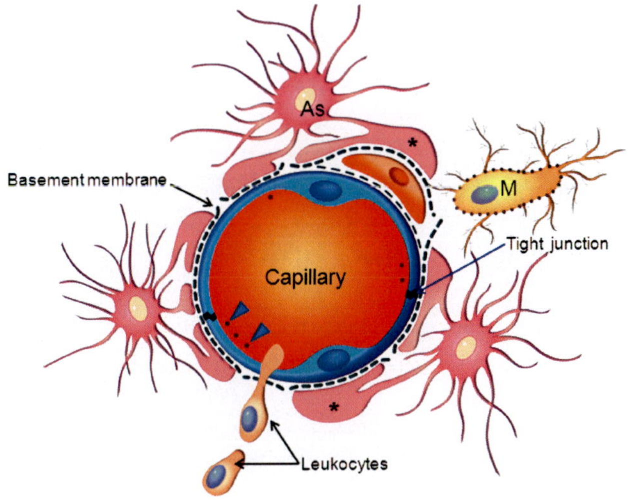

Figure 6. Astrocytes (As), swollen astrocyte end feet (*), a disrupted basement membrane, opening of tight junctions, extravasation of leukocytes, upregulation of adhesion molecules (arrowheads) on endothelial cells and activation of microglial cells (M) represent features of a dysfunctional blood brain barrier.

Vascular Endothelial Growth Factor

VEGF is an angiogenic growth factor, also known as vascular permeability enhancing factor (Croll et al, 2004; Dobrogowska et al, 1998). It has been implicated in the pathogenesis of AD (Kalaria et al, 1998; Tarkowski et al, 2002; Chiappelli et al, 2006), Parkinson's disease (Rite et al, 2007), ischemic lesions (Zhang et al, 2000; Zhang and Chopp, 2002), multiple sclerosis (Argaw et al, 2006), brain injury (Nag et al, 1997) and many other neurodegenerative disorders. Increased VEGF expression has been reported to breach the integrity of the BBB, causing brain edema and secondary injury. A recent study has shown that intranigral injections of VEGF resulted in disruption of the BBB suggesting that disruption of the BBB may be a causative factor for degeneration of nigral dopaminergic neurons (Rite et al, 2007). Hypoxia associated with the cerebral tissues in AD (Sun et al, 2006), stroke (Sun et al, 2008), multiple sclerosis (Brück and Stadelmann, 2005) and many other disorders such as carbon monoxide poisoning (smoke inhalation), cardiac arrest, stroke, accidental alcohol and drug overdose, partial drowning, suffocation and respiratory arrest following prolonged status epilepticus as well as respiratory arrest due to severe pneumonia (Wilson et al, 2003) may be one of the factors responsible for BBB dysfunction. Hypobaric hypoxia experienced at high altitude also results in cerebral edema (Basnyat, 2005; Clark, 2006; Wright, 2006) and altered cerebral hemodynamics (Van Osta et al, 2005; Palma et al, 2006). It has been reported that hypoxia leads to disruption of endothelial TJ resulting in increased permeability of the BBB (Abbruscato and Davis, 1999a, b; Fischer et al, 1999; Mark and Davis, 2002; Josko and Knefel, 2003). It may also increase permeability via the transcellular route (Plateel et al,. 1997; Cipolla et al, 2004). The expression of VEGF is potentiated in response to hypoxia (Figure. 7) and is considered an important pathogenic factor for induction of vascular leakage in the brain (Mayhan,1999; Pichiule et al, 1999; Sinor et al, 1998; Walter et al, 2001; Schoch et al, 2002; Kaur et al, 2006) leading to the formation of cerebral oedema.

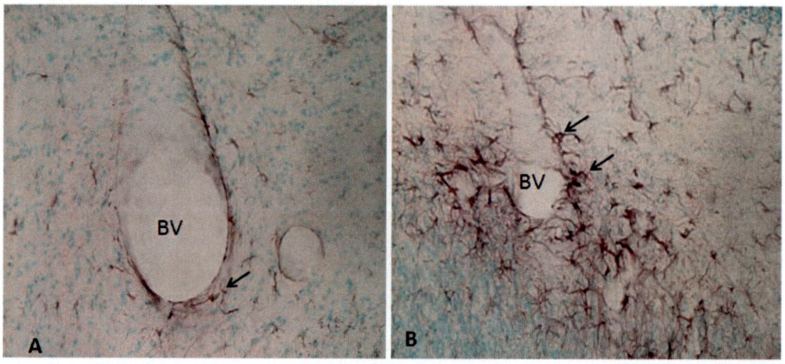

Figure 7. Blood vessels (BV) in the cerebellum of a control (A) and a hypoxic (B) rat are surrounded by VEGF expressing astrocytes (arrows). The expression of VEGF is markedly enhanced in B following the hypoxic insult.

The precise mechanism by which VEGF increases vascular permeability is not known but it has been reported that hypoxia-induced hyperpermeability in the brain microvessels involves VEGF-mediated changes in the expression of ZO-1 at the TJ of the endothelial cells

(Fischer et al, 2002). VEGF is also known to induce changes such as appearance of interendothelial gaps, fragmentation of the endothelium, fenestration of the endothelial cells and degenerative changes in endothelial basement membrane which affect the structural integrity of the microvessels leading to extravasation of plasma proteins including albumin (Dobrogowska et al, 1998).

Besides increasing the vascular permeability, VEGF may also be involved in inducing inflammatory changes observed in many CNS disorders. VEGF modulates immune responses in the CNS by increasing vascular permeability and BBB breakdown allowing contact of normally sequestered CNS antigens with blood-borne immune mediators ,and hence, altering the immune privileged status of the brain (Proescholdt et al, 1999). Because of its proinflammatory actions, VEGF enhances the adhesion of leukocytes to vascular walls by increasing ICAM-1 and VCAM-1 expression (Min et al, 2005). Overexposure of normal brain to VEGF has been shown to enhance ICAM-1, MHC I and MHC II expression (Proescholdt et al, 1999).

Nitric Oxide

NO is synthesized by the enzyme nitric oxide synthase (NOS) from L-arginine. NOS from neurons (nNOS) and endothelial cells (eNOS) are constitutively expressed enzymes, the activities of which are stimulated by increases in intracellular calcium. Inducible nitric oxide synthase (iNOS) is calcium-independent, and NO generated from this isoform is known to mediate immune functions. Many studies have shown that increased NO biosynthesis occurs in neurological disorders such as AD (Lüth et al, 2002; Malinski, 2007), Parkinson's disease (He et al, 2003), multiple sclerosis (Koch et al, 2008), stroke (Taffi et al, 2008), amyotrophic lateral sclerosis (Babu et al, 2008), traumatic brain injury (Hüttemann et al, 2008) and many other CNS pathologies.

NO has been reported to modulate the transport of ions, nutrients, and other molecules the and, hence, regulate the function of BBB (Janigro et al, 1994). Excess production of NO, however, increases the blood flow and permeability of the BBB allowing substances to enter into the brain passively (Shukla et al, 1996; Thiel and Audus, 2001; Mark et al, 2004). Vasodilation occurring after hypoxic-ischemic episodes is mediated by eNOS (Bolanos and Almeida, 1999) leading to increased blood flow. Besides vasodilatation and increasing the blood flow, a predominant role for eNOS has been proposed in VEGF induced vascular hyperpermeability (Fukumura et al, 2001).

Inflammatory Cytokines

Many CNS conditions, especially hypoxic-ischemic, are known to induce an inflammatory response in the CNS (Danton and Dietrich, 2003; Saleh et al, 2004) resulting in disruption of the BBB (Yang et al, 1999). Microglial cells and astrocytes are activated in response to hypoxia-ischemia (Kato et al, 2003; Lu et al, 2006; Yenari et al, 2006). Activated glia and endothelial cells produce chemokines and cytokines that enhance the permeability of the blood vessels and increase lymphocyte migration across the BBB (Zach et al, 1997; Gong et al, 1998; Weiss et al, 1998; Zhang et al, 2000; Prat et al, 2001). *In vitro* studies have also shown that cytokines such as TNF-α, IFN-γ, IL-1β, and IL-6 produced by perivascular microglia and astrocytes after injury or inflammation breakdown the BBB by disrupting the endothelial TJ (de Vries et al, 1996). TNF- α is known to affect paracellular permeability of the BBB by altering the endothelial cytoskeleton (Mark et al, 2001) and TJ protein expression (Mazzon and Cuzzocrea, 2007). TNF- α also induces cycloxygenase-2 expression which affects the endothelial cytoskeleton (Mark et al, 2001). IL-1β also affects the BBB permeability as it causes loss of TJ proteins (Bolton et al, 1998). In addition to the endothelial changes, increased adhesion of leukocytes to endothelial cells and their transmigration across the endothelium occurs under the influence of cytokines (Harhaj and Antonetti, 2004). IL-1β plays a significant role in leukocyte recruitment to the CNS through the disrupted BBB (Shaftel et al, 2007). Injection of TNF- α and IL-1β in rodents has been shown to initiate inflammatory responses such as adhesion and transmigration of leukocytes through vascular walls (Rhodin et al, 1999). Glial cells also produce chemokines such as monocyte chemoattractant protein (MCP)-1, macrophage inflammatory protein (MIP)-1α and interferon γ inducible protein in multiple sclerosis and experimental autoimmune encephalomyelitis (Berman et al, 1996; McManus et al, 1998; Simpson et al, 1998, 2000; Sorensen et al, 1999; Babcock and Owens, 2003). These chemokines have been implicated as key mediators of leukocyte entry to CNS (Fuentes et al, 1995; Huang et al, 2001).

In addition to the cytokines, T cell migration across the endothelium is also mediated by adhesion molecules like ICAM-1 and VCAM-1, moderate levels of which are expressed constitutively by brain endothelial cells (Prat et al, 2001). ICAM-1 and VCAM-1 expression is upregulated in neurological disorders, brain infections and injuries (Clark et al, 1995; del Zoppo, 1997; del Zoppo and Mabuchi, 2003; MacIntyre et al, 2003; Rentzos et al, 2005; Blum et al, 2006; Huang et al, 2006; Clausen et al, 2007) mediating leukocyte-endothelial cell adhesion (Oppenheimer-Marks et al, 1991). ICAM-1 binds to its leukocyte ligands and is essential for transendothelial migration of activated leukocytes into the CNS (Reiss et al, 1998; Dietrich, 2002). VCAM-1 also mediates adhesion and activation of lymphocytes by interacting with its counter receptor, very-late antigen (VLA)-4, a member of integrin alpha 4 β1 (Burkly et al, 1991). Migration of T cells across the endothelium at the disrupted BBB is followed by other inflammatory cells such as the monocytes which add to the augmentation of the inflammatory reaction and CNS tissue damage (Patcher et al, 2003).

Free Radicals

Overproduction of free radicals is a hallmark of neurological disorders including Parkinson's disease (Jenner and Olanow, 1998), AD (Rottkamp et al, 2001), ischemia (Flamm et al, 1978), stroke (Ferretti et al, 2008) and multiple sclerosis (Gonsette, 2008). Free radicals including the hydroxyl radical (OH), hydrogen peroxide (H_2O_2), singlet oxygen ($^1O_2$), hypochlorous acid (HOCl), peroxynitrite anion (ONOO(-)) and/or peroxynitrous acid (ONOOH) are mainly derived from oxygen (reactive oxygen species/ROS) and nitrogen (reactive nitrogen species/RNS). Aldehydes such as malondialdehyde (MDA) and 4-hydroxy-

2-nonenal (4- HNE) formed during lipid peroxidation also damage the tissues by augmenting free radical events (Esterbauer et al, 1991). Disruption of BBB by free radicals has been shown *in vivo* in experimental animal models (Parathath et al. 2006) as well as in *vitro* studies (Blasig et al. 2002). ROS contribute to dysfunction of the BBB by altering the distribution or disappearance of TJ proteins claudin-5 and occludin (Schreibelt et al, 2007). Loss of brain endothelium stability and increase in BBB permeability via degradation of basement membrane proteins by activated MMPs and by protein tyrosine kinase -mediated TJ protein phosphorylation has also been reported to be mediated by ROS (Gasche et al. 1999; Kim et al. 2003; Machado et al. 2006; Haorah et al, 2007). MMPs activation is also associated with disruption the TJ (Gursoy-Ozdemir et al. 2004; Sanchez-del-Rio and Reuter 2004). It has been suggested that ONOO(-) may be a direct trigger for increasing BBB permeability in CNS inflammation (Phares et al, 2007). The involvement of ONOO(-) in inducing BBB damage is evidenced by many studies which report that uric acid , a product of purine metabolism and a known scavenger of ONOO(-), inactivates ONOO(-) and reduces BBB permeability and immune cell invasion into the CNS (Hooper et al, 2000; Kean et al, 2000). Increased MDA levels in traumatic brain injury, infections and with increasing age have been found in the brain (Das et al, 1991; Mooradian and Uko-eninn, 1995; Ates et al, 2008). Lipid peroxidation has been reported to increase capillary permeability and cause formation of oedema (Das et al, 1991).

BBB Protective Agents

Antioxidants such as melatonin have been reported to be effective in reducing cerebral edema formation in ischemic animals (Kondoh et al, 2002). Melatonin reduces increased vascular permeability through modulation of endothelial–neutrophil interactions (Lotufo et al., 2001), direct effect on endothelial cells (Lotufo et al, 2006) and antioxidant actions (Bilici et al., 2002; Cuzzocrea et al., 1997, 1999). It also has a suppressive effect on the tissue concentration of VEGF (Kaur et al, 2006, Kaur and Ling, 2008) resulting in reduced vascular permeability and edema in many parts of the CNS (Kaur et al, 2006). Melatonin also suppressed the production of NO (Cuzzocrea et al, 2000; Kaur et al, 2006) and AQ4 (Kaur et al, 2006) in hypoxic brains and also reduced edema formation (Torii et al, 2004). It has been shown to reverse the inflammatory response by suppressing the production of inflammatory cytokines (Pei and Cheung, 2004; Lee et al, 2007).

Other agents reported to prevent damage to the BBB in ischemic conditions are curcumin (Jiang et al, 2007), simvastatin (Nagaraja et al, 2006), minocycline (Yenari et al, 2006), cyclosporine A and methylprednisolone (Akdemir et al, 2005). Minocycline, an antibiotic belonging to the tetracycline family, has been reported to ameliorate the brain damage by reducing extravasation of plasma proteins and, hence, edema formation (Wasserman and Schlichter, 2007). Inhibition of microglial activation by minocycline has been proven to be useful in ameliorating BBB disruption in ischemic (Yenari et al, 2006) and inflammatory (Tomás-Camardiel et al, 2004) conditions. As mentioned above, uric acid inactivates ONOO(-) and reduces BBB permeability and immune cell invasion into the CNS (Hooper et al, 2000; Kean et al, 2000). A recent study has shown that the dietary provitamin pantethine, a low-molecular-weight thiol, preserves the BBB in cerebral malaria (Penet et al, 2008). Edaravone (3-methyl-1-phenyl-2-pyrazolin-5-one), a free radical scavenger, reduces VEGF expression and brain edema in stroke patients (Ishikawa et al, 2007). Natalizumab, a humanized monoclonal antibody directed against alpha 4-integrin, binds to VLA-4 on leukocytes and blocks their interaction with endothelial cells inhibiting their migration through the BBB in multiple sclerosis (Kümpfel et al., 2002).

Conclusion

Disruption of the BBB is a hallmark of many conditions such as stroke, multiple sclerosis, Alzheimer's disease and head injury. Swelling of astrocytic end feet associated with the capillaries, activation of microglia, disruption of TJ and pericyte loss are associated with dysfunction of the BBB which results in cerebral edema. Many factors such as enhanced production of VEGF, NO, degradation of extracellular matrix, free radicals, inflammatory cytokines and chemokines may play a role in BBB breakdown. Although future research will likely lead to the discovery of new therapeutic strategies to improve the functioning of BBB in CNS disorders, experimental studies so far have reported beneficial effect of melatonin, edaravone, minocycline and natalizumab among many other drugs in suppressing the increased BBB permeability.

Acknowledgements

This study was supported by research grants (R181-000-065-112 and R-181-000-098-112) from the National University of Singapore. The technical assistance of Ms Y.G. Chan and Dr V. Sivakumar is gratefully acknowledged.

References

Abbott NJ, Ronnback L, Hansson E (2006) Astrocyte-endothelial interactions at the blood-brain barrier, *Nat. Rev. Neurosci. 7*:41–53.

Abbott NJ. (2002) Astrocyte-endothelial interactions and blood-brain barrier permeability. *J Anat 200*:629-638.

Abbruscato TJ and Davis TP (1999a) Combination of hypoxia/aglycemia compromises in vitro blood-brain barrier integrity. *J Pharmacol Exp The 289:* 668 675.

Abbruscato TJ and Davis TP (1999b) Protein expression of brain endothelial cell E-cadherin after hypoxia/aglycemia: influence of astrocyte contact. *Brain Res 842:* 277-286.

Abrahamson DR. (1986). Recent studies on the structure and pathology of basement membranes. *J Patho 149*: 257–278

Akdemir G, Ergungor MF, Sezer M, Albayrak L, Daglioglu E, Kilinc K (2005). Therapeutic efficacy of intraventricular cyclosporine A and methylprednisolone on a global cerebral ischemia model in rats. *Neurol Res 27*: 827-834.

Allt G, Lawrenson JG (2001). Pericytes: cell biology and pathology. *Cells Tissues Organs 169*:1-11.

Argaw AT, Zhang Y, Snyder BJ, Zhao ML, Kopp N, Lee SC, Raine CS, Brosnan CF, John GR (2006) IL-1beta regulates blood-brain barrier permeability via reactivation of the hypoxia-angiogenesis program. *J Immunol. 177*:5574-84

Arthur FE, Shivers RR, Bowman PD (1987). Astrocyte-mediated induction of tight junctions in brain capillary endothelium: an efficient in vitro model. *Dev. Brain Res 36* : 155–159

Ates O, Cayli S, Altinoz E, Gurses I, Yucel N, Sener M, Kocak A, Yologlu S.(2007) Neuroprotection by resveratrol against traumatic brain injury in rats. *Mol Cell Biochem. 294*: 137-144.

Babcock A, Owens T (2003) Chemokines in experimental autoimmune encephalomyelitis and multiple sclerosis. *Adv Exp Med Biol 520*: 120-132.

Babu GN, Kumar A, Chandra R, Puri SK, Kalita J, Misra UK. (2008) Elevated Inflammatory Markers in a Group of Amyotrophic Lateral Sclerosis Patients from Northern India. *Neurochem Res. (In press)*

Balabanov R, Dore-Duffy P (1998). Role of the CNS microvascular pericyte in the blood-brain barrier. *J Neurosci Res. 53* 637-644

Balda MS, Anderson JM (1993). Two classes of tight junctions are revealed by ZO-1 isoforms. *Am. J. Physiol 264* : C918–C924

Balda MS, Gonzalez-Mariscal L, Matter K, Cereijido M, Anderson JM (1993) Assembly of the tight junction: the role of diacylglycerol. *J Cell Biol 123*:293–302

Ballabh P, Braun A, Nedergaard M. (2004) The blood-brain barrier: an overview: structure, regulation, and clinical implications. *Neurobiol Dis. 16*:1-13.

Banks WA, Jaspan JB, Kastin AJ. (1997) Effect of diabetes mellitus on the permeability of the blood-brain barrier to insulin. *Peptides. 18*: 1577–1584

Barber AJ, Lieth E (1997). Agrin accumulates in the brain microvascular basal lamina during development of the blood–brain barrier. *Dev. Dyn 208*: 62–74.

Basnyat B (2005). High altitude cerebral and pulmonary edema. *Travel Med Infect Dis 3*:199-211.

Beck, L, D'Amore, P. A. (1997) Vascular development: Cellular and molecular regulation. *FASEB J. 11*:365–373

Benjamin L.E., Hemo I, Keshet E 91998) A plasticity window for blood vessel remodeling is defined by pericyte coverage of the preformed endothelial network and is regulated by PDGF-B and VEGF. *Development 125*:1591–1598

Bentzel CJ, Hainau B, Edelman A, Anagnostopoulos T, Benedetti EL. (1976) Effect of plant cytokinins on microfilaments and tight junction permeability. *Nature. 264*:666-668.

Benveniste EN. (1997) Role of macrophages/microglia in multiple sclerosis and experimental allergic encephalomyelitis. *J Mol Med. 75*:165-173

Bergers G, Song S (2005). The role of pericytes in blood-vessel formation and maintenance. *Neuro-oncol 7*: 452-464

Berman JW, Guida MP, Warren J, Amat J, Brosnan CF (1996) Localization of monocyte chemoattractant peptide-1 expression in the central nervous system in experimental autoimmune encephalomyelitis and trauma in the rat. *J Immunol 156*: 3017-3023

Bilici D, Akpinar E, Kiziltune A, (2002). Protective effect of melatonin in carrageenan-induced acute local inflammation. *Pharmacol. Res. 46*:133–139.

Blasig I. E., Mertsch K. and Haseloff R. F. (2002) Nitronyl nitroxides, a novel group of protective agents against oxidative stress in endothelial cells forming the blood-brain barrier. *Neuropharmacology 43*, 1006–1014.

Blum A, Khazim K, Merei M, Peleg A, Blum N, Vaispapir V. (2006) The stroke trial - can we predict clinical outcome of patients with ischemic stroke by measuring soluble cell adhesion molecules (CAM)? *Eur Cytokine Netw. 1*:295-298.

Blum MS, Toninelli E, Anderson JM, Balda MS, Zhou J, O'Donnell L, Pardi R, Bender JR (1997) Cytoskeletal rearrangement mediates human microvascular endothelial tight junction modulation by cytokines. *Am J Physiol. 273*: H286-294.

Bolanos JP, Almeida A (1999). Roles of nitric oxide in brain hypoxia-ischemia. *Biochim Biophys Acta 1411*:415-436.

Bolton S, Anthony D, Perry V (1998) Loss of tight junction proteins occludin and zonula occludens-1 from cerebral vascular endothelium during neurophil induced blood–brain barrier breakdown *in vivo. Neuroscience 86*:1245–1257

Bowman GL, Kaye JA, Moore M, Waichunas D, Carlson NE, Quinn JF. (2007) Blood-brain barrier impairment in Alzheimer disease: stability and functional significance. *Neurology. 68*:1809-1814.

Boyle PJ, Kempers SF, O'Connor AM, Nagy RJ (1995) Brain glucose uptake and unawareness of hypoglycemia in patients with insulin-dependent diabetes mellitus, *N. Engl. J. Med. 333* : 1726–1731.

Brown RC, Davis TP (2002). Calcium modulation of adherens and tight junction function: a potential mechanism for blood-brain barrier disruption after stroke. *Stroke. 33*:1706-1711

Bruce-Keller AJ. (1999). Microglial-neuronal interactions in synaptic damage and recovery. *J Neurosci Res 58*: 191-201.

Brück W, Stadelmann C (2005) The spectrum of multiple sclerosis: new lessons from pathology. *Curr Opin Neurol. 18*:221-224

Burkly LC, Jakubowski A, Newman BM, Rosa MD, Chi-Rosso G, Lobb RR (1991). Signaling by vascular cell adhesion molecule-1 (VCAM-1) through VLA-4 promotes CD3-dependent T cell proliferation. *Eur J Immunol. 21*:2871-2875.

Całka J, Wolf G (2003). An ultrastructural demonstration of NADPH-diaphorase/nitric oxide synthase activity in the rat striatal astroglia. *Folia Morphol (Warsz). 62*:251-253.

Castejón OJ, Castellano A, Arismendi GJ, Medina Z. (2005)The inflammatory reaction in human traumatic oedematous cerebral cortex. *J Submicrosc Cytol Pathol.* 37:43-52.

Chakravarthy U, Gardiner TA, Anderson P, Archer DB, Trimble ER (1992). The effect of endothelin 1 on the retinal microvascular pericyte. *Microvasc Res 43*: 241–254

Chakravarthy U, Gardiner TA (1999). Endothelium-derived agents in pericyte function/dysfunction. *Prog Retin Eye Res. 18*:511-527

Chao CC, Hu S, Molitor TW, Shaskan EG, Peterson PK (1992). Activated microglia mediate neuronal cell injury via a nitric oxide mechanism. *J Immunol. 149*:2736-2741

Chiappelli M, Borroni B, Archetti S, Calabrese E, Corsi MM, Franceschi M, Padovani A, Licastro F. (2006) VEGF gene and phenotype relation with Alzheimer's disease and mild cognitive impairment. *Rejuvenation Res. 9*:485-493.

Cipolla MJ, Crete R, Vitullo L, Rix RD (2004).Transcellular transport as a mechanism of blood-brain barrier disruption during stroke. *Front Biosci 9*:777-785.

Citi S, Sabanay H, Kendrick-Jones J,. Geiger B (1989). Cingulin: characterization and localization. *J Cell Sci 93* : 107–122

Clark WM, Lauten JD, Lessov N, Woodward W, Coull BM (1995). Time course of ICAM-1 expression and leukocyte subset infiltration in rat forebrain ischemia. *Mol Chem Neuropathol 26*:213-230.

Clarke C (2006). Acute mountain sickness: medical problems associated with acute and subacute exposure to hypobaric hypoxia. *Postgrad Med J 82:* 748-753.

Clausen F, Lorant T, Lewén A, Hillered L. (2007) T lymphocyte trafficking: a novel target for neuroprotection in traumatic brain injury. *J Neurotrauma. 24*:1295-1307.

Connell CJ, Mercer KL (1974). Freeze-fracture appearance of the capillary endothelium in the cerebral cortex of mouse brain. *Am J Anat 140*:595-599

Coomber BL, Stewart PA, Hayakawa EM, Farrell CL, Del Maestro RF (1988). A quantitative assessment of microvessel ultrastructure in C6 astrocytoma spheroids transplanted to brain and to muscle. *J Neuropathol Exp Neurol 47*: 29-40.

Cornford EM, Hyman S, Swartz BE (1994). The human brain GLUT1 glucose transporter: ultrastructural localization to the blood-brain barrier endothelia. *J Cereb Blood Flow Metab.* 14: 106-112.

Croll SD, Goodman JH, Scharfman HE (2004). Vascular endothelial growth factor (VEGF) in seizures: a double-edged sword. *Adv Exp Med Biol. 548*:57-68

Cuzzocrea S, Costantino G, Gitto E, Mazzon E, Fulia F, Serraino I, Cordaro S, Barberi I, De Sarro A, Caputi AP. (2000) Protective effects of melatonin in ischemic brain injury. *J Pineal Res. 29(4)*:217-227.

Cuzzocrea S, Costantino G, Mazzon E, Caputi AP (1999). Regulation of prostaglandin production in carrageenan-induced pleurisy by melatonin. *J. Pineal Res. 27*: 9–14.

Cuzzocrea S, Zingarelli B, Gilad E, Hake P, Salzman AL, Szabó C (1997). Protective effect of melatonin in carrageenan-induced models of local inflammation: relationship to its inhibitory effect on nitric oxide production and its peroxynitrite scavenging activity. *J. Pineal Res. 23*: 106–116.

Dallasta LM, Pisarov LA, Esplen JE, Werley JV, Moses AV, Nelson JA, Achim CL (1999). Blood-brain barrier tight junction disruption in human immunodeficiency virus-1 encephalitis. *Am J Pathol. 155*:1915-1927

Danton GH, Dietrich WD (2003). Inflammatory mechanisms after ischemia and stroke. *J Neuropathol Exp Neurol 62*:127-136

Das BS, Mohanty S, Mishra SK, Patnaik JK, Satpathy SK, Mohanty D, Bose TK. (1991) Increased cerebrospinal fluid protein and lipid peroxidation products in patients with cerebral malaria. *Trans R Soc Trop Med Hyg. 85*:733-734

Davies CA, Loddick SA, Stroemer RP, Hunt J, Rothwell NJ. (1998) An integrated analysis of the progression of cell responses induced by permanent focal middle cerebral artery occlusion in the rat. *Exp Neurol. 154*:199-212.

de Vries HE, Blom-Roosemalen MC, van Oosten M, de Boer AG, van Berkel TJ, Breimer DD, Kuiper J (1996). The influence of cytokines on the integrity of the blood-brain barrier in vitro. *J Neuroimmunol 64*:37-43.

Deane R, Sagare A, Hamm K, Parisi M, LaRue B, Guo H, Wu Z, Holtzman DM, Zlokovic BV (2005) IgG-assisted age-dependent clearance of Alzheimer's amyloid beta peptide by the blood-brain barrier neonatal Fc receptor, *J. Neurosci. 25* : 11495–11503

Deane R, Wu Z, Zlokovic BV. (2004) RAGE (yin) versus LRP (yang) balance regulates alzheimer amyloid beta-peptide clearance through transport across the blood-brain barrier. *Stroke. 35*:2628-2631

Dehouck MP, Vigne P, Torpier G, Breittmayer JP, Cecchelli R, C. Frelin C (1997). Endothelin-1 as a mediator of endothelial cell-pericyte interactions in bovine brain capillaries. *J Cereb Blood Flow Metab 17*:464–469

del Zoppo GJ (1997). Microvascular responses to cerebral ischemia/inflammation. *Ann N Y Acad Sci 823*:132-147.

del Zoppo GJ, Mabuchi T (2003). Cerebral microvessel responses to focal ischemia. *J Cereb Blood Flow Metab 23*:879-894

Dermietzel R, Krause D. (1991) Molecular anatomy of the blood-brain barrier as defined by immunocytochemistry. *Int Rev Cytol. 127*:57-109.

Dheen ST, Kaur C, Ling EA. (2007) Microglial activation and its implications in the brain diseases. *Curr Med Chem. 14*(11):1189-1197

Diaz-Flores L, Gutierrez R, Varela H, Rancel N, Valladares F (1991). Microvascular pericytes: a review of their morphological and functional characteristics. *Histol Histopathol 6*:269-286.

Dietrich JB. (2002) The adhesion molecule ICAM-1 and its regulation in relation with the blood-brain barrier. *J Neuroimmunol. 128*:58-68.

Dietrich, WD, Alonso, O, Halley M (1994). Early microvascular and neuronal consequences oftraumatic brain injury: A light and electron microscopic study in rats. *J Neurotraum 11*:289-301.

Dobrogowska DH, Lossinsky AS, Tarnawski M, Vorbrodt AW (1998). Increased blood-brain barrier permeability and endothelial abnormalities induced by vascular endothelial growth factor. *J Neurocytol 27*:163-173.

Dore-Duffy P, Owen C, Balabanov R, Murphy S, Beaumont T, and Rafols JA (2000) Pericyte migration from the vascular wall in response to traumatic brain injury. *Microvasc Res 60:* 55-69

Ehrlich P (1885) Das sauerstufbudurfnis des organismus, in *Eine Farbenanalytische Studie*, Hirschwald, Berlin.

Eng LF, Ghirnikar RS, Lee YL (2000). Glial fibrillary acidic protein: GFAP-thirty-one years (1969-2000). *Neurochem Res 25*:1439-1451.

Esterbauer H, Schaur RJ, Zollner H (1991). Chemistry and biochemistry of 4-hydroxynonenal, malonaldehyde and related aldehydes. *Free Radic Biol Med.* 11:81-128

Farquhar MG , Palade GE (1963). Junctional complexes in various epithelia. *J Cell Biol 17*:375-412

Ferrari-Dileo G, Davis EB, Anderson DR (1996). Glaucoma, capillaries and pericytes. 3. Peptide hormone binding and influence on pericytes. *Ophthalmologica 210*: 269–275.

Ferretti G, Bacchetti T, Masciangelo S, Nanetti L, Mazzanti L, Silvestrini M, Bartolini M, Provinciali L. (2008) Lipid peroxidation in stroke patients. *Clin Chem Lab Med. 46*:113-117.

Fischer S, Clauss M, Wiesnet M, Renz D, Schaper W, and Karliczek GF (1999). Hypoxia induces permeability in brain microvessel endothelial cells via VEGF and NO. *Am J Physiol Cell Physiol 276*: C812–C820

Fischer S, Wobben M, Marti HH, Renz D, Schaper W (2002). Hypoxia-induced hyperpermeability in brain microvessel endothelial cells involves VEGF-mediated changes in the expression of zonula occludens-1. *Microvasc Res 63*:70-80.

Folkman J, D'Amore, PA. (1996) Blood vessel formation: What is its molecular basis? *Cell 87*:1153–1155

Frank RN, Turczyn TJ, Das A (1990). Pericyte coverage of retinal and cerebral capillaries. *Invest Ophthalmol Vis Sci. 31*:999-1007

Fuentes M, Durham S, Swerdel M, Lewin A, Barton D, Megill J, Bravo R, Lira S (1995) Controlled recruitment of monocytes and macrophages to specific organs through transgenic expression of monocyte chemoattractant protein-1. *J Immunol 155*: 5769-5776

Fujimoto K (1995). Pericyte-endothelial gap junctions in developing rat cerebral capillaries: A fine structural study. *Anat Rec 242*:562–565

Fukumura D, Gohongi T, Kadambi A, Izumi Y, Ang J, Yun CO, Buerk DG, Huang PL, Jain RK (2001). Predominant role of endothelial nitric oxide synthase in vascular endothelial growth factor-induced angiogenesis and vascular permeability. *Proc Natl Acad Sci U S A 98*:2604-2609.

Furuse M, Fujita K, Hiiragi T, Fujimoto K, Tsukita S (1998). Claudin-1 and -2: novel integral membrane proteins localizing at tight junctions with no sequence similarity to occludin. *J Cell Biol 141*:1539-1550

Furuse M, Hirase T, Itoh M, Nagafuchi A, Yonemura S, Tsukita S, Tsukita S (1993). Occludin: a novel integral membrane protein localizing at tight junctions. *J Cell Biol 123*:1777-1788

Furuse M, Sasaki H, Tsukita S (1999). Manner of interaction of heterogeneous claudin species within and between tight junction strands. *J Cell Biol 147*:891-903

Gardner TW, Lieth E, Khin SA, Barber AJ, Bonsall DJ, Lesher T, Rice K, Brennan WA Jr. (1997) Astrocytes increase barrier properties and ZO-1 expression in retinal vascular endothelial cells. *Invest Ophthalmol Vis Sci. 38*:2423-2427.

Gasche Y, Soccal PM, Kanemitsu M, Copin JC (2006). Matrix metalloproteinases and diseases of the central nervous system with a special emphasis on ischemic brain. *Front Biosci 11*:1289-1301.

Gasche Y., Fujimura M., Morita-Fujimura Y., Copin J. C., Kawase M., Massengale J. and Chan P. H. (1999) Early appearance of activated matrix metalloproteinase-9 after focal cerebral ischemia in mice: a possible role in blood-brain barrier dysfunction. J. Cereb. *Blood Flow Metab. 19*, 1020–1028.

Gehrmann J, Matsumoto Y, Kreutzberg GW. (1995) Microglia: intrinsic immuneffector cell of the brain. *Brain Res Brain Res Rev. 20*:269-287.

Gerhart DZ, Djuricic B, Drewes LR, (1991) Quantitative immunocytochemistry (image analysis) of glucose transporters in the normal and postischemic rodent hippocampus, *J. Cereb. Blood Flow Metab. 11*: 440–448

Gladson CL (1999). The extracellular matrix of gliomas: modulation of cell function. *J Neuropathol Exp Neurol 58*:1029–1040.

Gloor SM, Wachtel M, Bolliger MF, Ishihara H, Landmann R, Frei K. (2001) Molecular and cellular permeability control at the blood-brain barrier. *Brain Res Brain Res Rev. 36*:258-264

Goldmann EE (1913) Vitalfarbung am zentralnervensystem. *Abhandl Konigl preuss Akad Wiss 1:* 1-60.

Gong C, Qin Z, Betz AL, Liu XH, Yang GY (1998). Cellular localization of tumor necrosis factor alpha following focal cerebral ischemia in mice. *Brain Res. 801*:1-8.

Gonsette RE. (2008) Oxidative stress and excitotoxicity: a therapeutic issue in multiple sclerosis? *Mult Scler. 14*: 22-34.

Gonul E, Duz B, Kahraman S, Kayali H, Kubar A, and Timurkaynak E (2002). Early pericyte response to brain hypoxia in cats: an ultrastructural study. *Microvasc Res 64:* 116-119

Gonzalez-Scarano F, Baltuch G. (1999). Microglia as mediators of inflammatory and degenerative diseases. *Annu Rev Neurosci 22*:219–240.

Graeber MB, Streit WJ, Kiefer R, Schoen SW, Kreutzberg GW (1990) New expression of myelomonocytic antigens by microglia and perivascular cells following lethal motor neuron injury. *J. Neuroimmunol. 27*:121–132.

Grossmann R, Stence N, Carr J, Fuller L, Waite M, Dailey ME. (2002) Juxtavascular microglia migrate along brain microvessels following activation during early postnatal development. *Glia. 37*:229-240

Gumbiner BM (1996). Cell adhesion: the molecular basis of tissue architecture and morphogenesis. *Cell 84*:345-357.

Gursoy-Ozdemir Y., Qiu J., Matsuoka N., Bolay H., Bermpohl D., Jin H., Wang X., Rosenberg G. A., Lo E. H. and Moskowitz M. A. (2004) Cortical spreading depression activates and upregulates MMP-9. *J. Clin. Invest. 113*, 1447–1455.

Guthrie PB, Knappenberger J, Segal M, Bennett MV, Charles AC, Kater SB. (1999) ATP released from astrocytes mediates glial calcium waves. *J Neurosci. 19*:520-528.

Ha SK, Lee P, Park JA, Oh HR, Lee SY, Park JH, Lee EH, Ryu JH, Lee KR, Kim SY. (2008) Apigenin inhibits the production of NO and PGE(2) in microglia and inhibits neuronal cell death in a middle cerebral artery occlusion-induced focal ischemia mice model. *Neurochem Int. 52*:878-886.

Hamann GF, Okada Y, Fitridge R, del Zoppo GJ (1995). Microvascular basal lamina antigens disappear during cerebral ischemia and reperfusion. *Stroke 26*:2120-2126

Hamann GF, Liebetrau M, Martens H, Burggraf D, Kloss CU, Bültemeier G, Wunderlich N, Jäger G, Pfefferkorn T (2002). Microvascular basal lamina injury after experimental focal cerebral ischemia and reperfusion in the rat. *J Cereb Blood Flow Metab. 22*:526-533

Hamm S, Dehouck B, Kraus J, Wolburg-Buchholz K, Wolburg H, Risau W, Cecchelli R, Engelhardt B, Dehouck MP (2004). Astrocyte mediated modulation of blood-brain barrier permeability does not correlate with a loss of tight junction proteins from the cellular contacts. *Cell Tissue Res 315*:157-166.

Han HS, Qiao Y, Karabiyikoglu M, Giffard RG, Yenari MA.(2002) Influence of mild hypothermia on inducible nitric oxide synthase expression and reactive nitrogen production in experimental stroke and inflammation. *J Neurosci. 22*:3921-3928.

Haorah J, Ramirez SH, Schall K, Smith D, Pandya R, Persidsky Y (2007) Oxidative stress activates protein tyrosine kinase and matrix metalloproteinases leading to blood-brain barrier dysfunction. *J Neurochem. 101*:566- 576

Haorah J, Schall K, Ramirez SH, Persidsky Y. (2008) Activation of protein tyrosine kinases and matrix metalloproteinases causes blood-brain barrier injury: Novel mechanism for neurodegeneration associated with alcohol abuse. *Glia. 56*:78-88.

Harhaj NS, Antonetti DA (2004). Regulation of tight junctions and loss of barrier function in pathophysiology. *Int J Biochem Cell Biol 36*:1206-1237.

Haskins J, Gu L, Wittchen ES, Hibbard J, Stevenson BR (1998). ZO-3, a novel member of the MAGUK protein family found at the tight junction, interacts with ZO-1 and occludin. *J Cell Biol 141*:199-208.

Hayashi K, Nakao S, Nakaoke R, Nakagawa S, Kitagawa N, Niwa M (2004). Effects of hypoxia on endothelial/pericytic co-culture model of the blood-brain barrier. *Regul Pept 123*:77-83.

He Y, Imam SZ, Dong Z, Jankovic J, Ali SF, Appel SH, Le W (2003) Role of nitric oxide in rotenone-induced nigro-striatal injury. *J Neurochem. 86*:1338-1345.

Hellstrom M, Gerhardt H, Kalen M, Li X, Eriksson U, Wolburg H, Betsholtz C (2001). Lack of pericytes leads to endothelial hyperplasia and abnormal vascular morphogenesis. *J Cell Biol 153*:543-553.

Herman IM, D'Amore PA. (1985) Microvascular pericytes contain muscle and nonmuscle actins. *J Cell Biol. 101*:43-52

Heyen JR, Ye S, Finck BN, Johnson RW (2000). Interleukin (IL)-10 inhibits IL-6 production in microglia by preventing activation of NF-kappaB. *Brain Res Mol Brain Res. 77*:138-147

Hickey WF, Vass K, Lassmann H (1992). Bone marrow-derived elements in the central nervous system: an immunohistochemical and ultrastructural survey of rat chimeras. *J. Neuropathol. Exp. Neurol. 51* : 246–256

Hirano, A, Kawanami T, Llena J F (1994). Electron-microscopy of the blood–brain-barrier in disease. *Microsc Res Techniq 27*:543–556.

Hirase T, Staddon JM, Saitou M, Ando-Akatsuka Y, Itoh M, Furuse M, Fujimoto K, Tsukita S, Rubin LL (1997). Occludin as a possible determinant of tight junction permeability in endothelial cells. *J Cell Sci 110*:1603-1613.

Ho KL (1985). Ultrastructure of cerebellar capillary hemangioblastoma. IV. Pericytes and their relationship to endothelial cells. *Acta Neuropathol 67* : 254–264.

Hooper DC, Scott GS, Zborek A, Mikheeva T, Kean RB, Koprowski H, Spitsin SV (2000). Uric acid, a peroxynitrite scavenger, inhibits CNS inflammation, blood-CNS barrier permeability changes, and tissue damage in a mouse model of multiple sclerosis. *FASEB J. 14*:691-698.

Huang DR, Wang J, Kivisakk P, Rollins BJ, Ransohoff RM (2001). Absence of monocyte chemoattractant protein 1 in mice leads to decreased local macrophage recruitment and antigen-specific T helper cell type 1 immune response in experimental autoimmune encephalomyelitis. *J Exp Med. 193*:713-726.

Huang J, Upadhyay UM, Tamargo RJ (2006). Inflammation in stroke and focal cerebral ischemia. *Surg Neurol 66*:232-245.

Hüttemann M, Lee I, Kreipke CW, Petrov T (2008). Suppression of the inducible form of nitric oxide synthase prior to traumatic brain injury improves cytochrome c oxidase activity and normalizes cellular energy levels. *Neuroscience. 151*:148-154

Ishikawa A, Yoshida H, Metoki N, Toki T, Imaizumi T, Matsumiya T, Yamashita K, Taima K, Satoh K (2007). Edaravone inhibits the expression of vascular endothelial growth factor in human astrocytes exposed to hypoxia. *Neurosci Res. 59*:406-412.

Jakobsen J, Knudsen GM, Juhler M (1987). Cation permeability of the blood-brain barrier in streptozotocin-diabetic rats. *Diabetologia. 30*:409-413

Jander S, Kraemer M, Schroeter M, Witte OW, Stoll G (1995). Lymphocytic infiltration and expression of intercellular adhesion molecule-1 in photochemically induced ischemia of the rat cortex. *J Cereb Blood Flow Metab. 15*:42-51.

Janigro D (1999). Blood–brain barrier, ion homeostatis and epilepsy: possible implications towards the understanding of ketogenic diet mechanisms, *Epilepsy Res. 37*: 223–232.

Janigro D, West GA, Nguyen TS, Winn HR (1994). Regulation of blood-brain barrier endothelial cells by nitric oxide. *Circ Res 75*:528-538.

Janzer RC, Raff MC (1987). Astrocytes induce blood-brain barrier properties in endothelial cells. *Nature 325*:253-257.

Jefferies WA, Brandon MR, Hunt SV, Williams AF, K.C. Gatter KC, Mason DY (1984). Transferrin receptor on endothelium of brain capillaries, *Nature 312*: 162–163.

Jenner P, Olanow CW (1998). Understanding cell death in Parkinson's disease. *Ann Neurol. 44*:S72-84

Jesaitis LA, Goodenough DA (1994). Molecular characterization and tissue distribution of ZO-2, a tight junction protein homologous to ZO-1 and the Drosophila discs large tumor suppressor protein. *J Cell Biol 124* : 949–962

Jiang J, Wang W, Sun YJ, Hu M, Li F, Zhu DY (2007). Neuroprotective effect of curcumin on focal cerebral ischemic rats by preventing blood-brain barrier damage. *Eur J Pharmacol 561*:54-62.

Josko J, Knefel K (2003). The role of vascular endothelial growth factor in cerebral oedema formation. *Folia Neuropathol 41*:161-166.

Josko J, Mazurek M (2004). Transcription factors having impact on vascular endothelial growth factor (VEGF) gene expression in angiogenesis. *Med Sci Monit 10*:RA89-98.

Kacem K, Lacombe P, Seylaz J, Bonvento G (1998). Structural organization of the perivascular astrocyte endfeet and their relationship with the endothelial glucose transporter: a confocal microscopy study. *Glia 23*:1–10.

Kalaria RN, Harik SI (1989).Reduced glucose transporter at the blood–brain barrier and in cerebral cortex in Alzheimer disease, *J. Neurochem. 53* : 1083–1088

Kalaria RN, Cohen DL, Premkumar DR, Nag S, LaManna JC, Lust WD (1998). Vascular endothelial growth factor in Alzheimer's disease and experimental cerebral ischemia. *Brain Res Mol Brain Res. 62*:101-105

Kalaria RN (1996). Cerebral vessels in ageing and Alzheimer's disease. *Pharmacol Ther. 72*:193-214

Kalaria RN (1999). The blood-brain barrier and cerebrovascular pathology in Alzheimer's disease. *Ann N Y Acad Sci. 893*: 113–125

Kato H, Takahashi A, Itoyama Y (2003). Cell cycle protein expression in proliferating microglia and astrocytes following transient global cerebral ischemia in the rat. *Brain Res Bull* 2003 *60*:215-221.

Kaur C, Ling EA (1992). Activation and re-expression of surface antigen in microglia following an epidural application of kainic acid in the rat brain. *J Anat. 180*:333-342

Kaur C, Ling EA (2008). Blood brain barrier in hypoxic-ischemic conditions. *Curr Neurovasc Res. 5*:71-81.

Kaur C, Sivakumar V, Zhang Y, Ling EA (2006). Hypoxia-induced astrocytic reaction and increased vascular permeability in the rat cerebellum. *Glia 54*:826-839.

Kawanokuchi J, Mizuno T, Takeuchi H, Kato H, Wang J, Mitsuma N, Suzumura A (2006). Production of interferon-gamma by microglia. *Mult Scler. 12*:558-564

Kean RB, Spitsin SV, Mikheeva T, Scott GS, Hooper DC (2000). The peroxynitrite scavenger uric acid prevents inflammatory cell invasion into the central nervous system in experimental allergic encephalomyelitis through maintenance of blood-central nervous system barrier integrity. *J Immunol. 165*:6511-6518

Kida S, Steart PV, Zhang ET, Weller RO (1993) Perivascular cells act as scavengers in the cerebral perivascular spaces and remain distinct from pericytes, microglia and macrophages. *Acta Neuropathol. 85* : 646–652

Kim Y, Imdad RY, Stephenson AH, Sprague RS, Lonigro AJ (1998). Vascular endothelial growth factor mRNA in pericytes is upregulated by phorbol myristate acetate. *Hypertension.* 31:511-515.

Kim G. W., Gasche Y., Grzeschik S., Copin J. C., Maier C. M. and Chan P. H. (2003) Neurodegeneration in striatum induced by the mitochondrial toxin 3-nitropropionic acid: role of matrix metalloproteinase-9 in early blood-brain barrier disruption *J. Neurosci. 23*, 8733–8742.

Kirk J, Plumb J, Mirakhur M, McQuaid S (2003). Tight junctional abnormality in multiple sclerosis white matter affects all calibres of vessel and is associated with blood-brain barrier leakage and active demyelination. *J Pathol. 201*:319-327.

Koch M, Mostert J, Arutjunyan A, Stepanov M, Teelken A, Heersema D, De Keyser J (2008). Peripheral blood leukocyte NO production and oxidative stress in multiple sclerosis. *Mult Scler. 14*:159-165.

Kondoh T, Uneyama H, Nishino H, Torii K (2002). Melatonin reduces cerebral edema formation caused by transient forebrain ischemia in rats. *Life Sci 72*:583-590.

Koprich JB, Reske-Nielsen C, Mithal P, Isacson O (2008). Neuroinflammation mediated by IL-1 beta increases susceptibility of dopamine neurons to degeneration in an animal model of Parkinson's disease. *J Neuroinflammation. 5*:8

Kortekaas R, Leenders KL, van Oostrom JC, Vaalburg W, Bart J, Willemsen AT, Hendrikse NH . (2005) Blood-brain barrier dysfunction in parkinsonian midbrain *in vivo*. *Ann. Neurol. 57*, 176–179.

Koto T, Takubo K, Ishida S, Shinoda H, Inoue M, Tsubota K, Okada Y, Ikeda E (2007). Hypoxia Disrupts the Barrier Function of Neural Blood Vessels through Changes in the Expression of Claudin-5 in Endothelial Cells. *Am J Pathol 170*:1389-1397.

Krum JM, Kenyon KL, and Rosenstein JM (1997) Expression of blood-brain barrier characteristics following neuronal loss and astroglial damage after administration of anti-Thy-1 immunotoxin. *Exp Neurol 146:* 33-45

Kümpfel T, Heydari N, Hohlfeld R (2002). Antegren (natalizumab). A promising new approach to therapy of multiple sclerosis. *Nervenarzt. 73*:552-555

Lai CH, Kuo KH (2005). The critical component to establish in vitro BBB model: Pericyte. *Brain Res Brain Res Rev 50*:258-265.

Lampugnani MG, Dejana E (1997). Interendothelial junctions: structure, signalling and functional roles. *Curr Opin Cell Biol 9*:674-682.

Larson DM, Carson MP, Haudenschild CC (1987). Junctional transfer of small molecules in cultured bovine brain microvascular endothelial cells and pericytes. *Microvasc. Res. 34* : 184–199

Lee MY, Kuan YH, Chen HY, Chen TY, Chen ST, Huang CC, Yang IP, Hsu YS, Wu TS, Lee EJ (2007). Intravenous administration of melatonin reduces the intracerebral cellular inflammatory response following transient focal cerebral ischemia in rats. *J Pineal Res 42*:297-309.

Lee TS, Hu KQ, Chao T, King GL (1989). Characterization of endothelin receptors and effects of endothelin on diacylglycerol and protein kinase C in retinal capillary pericytes. *Diabetes 38*:1643–1646.

Lee WH, Bondy CA (1993). Ischemic injury induces brain glucose transporter gene expression, *Endocrinology 133* : 2540–2544.

Liebner S, FischmannA, Rascher G, Duffner F, Grote EH, Wolburg H (2000a). Claudin-1 expression and tight junction morphology are altered in blood vessels of human glioblastoma multiforme. *Acta Neuropathol 100*:323–331.

Liebner S, Kniesel U, Kalbacher H,. Wolburg H (2000b). Correlation of tight junction morphology with the expression of tight junction proteins in blood–brain barrier endothelial cells. *Eur J Cell Biol 79*: 707–717

Lippoldt A, Kniesel U, Liebner S, Kalbacher H, Kirsch T, Wolburg H, Haller H (2000). Structural alterations of tight junctions are associated with loss of polarity in stroke-prone spontaneously hypertensive rat blood–brain barrier endothelial cells. *Brain Res 885*: 251–261.

Lotufo CM, Lopes C, Dubocovich ML, Farsky SH, Markus RP (2001). Melatonin and N-acetylserotonin inhibit leukocyte rolling and adhesion to rat microcirculation. *Eur J Pharmacol.* 430:351-357.

Lotufo CM, Yamashita CE, Farsky SH, Markus RP (2006). Melatonin effect on endothelial cells reduces vascular permeability increase induced by leukotriene B4. *Eur J Pharmacol. 534*:258-263.

Lu DY, Liou HC, Tang CH, Fu WM (2006). Hypoxia-induced iNOS expression in microglia is regulated by the PI3-kinase/Akt/mTOR signaling pathway and activation of hypoxia inducible factor-1alpha. *Biochem Pharmacol 72*:992-1000.

Lukes A, Mun-Bryce S, Lukes M, Rosenberg GA (1999). Extracellular matrix degradation by metalloproteinases and central nervous system diseases. *Mol Neurobiol 19*:267-284.

Lüth HJ, Münch G, Arendt T (2002). Aberrant expression of NOS isoforms in Alzheimer's disease is structurally related to nitrotyrosine formation. *Brain Res.* 953:135-143.

Machado L. S., Kozak A., Ergul A., Hess D. C., Borlongan C. V. and Fagan S. C. (2006) Delayed minocycline inhibits ischemia-activated matrix metalloproteinases 2 and 9 after experimental stroke. *BMC Neurosci. 7*, 56.

MacIntyre A, Abramov R, Hammond CJ, Hudson AP, Arking EJ, Little CS, Appelt DM, Balin BJ (2003). Chlamydia pneumoniae infection promotes the transmigration of monocytes through human brain endothelial cells. *J Neurosci Res. 71*:740-750

Malinski T (2007). Nitric oxide and nitroxidative stress in Alzheimer's disease. *J Alzheimers Dis. 11*:207-218.

Man S, Ubogu EE, Ransohoff RM (2007). Inflammatory cell migration into the central nervous system: a few new twists on an old tale. *Brain Pathol. 17*:243-250

Mandal M, Mandal A, Das S, Chakraborti T, Sajal C (2003). Clinical implications of matrix metalloproteinases. *Mol Cell Biochem 252*:305-329

Mark KS and Davis TP (2002). Cerebral microvascular changes in permeability and tight junctions induced by hypoxia-reoxygenation. *Am J Physiol Heart Circ Physiol 282*: H1485–H1494

Mark KS, Burroughs AR, Brown RC, Huber JD, Davis TP (2004). Nitric oxide mediates hypoxia-induced changes in paracellular permeability of cerebral microvasculature. *Am J Physiol Heart Circ Physiol* 286:H174-80.

Mark KS, Trickler WJ, Miller DW (2001). Tumor necrosis factor-alpha induces cyclooxygenase-2 expression and prostaglandin release in brain microvessel endothelial cells. *J Pharmacol Exp Ther. 297*:1051-1058

Martin-Padura I, Lostaglio S, Schneemann M, Williams L, Romano M, Fruscella P, Panzeri C, Stoppacciaro A, Ruco L, Villa A, Simmons D, Dejana E (1998). Junctional adhesion molecule, a novel member of the immunoglobulin superfamily that distributes at intercellular junctions and modulates monocyte transmigration. *J Cell Biol 142*:117-127.

Mato M, Ookawara S, Sakamoto A, Aikawa E, Ogawa T, Mitsuhashi U, Masuzawa T, Suzuki H, Honda M, Yazaki Y, Watanabe E, Luoma J, Yla-Herttuala S, Fraser I, Gordon S, Kodama T (1996). Involvement of specific macrophage-lineage cells surrounding arterioles in barrier and scavenger function in brain cortex. *Proc Natl Acad Sci U S A 93*:3269-3274.

Matsugi T, Chen Q, Anderson DR (1997). Contractile responses of cultured bovine retinal pericytes to angiotensin II. *Arch Ophthalmol 115*:1281–1285.

Mayhan WG (1999). VEGF increases permeability of the blood-brain barrier via a nitric oxide synthase/cGMP-dependent pathway. *Am J Physiol 276*:C1148-C1153.

Mazzon E, Cuzzocrea S (2007). Role of TNF-alpha in lung tight junction alteration in mouse model of acute lung inflammation. *Respir Res. 8*:75

McGeer PL, McGeer EG (1995). The inflammatory response system of brain: implication for therapy of Alzheimer and other neurodegenerative diseases. *Brain Res Brain Res Rev 21*:195–218.

McManus C, Berman JW, Brett FM, Staunton H, Farrell M, Brosnan CF (1998) MCP-1, MCP-2 and MCP-3 expression in multiple sclerosis lesions: an immunohistochemical and in situ hybridization study. *J Neuroimmunol 86*: 20-29

Meresse S, Delbart C, Fruchart JC, Cecchelli R (1989). Low-density lipoprotein receptor on endothelium of brain capillaries, *J. Neurochem. 53*: 340–345.

Min JK, Lee YM, Kim JH, Kim YM, Kim SW, Lee SY, Gho YS, Oh GT, Kwon YG (2005). Hepatocyte growth factor suppresses vascular endothelial growth factor-induced expression of endothelial ICAM-1 and VCAM-1 by inhibiting the nuclear factor-kappaB pathway. *Circ Res*. 96:300-307.

Minagar A, Alexander JS (2003). Blood-brain barrier disruption in multiple sclerosis. Mult Scler. 9:540-549.

Mooradian AD, Chung HC, Shah GN (1997). GLUT-1 expression in the cerebra of patients with Alzheimer's disease, *Neurobiol. Aging 18* : 469–474

Mooradian AD, Uko-eninn A (1995. Age-related changes in the antioxidative potential of cerebral microvessels. *Brain Res. 671*:159-163.

Morgan L, Shah B, Rivers LE, Barden L, Groom AJ, Chung R, Higazi D, Desmond H, Smith T, Staddon JM (2007). Inflammation and dephosphorylation of the tight junction protein occludin in an experimental model of multiple sclerosis. *Neuroscience. 147*:664-673.

Morioka T, Kalehua AN, Streit WJ 91993). Characterization of microglial reaction after middle cerebral artery occlusion in rat brain. *J Comp Neurol. 327*:123-132

Morita K, Sasaki H, Fujimoto K, Furuse M, M. Tsukita M (1999). Claudin-11/OSP-based tight junctions of myelin sheaths in brain and Sertoli cells in testis. *J Cell Biol 145*:579–588.

Mulligan SJ, MacVicar BA (2004). Calcium transients in astrocyte endfeet cause cerebrovascular constrictions. *Nature. 431*:195-199.

Nag S (2003). Morphology and molecular properties of cellular components of normal cerebral vessels. In: *The blood-brain barrier*. Ed. S. Nag. Humana Press, pp 3-36.

Nag S, Robertson DM, Dinsdale HB (1978). Cytoplasmic filaments in intracerebral cortical vessels. Ann Neurol. 3:555-559.

Nag S, Takahashi JL, Kilty DW (1997). Role of vascular endothelial growth factor in blood-brain barrier breakdown and angiogenesis in brain trauma. *J Neuropathol Exp Neurol. 56*:912-921

Nag S (1995). Role of the endothelial cytoskeleton in blood-brain-barrier permeability to protein. *Acta Neuropathol. 90*:454-460.

Nagaraja TN, Knight RA, Croxen RL, Konda KP, Fenstermacher JD (2006). Acute neurovascular unit protection by simvastatin in transient cerebral ischemia. *Neurol Res 28*:826-830.

Nagy JI, Patel D, Ochalski PA, Stelmack GL (1999). Connexin30 in rodent, cat and human brain: selective expression in gray matter astrocytes, co-localization with connexin43 at gap junctions and late developmental appearance. *Neuroscience. 88*:447-468

Naik UP, Eckfeld K (2003). Junctional adhesion molecule 1 (JAM-1). *J Biol Regul Homeost Agents 17*:341-347.

Nakagawa Y, Fujimoto N, Matsumoto K, Cervos-Navarro J (1990). Morphological changes in acute cerebral ischemia after occlusion and reperfusion in the rat. *Adv Neurol 52*:21-27.

Neuhaus J, Risau W, Wolburg H (1991). Induction of blood-brain barrier characteristics in bovine brain endothelial cells by rat astroglial cells in transfilter coculture. *Ann N Y Acad Sci 633*:578-580.

Nicchia GP, Frigeri A, Liuzzi GM, Santacroce MP, Nico B, Procino G, Quondamatteo F, Herken R, Roncali L, Svelto M (2000). Aquaporin-4-containing astrocytes sustain a temperature- and mercury-insensitive swelling in vitro. *Glia. 31*:29-38.

Nomura M , Yamagishi S, Harada S , Hayashi Y, Yamashima T, J. Yamashita J, Yamamoto H (1995). Possible participation of autocrine and paracrine vascular endothelial growth factors in hypoxia-induced proliferation of endothelial cells and pericytes. *J. Biol. Chem. 270* : 28316–28324

O'Donnell ME (1993). Role of Na-K-Cl cotransport in vascular endothelial cell volume regulation. *Am J Physiol. 264*: C1316-1326.

Oldendorf WH, Cornford ME, Brown WJ (1977). The large apparent work capability of the blood–brain barrier: a study of the mitochondrial content of capillary endothelial cells in brain and other tissues of the rat. *Ann Neurol 1*:409–417

Oppenheimer-Marks N, Davis LS, Bogue DT, Ramberg J, Lipsky PE (1991).. Differential utilization of ICAM-1 and VCAM-1 during the adhesion and transendothelial migration of human T lymphocytes. *J Immunol, 147*: 2913–2921

Pachter JS, de Vries HE, Fabry Z (2003). The blood-brain barrier and its role in immune privilege in the central nervous system. *J Neuropathol Exp Neurol 62*:593-604.

Pachter JS, de Vries HE, Fabry Z (2003). The blood-brain barrier and its role in immune privilege in the central nervous system. *J Neuropathol Exp Neurol. 62*:593-604.

Palma J, Macedonia C, Deuster P, Olsen C, Mozayeni BR, Crutchfield KE (2006). Cerebrovascular dynamics and vascular endothelial growth factor in acute mountain sickness. *Wilderness Environ Med 17*:1-7

Pan W, Banks WA, Kennedy MK, Gutierrez EG, Kastin AJ (1996). Differential permeability of the BBB in acute EAE: enhanced transport of TNF-α. *Am J Physiol. 271*: E636–E642

Panickar KS, Norenberg MD (2005). Astrocytes in cerebral ischemic injury: morphological and general considerations. *Glia 50*:287-298.

Papadopoulos MC, Krishna S, Verkman AS (2002). Aquaporin water channels and brain edema. *Mt Sinai J Med 69*:242-248.

Papadopoulos MC, Manley GT, Krishna S, Verkman AS (2004a). Aquaporin-4 facilitates reabsorption of excess fluid in vasogenic brain edema. *FASEB J 18*:1291-1293.

Papadopoulos MC, Saadoun S, Binder DK, Manley GT, Krishna S, Verkman AS. (2004 b). Molecular mechanisms of brain tumor edema. *Neuroscience 129*:1011-1020.

Papadopoulos MC, Krishna S, Verkman AS (2002).Aquaporin water channels and brain edema. *Mt Sinai J Med. 69*:242-248

Papadopoulos MC, Manley GT, Krishna S, Verkman AS (2004a). Aquaporin-4 facilitates reabsorption of excess fluid in vasogenic brain edema. *FASEB J. 18*:1291-1293

Papadopoulos MC, Saadoun S, Binder DK, Manley GT, Krishna S, Verkman AS (2004b).Molecular mechanisms of brain tumor edema. *Neuroscience. 129*:1011-1020

Papadopoulos MC, Verkman AS (2005). Aquaporin-4 gene disruption in mice reduces brain swelling and mortality in pneumococcal meningitis. *J Biol Chem 280*:13906-13912.

Parathath SR, Parathath S, Tsirka SE (2006). Nitric oxide mediates neurodegeneration and breakdown of the blood-brain barrier in tPA-dependent excitotoxic injury in mice. *J Cell Sci.* 119:339-349

Pardridge WM (1999). Blood-brain barrier biology and methodology. *J Neurovirol 5*:556-569

Pardridge WM (2005). Molecular biology of the blood-brain barrier. *Mol Biotechnol.* 2005 30:57-70

Parton RG, Richards AA (2003). Lipid rafts and caveolae as portals for endocytosis: new insights and common mechanisms. *Traffic.* 4:724-38.

Paspalas CD, Papadopoulos GC (1996). Ultrastructural relationships between noradrenergic nerve fibers and non-neuronal elements in the rat cerebral cortex. *Glia. 17*:133-146.

Pei Z, Cheung RT (2004). Pretreatment with melatonin exerts anti-inflammatory effects against ischemia/reperfusion injury in a rat middle cerebral artery occlusion stroke model. *J Pineal Res 37*:85-91.

Pekny M, Nilsson M (2005). Astrocyte activation and reactive gliosis. *Glia 50*:427-434

Penet MF, Abou-Hamdan M, Coltel N, Cornille E, Grau GE, de Reggi M, Gharib B (2008). Protection against cerebral malaria by the low-molecular-weight thiol pantethine. *Proc Natl Acad Sci U S A. 105*: 1321-1326

Persidsky Y, Heilman D, Haorah J, Zelivyanskay M, Persidsky R, Weber G, Shimokawa H, Kaibuchi K, Ikezu T (2006) Rho-mediated regulation of tight junctions during monocyte migration across blood–brain barrier in HIV-1 encephalitis (HIVE). *Blood 107*:4720–4730

Persidsky Y, Zheng J, Miller D, Gendelman HE (2000) Mononuclear phagocytes mediate blood–brain barrier compromise and neuronal injury during HIV-1-associated dementia. *J Leukoc Biol 68*:413–422

Petito CK (1979). Early and late mechanisms of increased vascular permeability following experimental cerebral infarction. *J Neuropathol Exp Neurol 38*:222-234.

Petty MA, Lo EH (2002). Junctional complexes of the blood-brain barrier: permeability changes in neuroinflammation. *Prog Neurobiol 68*:311-323.

Phares TW, Fabis MJ, Brimer CM, Kean RB, Hooper DC (2007). A peroxynitrite-dependent pathway is responsible for blood-brain barrier permeability changes during a central nervous system inflammatory response: TNF-alpha is neither necessary nor sufficient. *J Immunol. 178*: 7334-7343.

Pichiule P, Chavez JC, Xu K, LaManna JC (1999). Vascular endothelial growth factor upregulation in transient global ischemia induced by cardiac arrest and resuscitation in rat brain. *Brain Res Mol Brain Res 74*:83-90.

Planas AM, Sole S, Justicia C (2001). Expression and activation of matrix metalloproteinase-2 and -9 in rat brain after transient focal cerebral ischemia *Neurobiol Dis 8*:834-846.

Plateel M, Teissier E, and Cecchelli R (1997) Hypoxia dramatically increases the nonspecific transport of blood-borne proteins to the brain. *J Neurochem 68:* 874-877

Plumb J, McQuaid S, Mirakhur M, Kirk J (2002). Abnormal endothelial tight junctions in active lesions and normal-appearing white matter in multiple sclerosis. *Brain Pathol. 12*:154-169

Poritz LS, Garver KI, Tilberg AF, Koltun WA (2004). Tumor necrosis factor alpha disrupts tight junction assembly. *J Surg Res. 116*:14-18.

Prat A, Biernacki K, Wosik K, Antel JP (2001). Glial cell influence on the human blood-brain barrier. *Glia 36*:145-155.

Proescholdt MA, Heiss JD, Walbridge S, Muhlhauser J, Capogrossi MC, Oldfield EH, Merrill MJ (1999). Vascular endothelial growth factor (VEGF) modulates vascular permeability and inflammation in rat brain. *J Neuropathol Exp Neurol. 58*:613-627.

Queiroz G, Meyer DK, Meyer A, Starke K, von Kügelgen I (1999). A study of the mechanism of the release of ATP from rat cortical astroglial cells evoked by activation of glutamate receptors. *Neuroscience. 91*:1171-1181.

Qutub AA, Hunt CA (2005). Glucose transport to the brain: a systems model. *Brain Res Brain Res Rev. 49*:595-617.

Reiss Y, Hoch G, Deutsch U, Engelhardt B (1998). T cell interaction with ICAM-1-deficient endothelium in vitro: essential role for ICAM-1 and ICAM-2 in transendothelial migration of T cells. *Eur J Immunol. 28*:3086-3099.

Rentzos M, Michalopoulou M, Nikolaou C, Cambouri C, Rombos A, Dimitrakopoulos A, Vassilopoulos D (2005). The role of soluble intercellular adhesion molecules in neurodegenerative disorders. *J Neurol Sci. 228*:129-135.

Rhodin J, Thomas T, Bryant M, Clark L, Sutton ET (1999). Animal model of vascular inflammation. *J Submicrosc Cytol Pathol. 31*:305-311.

Risau W (1991). Induction of blood-brain barrier endothelial cell differentiation.*Ann N Y Acad Sci.* 633:405-419.

Risau, W (1997). Mechanisms of angiogenesis. *Nature 386* : 671–674

Rite I, Machado A, Cano J, Venero JL (2008). Intracerebral VEGF injection highly upregulates AQP4 mRNA and protein in the perivascular space and glia limitans externa. *Neurochem Int. 52*:897-903

Rite I, Machado A, Cano J, Venero JL (2007). Blood-brain barrier disruption induces in vivo degeneration of nigral dopaminergic neurons. *J Neurochem. 101*:1567-1582.

Rottkamp CA, Raina AK, Zhu X, Gaier E, Bush AI, Atwood CS, Chevion M, Perry G, Smith MA (2001). Redox-active iron mediates amyloid-beta toxicity. *Free Radic Biol Med. 30*:447-450.

Rubin LL, Barbu K, Bard F, Cannon C, Hall DE, Horner H, Janatpour M, Liaw C, Manning K, Morales J (1991). Differentiation of brain endothelial cells in cell culture. *Ann N Y Acad Sci 633*:420-425

Rucker HK, Wynder HJ, Thomas WE (2000). Cellular mechanisms of CNS pericytes. *Brain Res Bull. 51*:363-369.

Saija A, Princi P, De Pasquale R, Costa G, De Sarro GB (1992). Evaluation of local cerebral glucose utilization and the permeability of the blood–brain barrier in the genetically epilepsy-prone rat, *Exp. Brain Res. 88*: 151–157.

Saleh A, Schroeter M, Jonkmanns C, Hartung HP, Modder U, Jander S (2004). In vivo MRI of brain inflammation in human ischaemic stroke. *Brain 127*:1670-1677.

Sanchez-del-Rio M. and Reuter U. (2004) Migraine aura: new information on underlying mechanisms. *Curr. Opin. Neurol. 17*, 289–293.

Savettieri G, Di Liegro I, Catania C, Licata L, Pitarresi GL, D'Agostino S, Schiera G, De Caro V, Giandalia LI, Giannola LI, Cestelli A (2000). Neurons and ECM regulate occludin localization in brain endothelial cells. *NeuroReport 11*:1081–1084.

Schnitzer JE, Allard J, Oh P (1995). NEM inhibits transcytosis, endocytosis, and capillary permeability: implication of caveolae fusion in endothelia. *Am J Physiol. 268*:H48-55.

Schoch HJ, Fischer S, Marti HH (2002). Hypoxia-induced vascular endothelial growth factor expression causes vascular leakage in the brain. *Brain 125*:2549-2557.

Schreibelt G, Kooij G, Reijerkerk A, van Doorn R, Gringhuis SI, van der Pol S, Weksler BB, Romero IA, Couraud PO, Piontek J, Blasig IE, Dijkstra CD, Ronken E, de Vries HE (2007). Reactive oxygen species alter brain endothelial tight junction dynamics via RhoA, PI3 kinase, and PKB signaling. *FASEB J. 21*:3666-3676.

Shaftel SS, Carlson TJ, Olschowka JA, Kyrkanides S, Matousek SB, O'Banion MK (2007). Chronic interleukin-1beta expression in mouse brain leads to leukocyte infiltration and neutrophil-independent blood brain barrier permeability without overt neurodegeneration. *J Neurosci. 27*:9301-9309

Shepro D, Morel NML (1993). Pericyte physiology. *FASEB J. 7*:1031–1038

Shibuya M (2006). Vascular endothelial growth factor receptor-1 (VEGFR-1/Flt-1): a dual regulator for angiogenesis. *Angiogenesis 9*:225-230

Shivers RR, Edmonds CL, Del Maestro RF (1984). Microvascular permeability in induced astrocytomas and peritumor neuropil of rat brain. A high-voltage electron microscope-protein tracer study. *Acta Neuropathol (Berl) 64*:192-202.

Shukla A, Dikshit M, Srimal RC (1996). Nitric oxide-dependent blood-brain barrier permeability alteration in the rat brain. *Experientia 52*:136-140.

Simard M, Arcuino G, Takano T, Liu QS, Nedergaard M (2003). Signaling at the gliovascular interface. *J Neurosci. 23*:9254-9262.

Simionescu M (1988). Receptor-mediated transcytosis of plasma molecules by vascular endothelium. In: *Endothelial cell biology in health and disease.* Eds Simionescu N and Simionescu N. Plenum, New York. PP 69-104.

Simionescu M, Gafencu A, Antohe F (2002). Transcytosis of plasma macromolecules in endothelial cells: a cell biological survey. *Microsc Res Tech 57*:269-288

Simionescu M, Simionescu N, Palade GE (1974). Morphometric data on the endothelium of blood capillaries. *J Cell Biol 60*:128-152.

Simionescu M, Ghinea N, Fixman A, Lasser M, Kukes L, Simionescu N, Palade GE (1988). The cerebral microvasculature of the rat: structure and luminal surface properties during early development. *J Submicrosc Cytol Pathol.* 20:243-261.

Simpson IA, Chundu KR, Davies-Hill T, Honer WG, Davies P (1994). Decreased concentrations of GLUT1 and GLUT3 glucose transporters in the brains of patients with Alzheimer's disease, *Ann. Neurol. 35* : 546–551

Simpson JE, Newcombe J, Cuzner ML, Woodroofe MN (1998) Expression of monocyte chemoattractant protein-1 and other beta-chemokines by resident glia and inflammatory cells in multiple sclerosis lesions. *J Neuroimmunol 84*: 238-249

Simpson JE, Newcombe J, Cuzner ML, Woodroofe MN (2000) Expression of the interferon-gamma-inducible chemokines IP-10 and Mig and their receptor, CXCR3, in multiple sclerosis lesions. *Neuropathol Appl Neurobiol 26*: 133-142

Sims DE (1991). Recent advances in pericyte biology—Implications for health and disease. *Can. J. Cardiol. 7*: 431–443.

Sims DE (1986). The pericyte—A review. *Tissue Cell 18*:153–174

Sinor AD, Irvin SM, Cobbs CS, Chen J, Graham SH, Greenberg DA (1998). Hypoxic induction of vascular endothelial growth factor (VEGF) protein in astroglial cultures. *Brain Res 812*:289-291

Sinor AD, Irvin SM, Cobbs CS, Chen J, Graham SH, Greenberg DA (1998). Hypoxic induction of vascular endothelial growth factor (VEGF) protein in astroglial cultures. *Brain Res. 812*:289-291

Skalli O, Pelte MF, Peclet MC, Gabbiani G, Gugliotta P, Bussolati G, Ravazzola M, Orci L (1989). Alpha-smooth muscle actin, a differentiation marker of smooth muscle cells, is present in microfilamentous bundles of pericytes. *J Histochem Cytochem. 37*:315-321

Sorensen TL, Tani M, Jensen J, Pierce V, Lucchinetti C, Folcik VA, Qin S, Rottman J, Sellebjerg F, Strieter RM, Frederiksen JL, Ransohoff RM (1999) Expression of specific chemokines and chemokine receptors in the central nervous system of multiple sclerosis patients. *J Clin Invest 103*: 807-815

Stevenson BR, Siliciano JD, Mooseker MS, Goodenough DA (1986). Identification of ZO-1: a high molecular weight polypeptide associated with the tight junction (zonula occludens) in a variety of epithelia. *J Cell Biol 103*:755-766.

Stewart PA, Hayakawa K, Hayakawa E, Farrell CL, Del Maestro RF (1985). A quantitative study of blood-brain barrier permeability ultrastructure in a new rat glioma model. *Acta Neuropathol (Berl) 67*:96-102.

Stewart PA, Magliocco M, Hayakawa K, Farrell CL, Del Maestro RF, Girvin J, Kaufmann JC, Vinters HV, Gilbert J (1987). A quantitative analysis of blood-brain barrier ultrastructure in the aging human. *Microvasc Res 33*:270-282.

Stewart PA, Hayakawa K, Farrell CL (1994). Quantitation of blood-brain barrier ultrastructure. *Microsc Res Tech*. 27:516-527.

Streit WJ, Graeber MB, Kreutzberg GW (1989). Expression of Ia antigen on perivascular and microglial cells after sublethal and lethal motor neuron injury. *Exp. Neurol. 105* : 115–126

Sun D, Lytle C, O'Donnell ME (1995). Astroglial cell-induced expression of Na-K-Cl cotransporter in brain microvascular endothelial cells. *Am J Physiol. 269*: C150

Sun GY, Xu J, Jensen MD, Yu S, Wood WG, González FA, Simonyi A, Sun AY, Weisman GA (2005). Phospholipase A2 in astrocytes: responses to oxidative stress, inflammation, and G protein-coupled receptor agonists. *Mol Neurobiol. 31*:27-41

Sun L, Marti HH, Veltkamp R (2008). Hyperbaric oxygen reduces tissue hypoxia and hypoxia-inducible factor-1 alpha expression in focal cerebral ischemia. *Stroke. 39*:1000-1006.

Sun X, He G, Qing H, Zhou W, Dobie F, Cai F, Staufenbiel M, Huang LE, Song W (2006). Hypoxia facilitates Alzheimer's disease pathogenesis by up-regulating BACE1 gene expression. *Proc Natl Acad Sci U S A. 103*:18727-18732

Taffi R, Nanetti L, Mazzanti L, Bartolini M, Vignini A, Raffaelli F, Pasqualetti P, Vernieri F, Provinciali L, Silvestrini M (2008). Plasma levels of nitric oxide and stroke outcome. *J Neurol. 255*:94-98.

Takagi H, King GL, Robinson GS, Ferrara N, Aiello LP (1996). Adenosine mediates hypoxic induction of vascular endothelial growth factor in retinal pericytes and endothelial cells. *Invest Ophthalmol Vis Sci. 37*:2165-2176

Tao-Cheng JH, Nagy Z, Brightman MW (1987). Tight junctions of brain endothelium in vitro are enhanced by astroglia. *J Neurosci 7*:3293-3299.

Tarkowski E, Issa R, Sjögren M, Wallin A, Blennow K, Tarkowski A, Kumar P (2002). Increased intrathecal levels of the angiogenic factors VEGF and TGF-beta in Alzheimer's disease and vascular dementia. *Neurobiol Aging. 23*:237-243.

Tarkowski E (2002). Cytokines in dementias. *Curr Drug Targets Inflamm Allergy. 1*:193-200.

Thiel VE, Audus KL (2001). Nitric oxide and blood-brain barrier integrity. *Antioxid Redox Signal 3*:273-278.

Thomas WE. (1992). Brain microphages: evaluation of microglia and their functions. *Brain Res Brain Res Rev 17*:61–74.

Tilling T, Engelbertz C, Decker S, Korte D, Huwel S, and Galla HJ (2002) Expression and adhesive properties of basement membrane proteins in cerebral capillary endothelial cell cultures. *Cell Tissue Res 310:* 19-29

Tilling T, Korte D, Hoheisel D, and Galla HJ (1998) Basement membrane proteins influence brain capillary endothelial barrier function in vitro. *J Neurochem 71:* 1151-1157.

Tomás-Camardiel M, Rite I, Herrera AJ, de Pablos RM, Cano J, Machado A, Venero JL (2004). Minocycline reduces the lipopolysaccharide-induced inflammatory reaction, peroxynitrite-mediated nitration of proteins, disruption of the blood-brain barrier, and damage in the nigral dopaminergic system. *Neurobiol Dis. 16*:190-201

Torii K, Uneyama H, Nishino H, Kondoh T (2004). Melatonin suppresses cerebral edema caused by middle cerebral artery occlusion/reperfusion in rats assessed by magnetic resonance imaging. *J Pineal Res 36*:18-24.

van Horssen J, Bö L, Dijkstra CD, de Vries HE (2006). Extensive extracellular matrix depositions in active multiple sclerosis lesions. *Neurobiol Dis. 24*:484-4891.

van Horssen J, Brink BP, de Vries HE, van der Valk P, Bø L (2007).. The blood-brain barrier in cortical multiple sclerosis lesions. *J Neuropathol Exp Neurol. 66*:321-328.

van Horssen J, Dijkstra CD, de Vries HE (2007). The extracellular matrix in multiple sclerosis pathology. *J Neurochem. 103*:1293-301

van Meer G, Simons K (1986). The function of tight junctions in maintaining differences in lipid composition between the apical and the basolateral cell surface domains of MDCK cells. *EMBO J 5*:1455-1464

Van Osta A, Moraine JJ, Melot C, Mairbaurl H, Maggiorini M, Naeije R (2005). Effects of high altitude exposure on cerebral hemodynamics in normal subjects. *Stroke 36*:557-560.

Verbeek MM, Westphal JR, Ruiter DJ, de Waal RM (1995). T lymphocyte adhesion to human brain pericytes is mediated via very late antigen-4/vascular cell adhesion molecule-1 interactions. *J Immunol. 154*:5876-5884.

Vorbrodt AW, Dobrogowska DH (2003) Molecular anatomy of intercellular junctions in brain endothelial and epithelial barriers: electron microscopist's view. *Brain Res Rev 42*:221–242

Vorbrodt AW, Dobrogowska DH, Kim YS, Lossinsky AS and Wisniewski HM (1988). Ultrastructural studies of glycoconjugates in brain micro-blood vessels and amyloid plaques of scrapie-infected mice. *Acta Neuropathol (Berl) 75* : 277–287.

Walter R, Maggiorini M, Scherrer U, Contesse J, Reinhart WH (2001). Effects of high-altitude exposure on vascular endothelial growth factor levels in man. *Eur J Appl Physiol 85*:113-117.

Wang F, Graham WV, Wang Y, Witkowski ED, Schwarz BT, Turner JR (2005). Interferon-gamma and tumor necrosis factor-alpha synergize to induce intestinal epithelial barrier dysfunction by up-regulating myosin light chain kinase expression. *Am J Pathol. 166*:409-419

Wang CX, Shuaib A (2007). Critical role of microvasculature basal lamina in ischemic brain injury. *Prog Neurobiol.* 83:140-148

Wang X, Suzuki Y (2007). Microglia produce IFN-gamma independently from T cells during acute toxoplasmosis in the brain. *J Interferon Cytokine Res. 27*:599-605.

Wasserman JK, Schlichter LC (2007). Minocycline protects the blood-brain barrier and reduces edema following intracerebral hemorrhage in the rat. *Exp Neurol. 207*:227-237.

Wasserman JK, Zhu X, Schlichter LC (2007). Evolution of the inflammatory response in the brain following intracerebral hemorrhage and effects of delayed minocycline treatment. *Brain Res. 1180*:140-154

Weiss JM, Downie SA, Lyman WD, Berman JW (1998). Astrocyte-derived monocyte-chemoattractant protein-1 directs the transmigration of leukocytes across a model of the human blood-brain barrier. *J Immunol 161*:6896-6903.

Willis CL, Nolan CC, Reith SN, Lister T, Prior MJ, Guerin CJ, Mavroudis G, and Ray DE (2004) Focal astrocyte loss is followed by microvascular damage, with subsequent repair of the blood-brain barrier in the apparent absence of direct astrocytic contact. *Glia 45:* 325-337

Wilson FC, Harpur J, Watson T, Morrow JI (2003). Adult survivors of severe cerebral hypoxia--case series survey and comparative analysis. *NeuroRehabilitation 18*:291-298

Witt KA, Mark KS, Hom S, Davis TP (2003). Effects of hypoxia-reoxygenation on rat blood-brain barrier permeability and tight junctional protein expression. *Am J Physiol Heart Circ Physiol 285:* H2820-2831.

Wolburg H, Neuhaus J, Kniesel, U, Krauss B, Schmid EM,. Öcalan M, Farrell C , Risau W (1994). Modulation of tight junction structure in blood–brain barrier ECs. Effects of tissue culture, second messengers and cocultured astrocytes. *J Cell Sci 107*: 1347–1357.

Wright AD (2006). Medicine at high altitude. *Clin Med 6*:604-608.

Yamagishi S, Hsu CC, Kobayashi K, Yamamoto H (1993). Endothelin 1 mediates endothelial cell-dependent proliferation of vascular pericytes. *Biochem Biophy Res Commun 191* : 840–846

Yang GY, Gong C, Qin Z, Liu XH, Lorris Betz A (1999). Tumor necrosis factor alpha expression produces increased blood-brain barrier permeability following temporary focal cerebral ischemia in mice. *Brain Res Mol Brain Res 69*:135-143.

Yenari MA, Xu L, Tang XN, Qiao Y, Giffard RG (2006). Microglia potentiate damage to blood-brain barrier constituents: improvement by minocycline in vivo and in vitro. *Stroke 37*:1087-1093.

Youakim A, Ahdieh M (1999). Interferon-gamma decreases barrier function in T84 cells by reducing ZO-1 levels and disrupting apical actin. *Am J Physiol. 276*: G1279-1288

Yurchenko PD, Schittny JC (1990), Molecular architecture of basement membranes. *FASEB J 4* :1577–1590

Zach O, Bauer HC, Richter K, Webersinke G, Tontsch S, Bauer H (1997). Expression of a chemotactic cytokine (MCP-1) in cerebral capillary endothelial cells in vitro. *Endothelium 5*:143-153.

Zhang JM, Wang HK, Ye CQ, Ge W, Chen Y, Jiang ZL, Wu CP, Poo MM, Duan S (2003). ATP released by astrocytes mediates glutamatergic activity-dependent heterosynaptic suppression. *Neuron. 40*: 971-982.

Zhang W, Smith C, Howlett C, Stanimirovic D (2000). Inflammatory activation of human brain endothelial cells by hypoxic astrocytes in vitro is mediated by IL-1beta. *J Cereb Blood Flow Metab 20*:967-978.

Zhang Z, Chopp M (2002). Vascular endothelial growth factor and angiopoietins in focal cerebral ischemia. *Trends Cardiovasc Med. 12*:62-66.

Zhang ZG, Zhang L, Jiang Q, Zhang R, Davies K, Powers C, Bruggen N, Chopp M. (2000). VEGF enhances angiogenesis and promotes blood-brain barrier leakage in the ischemic brain. *J Clin Invest 106*:829-838.

Zhang ZG, Zhang L, Tsang W, Soltanian-Zadeh H, Morris D, Zhang R, Goussev A, Powers C, Yeich T, Chopp M (2002). Correlation of VEGF and angiopoietin expression with disruption of blood-brain barrier and angiogenesis after focal cerebral ischemia. *J Cereb Blood Flow Metab 22* :379-392.

Zipser BD, Johanson CE, Gonzalez L, Berzin TM, Tavares R, Hulette CM, Vitek MP, Hovanesian V, Stopa EG (2007). Microvascular injury and blood-brain barrier leakage in Alzheimer's disease. *Neurobiol Aging. 28*: 977-986

Zlokovic BV, Jovanovic S, Miao W, Samara S, Verma S, Farrell CL (2000). Differential regulation of leptin transport by the choroid plexus and blood-brain barrier and high affinity transport systems for entry into hypothalamus and across the blood-cerebrospinal fluid barrier. *Endocrinology*. 141:1434-1441.

Zlokovic BV (2002) Vascular disorder in Alzheimer's disease: role in pathogenesis of dementia and therapeutic targets. *Adv Drug Deliv Rev 54*:1553–1559

Zlokovic BV (2005) Neurovascular mechanisms of Alzheimer's neurodegeneration. *Trends Neurosci 28*:202–208

Zlokovic BV (2008). The blood-brain barrier in health and chronic neurodegenerative disorders. *Neuron. 57*:178-201.

In: The Blood-Brain Barrier
Editor: Tomas R. Helio
ISBN 978-1-60456-894-3

Chapter 2

TARGETING THE BLOOD-BRAIN BARRIER FOR MULTIPLE SCLEROSIS THERAPY

***Jorge Correale*[1,2,*] *and Andrés Villa*[3]**

[1]Department of Neurology, Institute for Neurological Research Dr. Raúl Carrea (FLENI), and [2]School of Biomedical Sciences, Austral University, Buenos Aires, Argentina; [3]Department of Neurology, José María Ramos Mejía Hospital, School of Medicine Buenos Aires University, Buenos Aires, Argentina.

ABSTRACT

Multiple Sclerosis (MS) is an inflammatory demyelinating disease of the Central Nervous System (CNS), characterized by multifocal perivascular infiltrates made up predominantly of lymphocytes and macrophages, in which lymphocyte recruitment into the brain across the blood-brain barrier (BBB) is critical to disease pathogenesis. Recent investigations have identified crucial components involved in leukocyte migration, providing new insights into mechanisms modulating these neuroinflammatory reactions, as well as novel targets for potential therapeutic strategies aimed at altering CNS inflammatory cell influx. Benefits of interferon β (IFN-β) and methylprednisolone treatment for example, have been associated with adhesion molecule (AM) pathway regulation. Likewise, monoclonal antibodies (mAb) against α_4 integrin have been shown to reduce clinical and MRI activity in experimental autoimmune encephalomyelitis (EAE), decreasing transmigration of lymphocytes to areas of inflammation, and reducing leukocyte activation and proliferation. Similarly, humanized mAb against α_4 integrin (natalizumab) has recently been successfully tested in MS patients. Interference in chemokine-chemokine receptor interactions may represent yet another new molecular target for novel MS therapies, such as IFN-β and statins. Beneficial effects of IFN-β in MS are mediated through T cell metalloproteinase (MMP) production suppression and

* Correspondence concerning this article should be addressed to: Jorge Correale, M.D, Institute for Neurological Research Dr Raúl Carrea, FLENI. Montañeses 2325 (1428), Buenos Aires, Argentina. Telephone: 54-11-5777-3200, Extension: 2704/2706; FAX: 54-11-5777-3209; Email:jcorreale@fleni.org.ar; bairesla@fibertel.com.ar.

increased transcription of inhibitory factors such as tissue inhibitor of metalloproteinase (TIMP). Recently minocycline for example, a tetracycline analogue, has demonstrated EAE severity attenuation through inhibition of MMP-2 and MMP-9 activity.

The presence of the BBB significantly limits therapeutic efficacy of anti-inflammatory molecules or neurotrophic factors administered systemically to patients affected by immune-mediated inflammatory diseases of the CNS like MS. Among some of the novel approaches attempting to overcome this barrier, current research has focused on the study of endogenous peptides that naturally cross it (e.g. insulin, and transferrin) through receptor-mediated endocytosis; the specific receptors involved in this process tend to preserve their transportation properties when linked to potential therapeutic agents, presenting an interesting new platform facilitating drug access into the CNS. Another alternative is the encapsulation of molecules into liposomes, which can then be directed to enter the brain. Under this approach, drugs, neurotrophic peptides, antisense oligonucleotides or genes would be incorporated into the centre of a liposome, and its surface then coated with polyethylene glycol (PEG) to prolong half-life. Current knowledge of cell-trafficking across BBB endothelium and into the CNS has increased significantly in recent years, promising further advances in the rational design of new therapeutic alternatives for the treatment of inflammatory neurological conditions such as MS.

Introduction

Multiple Sclerosis (MS) is an inflammatory demyelinating disease of the Central Nervous System (CNS), affecting an estimated 2 million people throughout the world, and representing the most common non-traumatic cause of disability in young adults. Although its etiology remains unknown, several lines of evidence support the notion that autoimmunity plays a major role in susceptibility to, and development of the disease [1-2]. MS and its animal model, experimental allergic encephalomyelitis (EAE), are both characterised at tissue level by multifocal perivascular infiltrates, predominantly of lymphocytes and macrophages. Interferon-γ (IFN-γ) secreting T lymphocytes (Th1) have long been considered the autoaggressive and disease-inducing CD4+ lymphocyte subset, triggered by circulating myelin antigen (Ag) recognition. However, research during the last decade has not only increased our knowledge of Th1 cell involvement in MS, but also shown that other immunological and neurodegenerative mechanisms within target tissues contribute to disease onset and propagation. For example, Th2 cells directed against myelin Ags and classically thought to be anti-inflammatory, have also been shown to induce destructive brain inflammation in both human and immunodeficient mice, in lieu of protecting the brain from disease [3-4]. Moreover, the range of CD4+ T cell lineages playing key roles in autoimmune disease development, including MS, has recently been expanded to include a new IL-17 producing subset identified as Th-17 [5-6], memory cells immunopositive for IL-17 were detected in highly infiltrated MS lesions, but not in normal appearing white matter or non inflamed brain specimens [7]. Demyelination in MS is characteristically most pronounced in areas bathed by CSF, where plaques tend to gather around small vessels [8]. Activated cell recruitment across blood-brain barrier endothelial cells (EC) seems to be an essential step in triggering CNS inflammation and subsequent tissue injury. Thus, elucidating molecular pathways through which different cell populations enter the CNS is crucial, not only to understand intrathecal immune reactivity, but also because it could make CNS inflammatory cell infiltration prevention a valid therapeutic strategy in disease control.

This chapter details the most important molecular mechanisms regulating immune cell invasion through the BBB in MS, and addresses how knowledge of trafficking determinants has impacted the development of new therapeutic strategies for effective treatment of inflammatory CNS diseases.

Cell Migration into the CNS

BBB structure is conformed by highly specialized ECs forming brain and spinal cord capillaries, in association with various perivascular cells such as smooth muscle cells, perycites, microglial cells and astrocytes [9-10]. ECs situated at the interface between the blood and the brain, perform essential biological functions, including nutrient transport, receptor mediated signaling, leukocyte trafficking, and osmoregulation. Electron microscopy studies of the BBB have identified distinct morphologic and metabolic characteristics in microvascular brain ECs, making them different from those present in peripheral tissues. The most important of these include: a) tight junctions (TJs) present along adjacent cell margins, produced by the interaction of transmembrane proteins such as claudins, occludins and junctional adhesion molecules[13], which projecting into the paracellular space effectively seal it, thus confining penetration across the brain endothelium to transcellular mechanisms [11-12]. b) Endothelial cytoplasm lacking the fenestrations typically present in peripheral-tissue capillaries [14]; c) Fewer pinocytotic vesicles compared to peripheral endothelial cells [15]; d) More mitochondria, suggesting important metabolic activity [16]; and e) Abluminally, a basement membrane and extracellular matrix composed of collagen, elastin, fibrillin, laminin and fibronectin [17-18].

In addition to the structural elements effectively sealing off the BBB, transport systems and drug-metabolizing enzymes provide an additional endothelial barrier [19-21]. Interestingly, quantitative chemical studies have demonstrated a polarity in the distribution of both transport systems and enzymes between luminal and abluminal EC membrane surfaces, further contributing to barrier function. Enzymes such as γ-glutamil transpeptidase (γGT), alkaline phosphatase (AP), and certain efflux transporters such as P-glycoprotein (P-gp) are present mainly on the luminal surface membrane, while ATP and the sodium-dependent amino acid transporter are found on the opposite endothelial surface [20-21].

Current evidence suggests that astrocytes may also influence particular BBB features leading to TJ formation, reducing functional gap area, as well distribution of polarized BBB transporters [22]. Recently, other cell types present on the BBB including pericytes, neurons and perivascular macrophages have also been shown to contribute to development and up-regulation of selective BBB functions [23-25]. For example, it has been suggested that the presence of perycites on blood vessels regulates EC proliferation, survival, migration, differentiation and vascular branching [26]. In addition, there is also evidence that perycites are able to mimic astrocytes in inducing BBB “tightness”. Interestingly, different studies have demonstrated that perycites migrate away from brain microvessels in response to hipoxia or brain trauma [27-28], conditions normally associated with increased BBB permeability. Perivascular macrophages occupy strategic positions allowing selective control of innate and adaptive immune responses. These bone-marrow derived cells, are found on the luminal side of brain vessel-associated basal membranes and replaced by monocytic precursor cells. In the human CNS, perivascular macrophages have been shown to express molecules involved in antigen recognition, antigen presentation and co-stimulation, supporting a possible role for these cells in perivascular inflammation regulation [29]. During pathological insults, the BBB is capable of modulating its own cyto-architecture, increasing permeability while retaining structural integrity, hence protecting the brain and maintaining homeostasis. This function however can be lost under extreme conditions, causing TJs to dissociate, leading to edema, decreased neuronal function and brain damage.

Leukocyte transmigration across the vascular endothelium is a highly regulated process. Under physiological conditions, immune surveillance limits the number of immune cells crossing the BBB and entering the CNS [30]. BBB dysfunction is associated with increased leukocyte trafficking into the CNS, resulting in intense perivascular leukocyte infiltration, a hallmark of MS lesions [8,31]. Some authors consider that activated T cells can penetrate the BBB and enter the perivascular or subarachnoid space, regardless of antigen specificity [32-33]. However, only those T cells encountering CNS antigens presented by perivascular or resident APCs are retained in brain parenchyma, triggering a local inflammatory process [33-34]. Molecular mechanisms leading to transendothelial leukocyte migration across the BBB involve a series of sequential and tightly controlled steps (Figure 1A) : a) weak adhesion of leukocytes to ECs through interaction between selectins and carbohydrate adhesion molecules; b) leukocyte activation through chemokine stimulation of G-protein linked receptors, resulting in functional activation of surface adhesion molecules (AM); c) interactions between activated AMs and endothelial molecules from the IgG superfamily, leading to firm leukocyte adhesion to EC, with subsequent matrix metalloproteinase (MMPs) expression, enabling basement membrane degradation; and finally d) migration of leukocytes across CNS endothelium into brain parenchyma, a process driven by chemokine-chemokine receptor interactions.

Leukocyte recruitment from the bloodstream in response to inflammatory stimuli is rapid but transient, requiring special mechanisms in order to establish cell contact. Selectins represent a specialized subgroup of adhesion molecules which, like lectins, bind carbohydrate ligands. Because the interaction mediated between selectins and their ligands is one of low-affinity, leukocytes can roll along the blood vessel wall and sense activating factors deposited on the endothelial cell surface such as chemokines. Experiments using intravital fluorescence videomicroscopy however, have shown T lymphocytes do not roll in non-inflamed spinal cord white matter, consequently selectins do not seem to participate in leukocyte trafficking across a healthy BBB [35]. Instead, it appears that T cells are arrested at the BBB endothelium level via α-4 integrin. This transient capture is followed by a G-protein dependent adhesion, strengthening T lymphocyte fixation to the microvascular VCAM-1 molecule. Likewise, recent studies of the blood-retina barrier have shown T lymphoblasts captured within retinal microvessels, through mechanisms resembling those observed in non-inflamed spinal cord tissue [36]. Carrithers and coworkers have demonstrated that activated CD4+ T cells can enter the brain in the absence of inflammation. However, in this model, T cell traffic is independent on α-4 integrin/VCAM-1 interactions, requiring increased surface expression of endothelial P selectin [37].

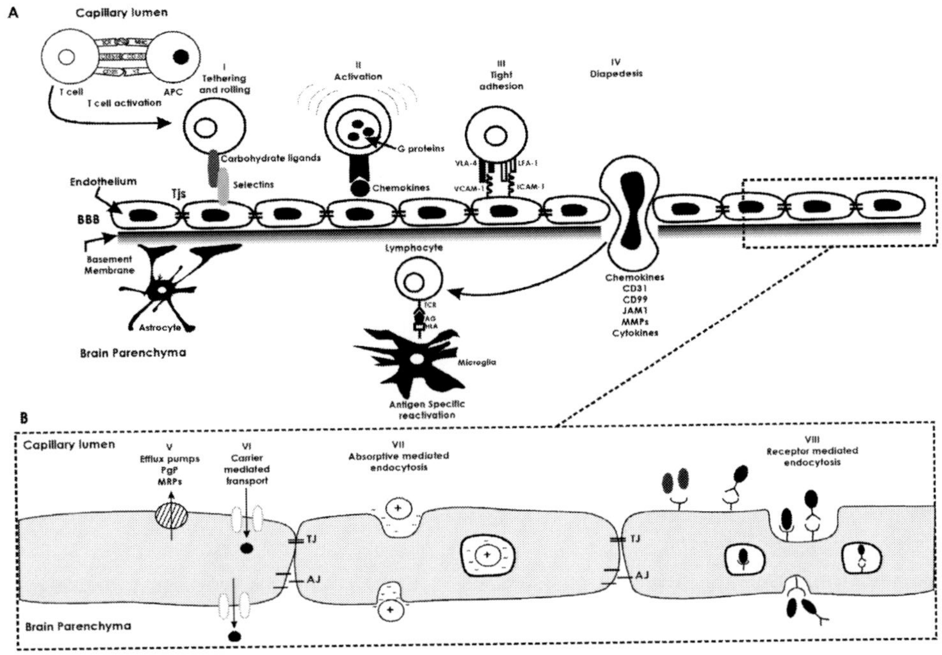

Figure 1. **A**. Physiological steps involved in leukocyte trafficking across the BBB. Selectins interact with their carbohydrate ligands, inducing the first step in leukocyte transmigration, a process referred to as tethering and rolling (I). The second step requires engagement of chemokines associated with the apical surface of the endothelium, and G-protein-coupled receptors expressed by leukocytes. This process triggers leukocyte activation (II), leading to increased avidity and modulation of integrin conformation, generating a state of high affinity and binding between members of the immunoglobulin superfamily expressed on endothelial cells. These interactions lead to tight adhesion, arrest and flattening of leukocytes (III). The final step in the transmigration process is diapedesis through the endothelium, usually at the intercellular junction (IV). This stage requires cytoskeletal reorganization of leukocytes, a process activated by chemokine-triggered signals. As referred in the text, T cells do not roll in non-inflamed spinal cord white matter, and consequently selectins are not involved in leukocytes trafficking across the BBB. Rather, T cells are arrested by α-4 integrin on endothelial VCAM-1.
B. Various physiological transport processes that may occur at the BBB. Efflux pumps (V) involve an energy dependent transporter and an energy independent exchanger at opposite poles of the capillary endothelium. Examples of this system include P-glycoprotein (Pgp), and the multidrug resistance proteins (MRPs). Carrier-mediated transport (VI) relies on molecular carriers present at both luminal and abluminal BBB membranes. These carriers tend to be highly stereospecific and are responsible for selective transport of small molecules. Absorptive mediated endocytosis (VII) relies on non-specific charge-based interactions. Large molecules such as lipoproteins, peptides or proteins can be transported across the BBB by receptor mediated endocytosis (VIII). This pathway involves three steps: receptor mediated endocytosis of the compound on the luminal (blood) side, movement through the endothelial cytoplasm and exocytosis of the drug on the abluminal (brain) side of the capillary endothelium. Examples of these systems include the transferrin receptor (TfR), the insulin receptor and the low density lipoprotein receptor (LPR1 and LPR2). Drug targeting of these receptors can be achieve either by using the endogenous ligand or by using an antibody directed against the specific receptor. TJ= tight junctions; AJ= adherent junctions.

Chemokines and their receptors play a central role in the recruitment of leukocytes and other cell types during inflammation, inducing leukocyte AM, which in turn mediate firm adhesion to the endothelium and establishes a chemotatic concentration that results in recruitment across the endothelial monolayer. Approximately fifty different human and mouse chemokines, and eighteen chemokine receptors have been identified to date, corresponding to four distinct families, subdivided on the basis of residue patterns close to the N-terminal of their products [38-39]. Marked redundancy in chemokine-chemokine receptor interaction exists, given that a single receptor may bind several chemokines, and individual chemokines may engage more than one receptor. Interestingly, recent characterization of the basement membrane has shown perivascular sulfated macromolecule deposits which can bind chemokines, therefore acting as chemokine reservoirs able to attract and maintain inflammatory infiltrates [40]. Numerous reports have analyzed the role of chemokines as well as their receptors in the intrathecal accumulation of leukocytes usually observed during MS, focusing in particular on CCR5 and CXCR3 as key Th1 receptors, and CCR3 and CCR4 in the case of Th2 . Using in situ hybridization, inflammatory cells present in perivascular MS foci were found to express chemokine CCL5 (RANTES) [41]. Likewise, chemokines CCL2 and CXCL10 (IP-10) have been detected predominantly in astrocytes within active MS plaques [42]. Furthermore, expression of the receptors CXCR3 (receptor for CXCL10) and CCR5 (for CCL5) has been demonstrated not only on leukocytes infiltrating active MS lesions, but also on microglia, macrophages, dendritic cells and astrocytes [43]. Interestingly, polyclonal expansion of CD4+CD25+ regulatory T cells in secondary lymphoid organs prevents pathological transmigration of encephalitogenic T cells into the CNS, by inhibiting IFN-γ production, as well through chemokine receptor CXCR-3 expression reduction [44]. Enrichment of CCR5 positive T cells in CSF from patients with active MS has also been detected, together with marked correlation between levels of T cells expressing CCR5 in blood and CSF. Overall, these findings suggest a major role for these two receptors in T cell recruitment during MS [45]. CSF CCL2 concentrations have been observed to decrease in MS patients during relapses, when compared to levels of non-inflammatory controls [46], and to correlate with likelihood of active lesion presence on MRI studies [47]. It has been tempting to speculate that these observations might reflect polarization of the immune response toward a Th1 cytokine profile, given the fact that CCL2 is associated with Th2-like responses in some experimental systems [48]. However, these findings contradict another recent study reporting that IL-17 promotes transmigration of human *ex vivo* CD4+ lymphocytes, most likely through enhanced BBB-EC-mediated secretion of CCL2 and CXCL8 [7]. CCL19 and CCL21 production by BBB endothelium has been observed during EAE [49]. These chemokines had previously been demonstrated in naïve lymphocyte recruitment into secondary lymphatic tissues [50]. Furthermore, *in vitro* they trigger adhesion of encephalitogenic CCR7+ lymphocytes to inflamed brain vessels. However, preliminary studies of MS tissues have been unable to confirm CCL19 or CCL21 expression on endothelial cells [51].

Depending upon their structure, three separate adhesion molecule (AM) families have been identified: selectins, integrins and members of the immunoglobulin (Ig) superfamiliy [52-55]. E-selectin expression is restricted to activated ECs, binding to sialylated molecules on neutrophils, monocytes and CD45RO+ T cells [56]. Through the action of selectins and their carbohydrate ligands, T cells initially establish loose reversible contact with ECs, often referred to as tethering, with subsequent interactions referred to as rolling [57]. Interactions between CD44 molecules expressed on the surface of activated T cells and proteoglycans expressed on ECs, may also contribute to this first contact [58], which is followed by firm and irreversible adhesion, mediated by activated leukocyte integrins and Ig superfamily members expressed on ECs [59-60]. Two main pairs of ligand/receptors have been defined during leukocyte migration into the CNS [61-62]. ICAM-1, which is expressed on ECs and leukocytes and recognizes the LFA-1 (integrin $\alpha_L\beta_2$) molecule expressed on leukocytes, and VCAM-1, another member of the Ig superfamily, which is expressed on ECs and macrophages and binds selectively to the VLA-4 (integrin $\alpha_4\beta_1$) molecule expressed on monocytes and lymphocytes. $\alpha_4\beta_1$ integrin-expressing leukocytes have also been shown to bind to the extracellular matrix molecule fibronectin and to Mad-CAM-1. Studies using immobilized ligands have suggested that this interaction is important for lymphocyte migration through the extracellular matrix towards sites of inflammation [63]. Under normal conditions, only ICAM- 1 has been detected on a small number of CNS microvessels [64]. In contrast, although E-selectin, and ICAM-1 are both expressed on brain microvessel ECs [62,64], VCAM-1 upregulation along microvessels is still a matter of debate [62,65]. Recently, using a lipid raft-based proteomic approach, a new AM member of the Ig superfamily was identified [66]. This new molecule called ALCAM was originally characterized as a ligand for CD6, a costimulatory molecule involved in lymphocyte activation and differentiation [67], as well as in various cell migration processes. ALCAM is expressed in brain ECs, and upregulated after exposure to proinflammatory cytokines along both BBB, and vessels infiltrated in active MS and EAE lesions. Moreover, *in vitro* experiments have demonstrated that ALCAM is involved in both human lymphoid (CD4+ or CD19+) and myeloid (Mac-1+ or CD14+) leukocyte transmigration across human BBB ECs. Interestingly, ALCAM blockade does not affect CD8+ T lymphocyte migration *in vivo* or *in vitro* [66].

Lymphocyte migration through the endothelium in tissues subject to inflammation is partially regulated by the ability of LFA-1 and α_4-integrins to alter their respective ligand affinity. Changes in affinity associated with conformational changes in extracellular domains are mediated, at least in part, by talin, a cytoskeleton protein linking integrins to cytoskeleton actin, thus remodeling TJs [68-69]. This phenomenon coincides with apico-basal leukocyte transmigration via specific interactions of ICAM-1 with its integrin, LFA-1 [70-71]. In addition, chemokines activate several signaling pathways (PI3K, PLC, RAS- and RHO-family GTPase, and MAPK) some of which have been implicated in the signaling that controls integrin affinity [68]

Cell migration into the CNS through the BBB involves degradation of the sub-endothelial basement membrane. This process is mediated by metalloproteinases (MMPs), a family made up of four groups of enzymes: collagenases, stromelysins, gelatinases, and membrane-type MMPs. MMPs are represented by at least 23 proteolytic enzymes involved in extracellular matrix remodeling during a variety of physiological and pathological conditions [72]. T cells and macrophages have been found to produce two closely related MMPs, MMP-2 and MMP-9. There is accumulating evidence that MMPs play a role in neuroinflammatory disease pathogenesis. MMP-9 deficient mice are less susceptible to EAE than wild-type mice

[73], consistent with the notion that loss of BBB integrity mediated by MMP-9 leads to CNS inflammation amplification. Among MS patients, CNS lesions show increased MMP-2, MMP-3, MMP-7 and MMP-9 expression [74] as well as increased MMP-9 in CSF and serum, correlating with greater disease activity as indicated by the development of new gadolinium enhancing lesions [75]. In addition to their effect on the extracellular matrix, recent investigations have demonstrated that MMPs regulate cell to cell contact disruption, and proteolysis of occludin in ECs, causing monocyte diapedesis through brain endothelium to increase [76]. Aside from their role as effector molecules in BBB disruption and cell infiltration, MMPs are also known to degrade myelin basic protein and cause axonal injury [72,77].

MMP activation is controlled at several levels [78-79]: a) most MMPs are not constitutively expressed, but gene transcription can be induced through different stimuli including cytokines, growth factors, and chemokines; b) MMPs are secreted as inactive pro-forms, subsequently activated through proteolytic reactions yielding active enzyme. One important physiological activator is plasmin, a proteinase generated from plasminogen through tissue or urokinase-plasminogen activator; and c) MMP activity is closely regulated by four tissue inhibitors (TIMPs), a group of antagonists that bind to the catalytic site of MMPs, and are expressed by macrophages and astrocytes.

Studies on T cell traffic into the CNS have focused on CD4+ T cells, given their importance in neuroinflammatory processes. This is changing however, and CD8+ T cells are now recognized as major players in different diseases, including MS, encephalitis, paraneoplastic CNS syndromes, and T cell-lymphotropic virus-associated myelopathy. Experiments recently conducted in animal models show that *in vivo* CD8+ T cell accumulation within the brain is the result of Ag-specific infiltration. This selective traffic of CD8+ T cells into the brain is dependent on luminal expression of MHC Class I antigens by cerebral endothelium [80], and independent of Ag presentation by perivascular macrophages, with full activation not considered to be an absolute prerequisite for CNS infiltration by CD8 T cells to occur [80].

Mechanisms governing monocyte migration through the BBB are not as well understood as those of lymphocytes. Because monocytes function mainly as effectors of inflammatory reactions, they are unlikely to reach healthy CNS tissue. The VCAM-1/VLA-4 pathway appears to play an important role during monocyte migration across microvascular ECs in the brain [81]. In addition, other Ig superfamily members may also participate in transendothelial migration of monocytes. For instance, in neuroinflammatory diseases interactions occur between the signal regulatory protein-α (SIRP-α) and the integrin-associated protein (CD47) contributing to the adhesion step during monocyte recruitment into brain tissue [82]. This process triggers cytoskeletal rearrangements in brain ECs, which in turn promote monocyte migration. Likewise, junctional proteins like JAM and CD99 also appear to aid monocyte migration through diapedesis enhancement at the tight junction level [83]. Moreover, integrin-mediated signaling promotes recruitment of peripheral blood-derived CD14+ monocytes, as well as their differentiation into functional DCs through TGF-β and GM-CSF secretion. These myeloid DCs, closely associated to microvascular BBB-ECs within acute MS lesions, secrete IL-12, TGF-β, and IL-6, all favoring CD4+ lymphocyte differentiation into IFN-γ or IL-17 secreting cells [84]. Chemokine receptors such as CCR5 may also play a major role in phagocytic cell recruitment in MS, as they are expressed both by macrophages and microglia in active lesions, as well as by monocytes present in CSF from MS patients [85]. Moreover, co-localization of various ligands for this receptor (CCL3, CCL4, CCL5 and CCL8) are also found in MS lesions [86-87], further suggesting these molecules play distinct roles in directing hematogenous monocytes and macrophages from the bloodstream into CNS tissue. Finally, CCR2 and one of its ligands CCL2 have also been associated with monocyte migration across the BBB. CCL2 or CCR2 deficient mice for example show resistance to active EAE induction, with significantly impaired recruitment of monocytes into the CNS [88].

Access of neutrophils into CNS tissues occurs only under extreme circumstances, however this migration across brain microvascular ECs has been associated with the vascular endothelial growth factor (VEGF) production, which in turn stimulates expression of IL-8, a neutrophil targeting chemokine [89]. Also, in different animal models, CXCR2 chemokine receptor induction and that of its ligand CXCL1, have been shown to significantly increase neutrophil infiltration into CNS parenchyma [90].

Therapeutic Implications

Migration of activated T cells and monocytes into the CNS is critical for MS onset as well as for disease progression to occur. Thus, all the molecular mechanisms previously described represent good potential targets for therapeutic strategies aimed at altering inflammatory cell influx into the CNS (Table 1). Benefits of interferon β (IFN-β) and methylprednisolone (MP) treatment have been associated with regulation of AM pathways. MS patients treated with IFN-β 1b have shown VLA-4 down-regulation on the surface of lymphocytes [91], a finding also correlated with prior increase in soluble VCAM-1(sVCAM-1) levels and a reduction in the number of contrast-enhancing lesions on MRI [92]. Soluble AMs interacting with their specific T cells ligands, may inhibit T cell attachment to BBB endothelium. Likewise, MP suppresses expression of LFA-1, VLA-4 and ICAM-1 on mononuclear cells obtained both from blood or CSF of MS patients, suggesting that MP inhibits the ability of immune cells to adhere to EC through AM expression reduction, thus restricting their entry into the brain [93]. These findings suggest that therapies specifically targeting AM should be considered as potential options for MS treatment.

Monoclonal antibodies against α_4 integrin have been shown to reduce clinical and MRI activity in EAE, decreasing transmigration of lymphocytes to areas of inflammation, reducing leukocyte activation and proliferation, and increasing T cell apoptosis [94-98]. Although migration of leukocytes across the BBB requires interaction between α-4 integrin expressing leukocytes and VCAM-1 molecules expressed on BBB ECs and glial cells, interaction between α-4 integrin also occurs with extracellular matrix molecules, such as fibronectin and ostopontin, further perpetuating the inflammatory cascade already triggered within the brain parenchyma [99-101]. Interestingly, recent studies have demonstrated that B cells and monocytes express a higher density of α-4 integrin than T cells [102]. Antibodies against this molecule can therefore inhibit both humoral and cellular immune responses within the nervous system. Recently, a humanized mAb against α_4 integrin (natalizumab) was tested in

MS patients. Initial trials showed significant reduction of both contrast-enhancing MRI lesions and clinical relapses [103-104]. These encouraging results led to two larger successful multicenter clinical trials, recently published [105-106]. Unfortunately however, the drug was later withdrawn from the market after reports of progressive multifocal leukoencephalopathy development (PML), an infection of CNS glia with human polyoma (JC) virus, often fatal, observed in two MS patients receiving natalizumab and IFN-β 1a [107-108]. An additional case of PML observed in a patient receiving natalizumab for Crohn's disease was also reported [109]. In response to these serious safety concerns, an independent committee investigated all patients receiving natalizumab as part of any clinical trial for signs of PML. Analysis of 3116 patients exposed to a mean of 17.9 monthly doses, failed to identify any further cases of the disease [110]. Investigators now estimate risk of PML development to be 1 case per 1000 patients treated. Based on these data, and on other recommendations made by the advisory committee, the FDA has approved reintroduction of natalizumab as monotherapy in relapsing remitting MS patients, albeit with restrictions, including a revised label and a new risk management plan defined under the TOUCH prescribing program [111]. The European Medicines Agency and the Canadian regulatory agency have also approved natalizumab with similar restrictions.

Although α-4 antibody therapy is now available, small molecule α-4 antagonists still seem a very attractive treatment alternative. These molecules could potentially represent less costly and more convenient dosing regimes, with greater efficacy and reduced side effects [112]. One recent study demonstrated that CT301, a small molecule α-4 integrin inhibitor, reduced clinical, pathological and MRI signs of acute EAE, thus preventing progressive changes in BBB permeability [113].

Statins are oral lipid-lowering drugs approved for dyslipidaemia treatment, that inhibit 3-hydroxy-3methyl-glutaryl coenzyme A (HMG-CoA) reductase, the enzyme which converts HMG-CoA to L-mevalonate, a key intermediate in cholesterol biosynthesis [114]. In recent years, statins have provided a new therapeutic opportunity for treating neuroinflammatory diseases, such as MS, because of their capacity to alter GTP-ase mediated signaling events [115-118]. The first evidence of the anti-inflammatory properties of statins came from studies reporting an association between decreased natural killer cell activity and cardiac transplantation success independent of cholesterol levels modification [119]. When prescribing statins for diseases of the CNS one should be aware that lipophilic statins, such as simvastatin and lovastatin, easily enter the CNS compartment [120] whereas more hydrophilic statins such as fluvastatin and parvastatin do not [121]. Seminal studies demonstrated that statins prevent the expression of inducible nitric oxide synthase as well as the TNF-α and IL-6 production in astrocytes and in microglia cultures [122]. Furthermore, different investigations provide evidence for a potent immunomodulatory action of statins on APC-T cell interactions by modulating the expression of MHC and co-stimulatory molecules [123-125]. In addition, statins exert profound dose-dependent changes on BBB permeability [126]. After stimulation, lovastatin binds directly to the extracellular domain of LFA-1 reducing lymphocyte adhesion capacity to ICAM-1 [127]. Likewise, *in vitro* lovastatin also inhibits monocyte expression of Mac-1, and subsequent binding to ECs [128]. Statins on ECs were shown to decrease the expression of ICAM-1 and VCAM-1, resulting in reduced transendothelial migration [129-131]. Thus, statins reduce leukocyte recruitment into the

CNS by suppressing AM expression in both activated leukocytes and ECs, and also significantly reduce MMP-9 secretion by monocytes [132-133], down-regulating the release of chemokines CCL2 and CXCL10 by BBB ECs, and decreasing leukocyte migration across biological membranes that resemble the BBB in MS patients [126].

Treatment of EAE with statins resulted in a significant drop in disease scores as well as in the number of new relapses once treatment had started [134-135]. Interestingly, in this mouse model part of the beneficial effect of statins has been linked to enhanced survival of OGD progenitor cells and their differentiation to remyelinating OGDs *in vivo* [136]. These results encouraged clinical trials in MS patients using statins. In one study beneficial effects of sinvastatin (80 mg daily) were demonstrated in a small open-label 6 month trial involving 28 patients with RR MS, where the number and volume of gadolinium-enhancing lesions were reduced by 44% and 41 % respectively [137]. A larger 152-patient, placebo controlled trial using atorvastatin is currently being conducted in patients with clinically isolated syndromes, the results of which are eagerly awaited [138]. Statins are attractive candidates for combined therapy studies. In EAE the combination of glatiramer acetate (GA) and atorvastatin synergistically ameliorated established clinical signs of the disease [139]. Based on these findings, clinical trials testing GA in combination with atorvastatin are anticipated. Conversely however, another recent study indicated that the combination of atorvastatin and high dose IFN-β 1a caused antagonistic effects, paradoxically generating increased MS activity [140].

EC dysfunction in inflammatory responses within the CNS is driven in part by IFN-γ and TNF-β action. IFN-γ significantly reduces occludin and cadherin expression, producing gaps in endothelial monolayers. TNF-β induces translocation of ZO-1 and ZO-2 proteins with random distribution within the cytoplasm, causing retraction of EC borders. Recently, different investigations have demonstrated that IFN-β treatment prevents IFN-γ- and TNF-β-induced disintegration of endothelial TJ molecules, thereby preserving barrier function [141-142]. These effects represent novel molecular mechanisms for therapeutic modifications of the BBB using IFN-β that could be applied to MS. Likewise, glucocorticoid administration induces the formation of the endothelial TJ protein occludin, further protecting functional integrity along the BBB [143-144].

Chemokines and their receptors, by virtue of their potential role as mediators of CNS inflammation in MS, also provide potential targets for pharmacological intervention [145-146]. After treatment with IFN-β, CXCL8 and CCL5 serum levels, as well as CXCR3 expression on T cells drop significantly in patients with MS [147-149]. This last finding is consistent with a key role for CXCR3 in encephalitogenic Th-1-like T cell recruitment and with the impact of IFN-β on cytokine secretion patterns during the course of disease. Recently published studies indicate a reduction in CCL5 serum levels, as well as in CCR5 receptor expression on blood T cells from MS patients receiving methylprednisolone [150]. Likewise, immunosuppressive therapy in RR MS patients with Cladribine reduced CCL5 levels both in serum and CSF, and CXCL8 level in CSF [151].

Recently, a greater number of treatment strategies specifically targeting chemokines have been proposed, including a) small molecule inhibitors blocking chemokine receptors; b) neutralizing Abs against receptors or neutralizing chemokines; and c) modified chemokines, disrupting normal function [146,152]. Small-molecule receptor antagonists against CCR1,

CCR2, CCR5, and CXCR3 could prove useful in MS. Data published after early clinical trials using an oral CCR1 antagonist had shown efficacy in treating rheumatoid arthritis [153], unfortunately in larger subsequent studies therapeutic endpoints were not met. A potent, novel, selective, orally available CCR1 antagonist, BX471, [154] was tested in patients with RR MS during a 16 week randomized, double-blind placebo controlled trial. The primary endpoint was the number of newly active lesions detected on serial MRI brain scans. Although the compound proved to be safe, no treatment effect was observed [155]. A small-molecule CCR2 antagonist INCB344, has also been shown to significantly reduce disease in mice with EAE, although it has not yet been tested for treatment of MS [156]. TAK779, another antagonist targeting both CCR5 and CXCR3, inhibits development of experimentally induced arthritis [157], making it potentially useful in MS. The number of small molecule inhibitors has expanded rapidly, nevertheless limitations to the approach still exist. First, the binding site for many of the chemokine receptors is still not known. Second, because these molecules block several ligands, it is not always possible to know which ligand to select in order to screen the system [158-159]. Finally, small molecule inhibitors show species selectivity, reducing the possibility of developing relevant pharmacological animal models to perform proof-of-principle experiments [160-161].

Neutralizing Abs to chemokines have shown efficacy blocking disease symptoms in different animal models [162-165]. For example, antibody-mediated blockade of CXCR3 suppresses Th-1 cell recruitment in inflammatory foci, and inhibits delayed-type hypersensitivity responses [166]. Interestingly, the pleiotropic effects of different chemokines such as CXCL9, CXCL10, and CXCL11 are mediated by a common receptor CXCR3, suggesting that inhibition of this pivotal receptor may be important in different disease conditions [167]. Furthermore, administration of anti-CCL5 antibodies in a viral MS model resulted in less leukocyte infiltration into the CNS, reduced severity of demyelination, and improvement in neurological function [168].

An alternative to Ab therapy is the use of modified chemokines. Truncated forms of CCL2 were shown to be efficacious in the MRL-lpr mice arthritis model [169]. Likewise, Met-CCL5 has shown efficacy in animal models of lung inflammation, nephritis, collagen induced arthritis, and chronic colitis [163,165,170-171]. In addition, a chemically modified CCL5 analogue, AOP-CCL5, has validated altering receptor trafficking. AOP-CCL5, a potent CCR5 agonist, was effective through its ability to remove the CCR5 receptor from the cell surface [172]. These results indicate that it is possible to interfere with receptor recycling, offering a new approach for future therapies.

Beneficial effects of IFN-β may also be mediated by an ability to suppress T cell MMP production, as well as increasing TIMP-s transcription, thus attenuating MMP over-activity observed in MS through a dual mechanism [173-175]. Treatment of peripheral blood mononuclear cells with statins reduces MMP-9 secretion, although this effect is less prominent than the one achieved with IFN-β 1b [176]. Likewise, mitoxantrone and perfosfamide (the active metabolite of cyclophosphamide), decrease monocytes and T cell migration across a fibronectin layer in an *in vitro* BBB model, through reduction of proteolytic activity in both MMP-9 and MMP-2, as well as by decreasing MMP-9 mRNA expression by mononuclear cells [177]. Glucocorticoids have been shown to increase TIMP-1 mRNA transcription in ECs, an effect mediated via the glucocorticoid receptor [178], and also to stabilize the BBB by altering the balance between MMP-9 and TIMP-1 [179]. MMPs inhibitors block the BBB disruption and have been proposed as candidates for the treatment of neuroinflammation [180-181]. Many MMP inhibitors have been engineered based on their capability to chelate Zn^{2+} at the active catalytic site, and contain a hydroxamate group for this purpose. One of the first hydroxamates developed was BB94, commonly used in laboratory experiments. However, its solubility is poor, making it unsuitable for oral or IV administration. Marimastat is a second generation hydroxamate with increased bioavailability after oral intake [181]. Several broad-spectrum inhibitors have been shown to block the opening of the BBB in EAE, bacterial meningitis, cerebral ischemia, and intracerebral hemorrhage [182-187]. Studies using broad-spectrum MMP inhibitors have shown attenuation of clinical EAE symptoms and partial BBB restoration, suggesting this therapeutic strategy corrects a specific pathogenic mechanism of the disease [186-187]. However, the situation in EAE is complex when considering use of MMP inhibitors, for two reasons: a) several MMPs change expression levels at different stages of the disease, and b) MMPs are also involved in different healing processes [181]. Therefore, when prolonged treatment is required, the risk of inhibiting physiological and repair MMP properties also increases. In this respect, it was shown recently that treatment with broad-spectrum inhibitors of MMPs for extended periods in rodents with stroke impaired healing, probably interfering with recovery through blocking of MMP-dependent angiogenesis and neurogenesis. [188-189]. Moreover, MMPs inhibitors can potentially have an effect on other types of proteases containing metal ions in their active sites. So far, early clinical use of MMPs inhibitors in a variety of cancer types has been largely unsuccessful, although side effects were not observed, therapeutic response was not achieved either [190]. Application of MMP inhibitors to treat MS requires careful balance between beneficial and detrimental effects, and the need for more selective inhibitors retaining the beneficial traits shown by MMPs in CNS physiology and recovery persists [191].

Minocycline, a tetracycline analogue, has recently been found to exert numerous immunomodulatory functions. The use of minocycline is of particular interest in CNS disorders because of its high oral bioavailability, high BBB penetration and good tolerance in humans, and has been used for decades to treat bacterial infections [192-193]. Proposed mechanisms of action include diverse effects on several cell types. Minocycline inhibits inducible nitric oxide synthase (iNOS) and cyclooxygenase 2 (COX-2) activity and impairs the production of cytokines such as TNF-α, and IL-1β [194-196]. In addition, it prevents BBB permeability increase. AM quantification studies have demonstrated increased sVCAM-1 levels after minocycline treatment [197]. As previously described for IFN-β, sVCAM-1 increase is thought to exert negative feedback on inflammation as it binds to VLA-4 integrin on inflammatory cells, hindering interaction between these cells and the BBB. Other critical targets of minocycline may be MMP-2 and MMP-9 inhibition, and reduced MMP-9 production [198]. Minocycline acts on MMP-9 as an uncompetitive inhibitor [199]. Upon formation of the minocycline-MMP complex permanent rearrangement of tertiary structure of the enzyme can occur, resulting in loss of activity. *In vitro* experiments have demonstrated that minocycline decreased T lymphocytes transmigration across a fibronectin matrix [198], and in recent years the drug has shown remarkable protective effect on the course of EAE [200]. In an open-label pilot study, 10 RR MS patients treated with minocycline, 100 mg twice daily for 24 months showed significant reduction in the number of MRI enhancing lesions, as well as reduction of MMP-9 activity [201], encouraging results certainly supporting further investigation of minocycline in MS.

Because it is impermeable to many drug molecules and protein biopharmaceuticals, the BBB constitutes a major hurdle in systemic administration of anti-inflammatory molecules or neurotrophic factors to patients affected by immune-mediated inflammatory diseases of the CNS like MS. Therefore, innovative drug delivery systems into the brain are needed to complement drug discovery efforts. Initial attempts to overcome this anatomical barrier were directed towards improving lipid-mediated entry. However thus far, reformulation of water-soluble drugs through chemical modifications such as lipidization have proven unsuccessful, failing in actual practice to convert a non-brain penetrating drug into a molecule crossing the BBB and reaching useful pharmacological concentrations.

Table 1. Therapeutic interventions on the blood-brain barrier during the course of Multiple Sclerosis

Molecular target	Therapeutic strategy	Mechanism of action	References
Adhesion molecules	IFN-β	Down-regulates VLA-4 and increases sVCAM-1	91,92
	Methylprednisolone	Suppresses LFA-1, VLA-4 and ICAM-1 expression on mononuclear cells	93
	Natalizumab	Reduces transmigration of lymphocytes to areas of inflammation, reduces activation and proliferation of leukocytes, and induces apoptosis of T cells.	94-96
	Alpha-4 integrin antagonists	Reduce transmigration of lymphocytes across the BBB	112-113
	Statins	Bind to LFA-1, reducing adhesion capacity to ICAM-1; Inhibition of Mac-1 expression on monocytes, and binding to endothelial cells; Decreased expression of ICAM-1 and VCAM-1 on ECs	119-123
	Minocycline	Increases sVCAM-1	189
Endothelial tight junction complex	IFN-β	Prevents IFN-γ and TNF-β disintegration of endothelial TJ molecules.	133-134
	Methylprednisolone	Induces the formation of the endothelial TJ protein occludin.	135-136
Chemokines	IFN-β	Decreases serum levels of CXCL8, CCL5 and expression of chemokines receptors CXCR3 and CCR5	139-142
	Statins	Down regulate the secretion of CCL2 and CXCL10 by BBB ECs	118
	Cladribine	Reduces serum levels of CCL5 and CSF levels of CCL5 and CXCL8	143
	Receptor antagonists	Block chemokine receptors	138,144, 146-149
	Antibodies against chemokine receptors	Block chemokine receptors	154-157
	Modified chemokines	Block chemokine receptors; Interfere with receptors recycling	161-164

Table 1. (Continued)

Molecular target	Therapeutic strategy	Mechanism of action	References
Matrix metalloproteinases	IFN-β	Suppress T cell MMPs production; increases transcription of TIMP-s	165-167
	Statins	Reduce MMP-9 secretion	168
	Mitoxantrone	Reduces proteolytic activity of MMP-9 and MMP-2; Reduces transcription of MMP-9	169
	Perfosfamide	Reduces proteolytic activity of MMP-9 and MMP-2; Reduces transcription of MMP-9	169
	Glucocorticoids	Increase transcription of TIMP-1 in ECs	170
	Minocycline	Inhibits MMP-2 and MMP-9 activity; Reduces production of MMP-9	190
	Inhibitors of metalloproteinases	Block the catalytic site	172-173
Active efflux transports (Pgp; MRP)	Co-drugs	Inhibition of active BBB efflux transports, consequently increasing brain penetration of therapeutic agent.	196-200
Receptor-mediated endocytosis (TfR; Insulin receptor; LPR1, LPR2)	Therapeutic agents linked to endogenous ligand: transferrin, insulin, low density lipoprotein. Therapeutic agents linked to antibodies against TfR or insulin receptor	Increased therapeutic agent penetration across the BBB by using receptor mediating endocytosis.	201-207
	Liposomes and immunoliposomes	Facilitate the delivery of therapeutic agents across the BBB; prolong half-life in circulation	197, 209-210

BBB= Blood-brain barrier; ECs= Endothelial cells; MMPs= metalloproteinases; LPR= Lipoprotein receptor; sVCAM-1= soluble VCAM-1; TfR= Transferrin receptor; TIMP-s= Tissue inhibitors of metalloproteinases; TJ= Tight junctions.

Because it is impermeable to many drug molecules and protein biopharmaceuticals, the BBB constitutes a major hurdle in systemic administration of anti-inflammatory molecules or neurotrophic factors to patients affected by immune-mediated inflammatory diseases of the CNS like MS. Therefore, innovative drug delivery systems into the brain are needed to complement drug discovery efforts. Initial attempts to overcome this anatomical barrier were directed towards improving lipid-mediated entry. However thus far, reformulation of water-soluble drugs through chemical modifications such as lipidization have proven unsuccessful, failing in actual practice to convert a non-brain penetrating drug into a molecule crossing the BBB and reaching useful pharmacological concentrations.

Brain ECs and astrocyte processes contain numerous transporters on both luminal and abluminal membranes of capillaries, regulating traffic of essential molecules between blood and the brain, as well as allowing efflux of potentially harmful substances (Figure 1B) [202-204]. An alternative strategy might therefore be to inhibit active efflux transport (AET) mechanisms mediated by members of the ATP-binding cassette family like P-glycoprotein (Pgp), and the multidrug resistance-associated protein family (MRP; also known as ABC1)

[205-206]. Reported Pgp substrates include structurally diverse compounds such as antineoplastic agents, immunosuppressive drugs, and antibiotics. Many compounds function as both Pgp substrates and inhibitors, and may interact with Pgp at more than one binding site [207]. MRP1 is the best characterized member of the MRP family, and has been also implicated in resistance to different anticancer agents [208]. Drugs that inhibit a BBB AET could be used as "codrugs" to increase brain penetration of a therapeutic drug normally excluded from the brain by BBB AET system. This strategy has been successfully used to enhance CNS uptake of several drugs. However, inhibition of efflux transport activity may allow entry of potential neurotoxins, producing unwanted side effects. Long-term use is therefore not advisable [207].

Endogenous peptides that cross the BBB (e.g. transferrin and insulin) use receptor-mediated endocytosis (RME). These specific receptors tend to have similar transport properties when linked to potential therapeutic agents, and might therefore serve as new transport vehicles to facilitate BBB passage. The transferrin receptor (TfR) is highly expressed in brain capillaries, and is the most widely characterized receptor-mediated transport system for targeting drugs to the brain. Drug targeting to the TfR can be achieved either by using the endogenous transferrin ligand or by using an Ab directed against TfR [209]. The use of TfR-Abs targeting of the BBB has been validated extensively as a brain delivery mechanism that can elicit pharmacological effects. For example, recombinant neurotrophic factors such as nerve growth factor (NGF) and brain-derived neurotrophic factor (BDNF) linked to the anti-transferrin receptor (TfR) antibody have been vector-delivered to the brain, limiting infarct size in a rat model of regional brain ischemia [210]. The insulin receptor, like the TfR, is found on the luminal membrane of brain capillary endothelial cells as well as on the plasma membrane of other brain cells [211], and can undergo receptor-mediated transport across the BBB endothelium [212]. As for TfR, Abs recognizing the insulin receptor have been used as BBB-targeting vectors [213]. Recently, fully humanized Abs against the insulin receptor have been created, in order to avoid immunogenic responses observed with murine Abs [214]. Low density lipoprotein receptor-related proteins 1 (LRP1) and 2 (LRP2) have also been used for targeted drug delivery. These receptors are structurally similar to the low density lipoprotein receptor (LDL) receptor, and are multifunctional RME systems with multiple ligands [215]. As such, there are reports of several BBB-targeting vectors that take advantage of the LPR1 and LPR2 RME system [209,216].

Liposomes are large complex constructs which can be made from a variety of chemical constituents, and offer a mechanism through which molecules can be encapsulated and then directed to enter the brain. Using this approach, drugs, neurotrophic peptides, antisense-oliogonucleotides or genes can be incorporated into the centre of a liposome, and its surface then coated with polyethylene glycol (PEG) to prolong half-life [205,217]. In addition, 1 to 2% of PEG strands are attached to mAbs that interact with the TfR, and effectively target immunoliposomes against tissues that have high TfR expression, such as the liver or the brain. If glial cell- or neuron-specific promoters are encapsulated together with the gene selected, then expression of gene therapeutics becomes confined to the CNS [218]. In addition, ligand dependent promoters, such as tetracycline inducible promoters, may control exogenous gene regulation or expression [219]. These approaches represent great promise for successful delivery of therapeutic agents across the previously impermeable BBB endothelium and into the brain.

Our knowledge of brain capillary biology and haematopoietic cells trafficking across the BBB and into the CNS had advanced significantly in recent years. Application of modern molecular and cell biology techniques, together with traditional structural ones, enables us to appreciate the barrier not only as a static anatomical entity, but also as a highly complex and active bi-directional interface. This improved knowledge heralds rapid advances in the rational design of new therapeutic alternatives for the treatment of inflammatory neurological diseases such as MS.

ACKNOWLEDGEMENTS

We thank Adriana Zufriategui for preparation of the Figure.

REFERENCES

[1] Noseworthy JH, Lucchinetti C, Rodriguez M, Weinshenker BG. Multiple sclerosis. *N Engl J Med* 2000;343:938-942.

[2] Sospedra M & Martin R. Immunology of multiple sclerosis. *Annu Rev Immunol* 2005;23:683-747.

[3] Bielekova B, Goodwin B, Richert N, Cortese I, Kondo T, Afshar G, Garn B, Eaton J, Antel J, Frank JA, McFarland HF, Martin R. Encephalitogenic potential of the myelin basic protein peptide (amino acids 83-99) in multiple sclerosis: results of a phase II clinical trial with an altered peptide ligand. *Nat Med* 2000; 6:1167-1175.

[4] Lafaille JJ, Keere FV, Hsu AL, Baron JL, Haas W, Raine CS, Tonegawa S. Myelin basic protein-specific T helper 2 (Th2) cells cause experimental autoimmune encephalomyelitis in immunodeficient hosts rather than protect them from the disease. *J Exp Med* 1997; 186:307-312.

[5] Weaver CT, Hatton RD, Mangan PR, Harrington LE. IL-17 family cytokines and the expanding diversity of effector T cell lineages. *Annu Rev Immunol* 2007; 25:821-852.

[6] Langrish CL, Chen Y, Blumenschein WM, Mattson J, Bashem B, Sedgwick JD, McClanahan T, Castelein RA, Cua DJ. IL-23 drives a pathogenic T cell population that induces autoimmune inflammation. *J Exp Med* 2005; 201:233-240.

[7] Kebir H, Kreymborg K, Ifergan I, Dodelet-Devillers A, Cayrol R, Bernard M, Giuliani F, Arbour N, Becher B, Prat A. Human Th17 lymphocytes promote blood-brain-barrier disruption and central nervous system inflammation. *Nat Med* 2007; 13:1173-1175.

[8] Raine CS. The Dale McFarlin memorial lecture: the immunology of multiple sclerosis lesions. *Ann Neurol* 1994;36:S61-S72.

[9] Pardridge WM. A morphological approach to the analysis of blood-brain-barrier transport function. In: Paulson O, Knudsen G, Moos T, editors. *Brain Barrier Systems.* Copenhagen: Munkgaard; 1999. p. 19-42.

[10] Begley D, Brightman MW. Structural and functional aspects of the blood-brain-barrier. In: Prokai L, Prokai-Tatrai K, editors. *Peptide transport and delivery into the Central Nervous System. Progress in Drug Research.* Basel: Birkhauser Verlag; 2003. p 39-78.

[11] Brightman MW & Reese TS. Junctions between intimately apposed cell membranes in the vertebrate brain. *J Cell Biol* 1969;40:648-677.

[12] Lane NJ, Reese TJ, Kacher B. Structural domains of the tight junctional intramembrane fibrils. *Tissue Cell* 1992;24:291-300.

[13] Huber JD, Egelton RD, Davis TP. Molecular physiology and patholophysiology of tight junctions in the blood-brain. *Trends Neurosci* 2001;24:719-725.

[14] Bearer EL & Orci L. Endothelial fenestral diaphragms: a quick-freeze, deep-etch study. *J Cell Biol* 1985;100:418-428.

[15] Dorovini-Zis K, Prameya R, Bowman PD. Culture and characterization of microvascular endothelial cells derived from human brain. *Lab Invest* 1991;64 :425-436.

[16] Villegas JC & Broadwell RD. Transcytosis of protein through the mammalian cerebral epithelium and endothelium. II. Adsorptive transcytosis of WGA-HRP and the blood-brain and blood-brain barriers. *J Neurocytol* 1993;22:67-80.

[17] Hayashi Y, Nomura M, Yamagishi S, Harada S, Yamashita J, Yamamoto H. Induction of various blood-brain barrier properties in non-neural endothelial cells by close apposition to co-cultured astrocytes. *Glia* 1997;19:13-26.

[18] Hurwitz AA, Berman JW, Rashbaum WK, Lyman WD. Human fetal astrocytes induce the expression of blood-brain barrier specific proteins by autologous endothelial cells. *Brain Res* 1993; 625:238-243.

[19] Pardridge WM. Molecular biology of the blood-brain barrier. *Mol Biotechnol* 2005;30:57-70.

[20] Lee G, Dallas S, Hong M, Bendayan R. Drug transporters in the central nervous system: brain barriers and brain parenchyma considerations. *Pharmacol Rev* 2001; 53:569-596.

[21] Leslie EM, Deeley RG, Cole SP. Multidrug resistance proteins: role of P-glycoprotein, MRP1, MRP2, and BCRP (ABCG2) in tissue defense. *Toxicol Appl Pharmacol* 2005; 204:216-237.

[22] Abbott NJ, Rönnbäck L, Hansson E. Astrocyte-endothelial interactions at the blood-brain barrier. *Nat Rev Neurosc* 2006;7:41-53.

[23] Ramsauer M, Krause D, Dermietzel R. Angiogenesis of the blood-brain barrier *in vitro* and the function of cerebral perycites. *FASEB J* 2002;16:1274-1276.

[24] Schiera G, Bono E, Raffa MP, Gallo A, Pitarresi GL, Di Ligero I, Savettieri G. Synergistic effects of neurons and astrocytes in the differentiation of brain capillary endotelial cells in culture. *J Cell Mol Med* 2003;7:165-170.

[25] Zenker D, Begley DJ, Bratzke H, Rübsamen-Waigmann H, von Briesen H. Human blood-derived macrophages enhance barrier function of cultured bovine and human brain capillary endothelial cells. *J Physiol* 2003;551:1023-1032.

[26] Lai CH & Kuo KH. The critical component to establish *in vitro* BBB model: pericyte. *Brain Res Dev* 2005;50:258-265.

[27] Gonul E, Duz B, Kahraman S, Kayali H, Kubar A, Timurkaynak E. Early pericyte response to brain hipoxia in cats: an ultrastructural study. *Microvasc Res* 2002;64:116-119.

[28] Dore-Duffy P, Owen C, Balabanov R, Murphy S, Beaumont T, Rafols JA. Pericyte migration from the vascular wall in response to traumatic brain injury. *Microvasc Res* 2000;60:55-69.

[29] Fabriek BO, van Haastert ES, Galea I, Polfliet MMJ, Döpp ED, van den Heuvel MM, van den Berg TK, De Groot CJA, van der Valk P, Dijstra CD. CD163-positive perivascular macrophages in the human CNS express molecules for antigen recognition and presentation. *Glia* 2005;51:297-305.

[30] Hickey WF. Leukocyte traffic in the central nervous system: the participants and their roles. *Semin Immunol* 1999;11:125-137.

[31] Lucchinetti C, Brück W, Parisi J, Scheithauer B, Rodriguez M, Lassman H. Heterogeneity of multiple sclerosis lesions: implications for the pathogenesis of demyelination. *Ann Neurol* 2000;47:707-717.

[32] Hickey WF. Migration of hematogeneous cells through the blood-brain barrier and the initiation of CNS inflammation. *Brain Pathol* 1991;1:97-105.

[33] Wekerle H, Linington C, Lassmann H, Meyermann R. Cellular immune reactivity within the CNS. *Trends Neurosc* 1986;9:271-277.

[34] Smodorodchenko A, Wuerfel J, Pohl EE, Vogt J, Tysiak E, Glumm R, Hnedrix E, Nitsch R, Zipp F, Infante-Duarte C. CNS-irrelevant T-cells enter the brain cause blood-brain barrier disruption but not glia pathology. *Eur J Neurosci* 2007;26:1387-1398.

[35] Vajkoczy P, Laschinger M, Engelhardt B. Alpha-4 integrin-VCAM-1 binding mediates G-protein-independent capture of encephalitogenic T cell blasts to CNS white matter microvessels. *J Clin Invest* 2001;108:557-565.

[36] Xu H, Manivannan A, Liversidge J, Sharp PF, Forrester JV, Crane IJ . Requirements for pasasage of T lymphocytes across non-inflamed retinal microvessels. *J Neuroimmunol* 2003;142:47-57.

[37] Carrithers MD, Visintin I, Kang SJ, Janeway CA Jr. Differential adhesion molecule requirements for immune surveillance and inflammatory recruitment. *Brain* 2000;123: 1092-1101.

[38] http://cytokine.medic.kumamoto-u-ac.jp/CFC/CK/Chemokine.html.

[39] http://www.gpcr.org.proxy2.lib.uwo.ca:2048/7tm/

[40] van Horssen J, Bö L, Vos CMP, Virtanen I, de Vries HE. Basement membrane proteins in multiple sclerosis-associated inflammatory cuffs: potential role in influx and transport of leukocytes. *J Neuropathol Exp Neurol* 2005;64:722-729.

[41] Hvas J, McLean C, Justesen J, Kannourakis G, Steinman L, Oksenberg JR, Bernard CC. Perivascular T cells express the pro-inflammatory chemokine RANTES mRNA in multiple sclerosis lesions. *Scand J Immunol* 1997;46:195-203.

[42] McManus C, Berman JW, Brett FM, Staunton H, Farrel M, Brosnan CF. MCP-1, MCP-2, and MCP-3 expression in multiple sclerosis lesions: an immunohistochemical and in situ hybridization study. *J Neuroimmunol* 1998;86:20-29.

[43] Sorensen TL, Tani M, Jensen J, Pierce V, Lucchinetti C, Folcik VA, Qin S, Rottman J, Sellebjerg F, Strieter RM, Frederiksen JL, Ransohoff RM. Expression of specific

chemokines and chemokine receptors in the central nervous system of multiple sclerosis patients. *J Clin Invest* 1999;103:807-815.

[44] Tischner D, Weishaupt A, van den Brandt J, Müller N, Beyersdorf N, Ip CW, Toyka KV, Huning T, Gold R, Kerkau T, Reichardt HM. Polyclonal expansion of regulatory T cells interferes with effector cell migration in a model of multiple sclerosis. *Brain* 2006;129:2635-2647.

[45] Sorensen TL, Ransohoff RM, Jensen J, Sellebjerg F. Evidence favoring the involvement of CC chemokine receptor (CCR) 5 in T-lymphocyte accumulation in optic neuritis. *Acta Neurol Scand* 2003;107:221-227.

[46] Sorensen TL, Sellebjerg F, Jensen CV, Strieter RM, Ransohoff RM. Chemokines CXCL10 and CCL2: differential involvement in intrathecal inflammation in multiple sclerosis. *Eur J Neurol* 2001;8:665-672.

[47] Sindern E, Niederkinkhaus Y, Henschel M, Ossege LM, Patzold T, Malin JP. Differential release of beta-chemokines in serum and CSF of patients with relapsing-remitting multiple sclerosis. *Acta Neurol Scand* 2001;104:88-91.

[48] Gu L, Tseng S. Horner RM, Tam C, Loda M, Rollins BJ. Control of TH2 polarization by the chemokine monocyte chemoatractant protein-1. *Nature* 2000;404: 407-411.

[49] Columba-Cabezas S, Serafini B, Ambrosini E, Aloisi F. Lymphoid chemokines CCL19 and CCL21 are expressed in the central nervous system during experimental autoimmune encepahlomyelitis: implications for the maintenance of chronic inflammation. *Brain Pathol* 2003;13:38-51.

[50] Alt C, Laschinger M, Engelhardt B. Functional expression of lymphoid chemokines CCL19 (ELC) and CCL21 (SLC) at the blood-brain barrier suggests their possible involvement in lymphocyte recruitment into the central nervous system during experimental autoimmune encephalomyelitis. *Eur J Immunol* 2002;32:2133-2144.

[51] Kivisakk P, Mahad DJ, Callahan MK, Sikora K, Trebst C, Tucky B, Wujek J, Ravid R, Staugaitis SM, Lassmann H, Ransohoff RM . Expression of CCR7 in multiple sclerosis: implications for CNS immunity. *Ann Neurol* 2004;55:627-638.

[52] Rössler K, Neuchrist C, Kitz K, Scheiner O, Kraft D, Lassman H. Expression of leukocyte adhesion molecules at the human blood-brain barrier (BBB). *J Neurosci Res* 1992;31:365-374.

[53] Engelhardt B, Conley FK, Butcher EC. Cell adhesion molecules on vessels during inflammation in the mouse central nervous system. *J Neuroimmunol* 1994;51:199-208.

[54] Wong D, Prameya R, Dorovini-Zis K. In vitro adhesion and migration of T lymphocytes across monolayers of human brain microvessel endothelial cells: regulation by ICAM-1, VCAM-1, E-selectin and PECAM-1. *J Neuropathol Exp Neurol* 1999;58:138-152.

[55] Zameer A & Hoffman SAA. Increased ICAM-1 and VCAM-1 expression in the brains of autoimmune mice. *J Neuroimmunol* 2003;142:67-74.

[56] Kansas GS (1996). Selectins and their ligands: current concepts and controversies. *Blood* 1996;88:3259-3287.

[57] Englehardt B & Ransohoff RM. The ins and outs of T-lymphocyte trafficking to the CNS: anatomical sites and molecular mechanisms. *Trends Immunol* 2005;26:485-495.

[58] Brennan FR, O'Neil JK, Allen SJ, Butter C, Nuki G, Baker D. CD44 is involved in selective leukocyte extravasation during inflammatory central nervous system disease. *Immunology* 1999;98:427-435.

[59] Archelos JJ, Previrtali SC, Hartung HP. The role of integrins in immune-mediated diseases of the nervous system. *Trends Neurosci* 1999;22:30-38.

[60] Springer TA. Traffic signals for lymphocyte recirculation and leukocyte emigration: the multistep paradigm. *Cell* 1994;76:301-314.

[61] Butcher E. Leukocyte-endothelial cell recognition: three (or more) steps to specificity and diversity. *Cell* 1991;67:1033-1036.

[62] Canella B & Raine CS. The adhesion molecule and cytokine profile of multiple sclerosis lesions. *Ann Neurol* 1995;37:424-435.

[63] Chan PY & Aruffo A. VLA-4 integrin mediates lymphocyte migration on the inducible endothelial cell ligand VCAM-1 and the extracellular matrix ligand fibronectin. *J Biol Chem* 1993;268 :24655-24664.

[64] Bö L, Peterson JW, Mork S, Hoffman PA, Gallatin WM, Ransohoff RM, Trapp BD . Distribution of immunoglobulin superfamily members ICAM-1,-2-,-3, and the β2 integrin LFA-1 in Multiple Sclerosis lesions. *J Neuropathol Exp Neurol* 1996;55:1060-1072.

[65] Peterson JW, Bo L, Mork S, Cahng A, Ransohoff RM, Trapp BD. VCAM-1 positive microglia target oligodendrocytes at the border of multiple sclerosis lesions. *J Neuropathol Exp Neurol* 2002;61:539-546.

[66] Cayrol R, Wosik K, Berard J, Dodelet-Devillers A, Ifergan I, Kebir H, Haqqani AS, Kreymborg K, Krug S, Moundjian R, Bouthillier A, Becher B, Arbour N, David S, Stanimirovic D, Prat A. Activated leukocyte cell adhesion molecule promotes leukocyte trafficking into the central nervous system. *Nat Immunol* 2008;9:137-145.

[67] Gimferrer I, Calvo M, Mittelbrunn M, Farnós M, Sarrias MR, Enrich C, Vives J, Sanchez-Madrid F, Lozano F. Relevance of CD6-mediated interactions in T cell activation and proliferation. *J Immunol* 2004;173:2262-2270.

[68] Hughes PE & Pfaff M. Integrin affinity modulation. *Trends Cell Biol* 1998;8: 359-364.

[69] Kinashi T. Intracellular signaling controlling integrin activation in lymphocytes. *Nature Rev Immunol* 2005;5:546-559.

[70] Carman CV & Springer TA. A transmigratory cup in leukocyte diapedesis both trough individual vascular endothelial cells and between them. *J Cell Biol* 2004;167:377-388.

[71] Hordijk PL. Endothelial signaling events during leukocyte transmigration. *FEBS J* 2006;273:4408-4415.

[72] Hartung HP & Kieseier BC. The role of metalloproteinases in auto-immune damage to the central and peripheral nervous system. *J Neuroimmunol* 2000;107:140-147.

[73] Dubois B, Masure S, Hurtenbach U, Paemen L, Heremans H, van den Oord J, Sciot R, Meinhardt T, Hämerling G, Opdenakker G, Arnold B. Resistance of young gelatinase-B deficient mice to experimental autoimmune encephalomyelitis and necrotizing tail lesions. *J Clin Invest* 1999;104:1507-1515.

[74] Cuzner ML & Opdenakker G. Plasminogen activators and matrix metalloproteinases mediators of extracellular proteolysis in inflammatory demyelinataion of the Central Nervous System. *J Neuroimmunol* 1999;94:1-14.

[75] Waubant E, Goodkin DE, Gee L, Bacchetti P, Sloan R, Stewart T, Andersson PB, Satbler G, Miller K. Serum MMP-9 and TIMP-1 levels are related to MRI activity in relapsing multiple sclerosis. *Neurology* 1999;53:1397-1401.

[76] Reijerkerk A, Kooij G, van der Pol SMA, Khazen S, Dijkstra CD, de Vries HE. Diapedesis of monocytes is associated with MMP-mediated occluding disappearance in brain endothelial cells. *FASEB J* 2006;20:E1901-E1909.

[77] Newman TA, Wooley St, Hughes PM, Sibson NR, Anthony DC, Perry VH. T-cell and macrophage-mediated axon damage in the absence of a CNS-specific immune response: involvement of metalloproteinases. *Brain* 2001;124:2203-2214.

[78] Xie B, Dong Z, Fidler IJ. Regulatory mechanisms for the expression of type IV collagenases/gelatinases in murine macrophages. *J Immunol* 1994;152:3637-3644.

[79] Zhou H, Bernhard EJ, Fox PC, Billings PC. Induction of metalloproteinase activity in human T-lymphocytes. *Biochem Biophys Acta* 1993;1177:174-178.

[80] Galea I, Bernardes-Silva M, Forse PA, van Rooijen N, Libalu RL, Perry VH. An antigen-specific pathway for CD8 T cells across the blood-brain barrier. *J Exp Med* 2007;204:2023-2030.

[81] Shang XZ, Lang BJ, Issekutz AC. Adhesion molecule mechanisms mediating monocyte migration through synovial fibroblast and endotelium barriers: Role for CD11/CD18, very late antigen-4 (CD49d/CD29), very late antigen-5 (CD49e/CD29), and vascular adhesión molecule-1 (CD106). *J Immunol* 1998;160:467-474.

[82] de Vries HE, Hendriks JJ, Honing H, De Lavalette CR, van der Pol SM, Hooijberg E, Dijkstra CD, van der Berg TK. Signal-regulatory protein alpha-CD47 interactions are required for the transmigration of monocytes across cerebral endothelium. *J Immunol* 2002;168:5832-5839.

[83] Martin-Padura I, Lotaglio S, Schneemann M, Williams L, Romano M, Fruscella P, Panzeri C, Stoppacciaro A, Ruco L, Villa A, Simmons D, Dejana E. Junctional adhesion molecule, a novel member of the immunoglobulin superfamily that distributes at intracellular junctions and modulates monocyte transmigration. *J Cell Biol* 1998;142: 117-127.

[84] Ifergan I, KébirH, Bernard M, Wosik K, Dodelet-Devillers A, Cayrol R, Arbour N, Prat A. The blood-brain barrier induces differentiation of migrating monocytes into Th17-polarizing dendritic cells. *Brain* 2008;131:785-799

[85] Trebst C, Sorensen TL, Kivisäkk P, Cathcart MK, Hesselgesser J, Horuk R, Sellebjerg F, Lassmann H, Ransohoff RM. CCR1/CCR5+ mononuclear phagocytes accumulate in the central nervous system of patients with multiple sclerosis. *Am J Pathol* 2001;159:1701-1710.

[86] Tanuma N, Sakuna H, Sasaki A, Matsumoto Y. Chemokine expression by astrocytes plays a role in microglia/macrophage activation and subsequent neurodegeneration in secondary progressive multiple sclerosis. *Acta Neuropathol (Berl)* 2006;112:195-204.

[87] dos Santos AC, Barsante MM, Esteves Arantes RM, Bernard CC, Teixeira MM; Carvalho-Tavares J. CCL2 and CCL5 mediate leukocyte adhesion in experimental autoimmune encephalomyelitis –an intravital microscopy study. *J Neuroimmunol* 2005;162:122-129.

[88] Izikson L, Klein RS, Charo IF, Weiner HL, Luster AD. Resistance to experimental autoimmune encephalomyelitis in mice lacking the CC chemokine receptor (CCR)2. *J Exp Med* 2000;192:1075-1080.
[89] Lee TH, Avraham H, Lee SH, Avraham S. Vascular endothelial growth factor modulates neutrophil transendothelial migration via up-regulation of interleukin-8 in human brain microvascular endothelial cells. *J Biol Chem* 2002;277:10445-10451.
[90] Tani M, Fuentes ME, Peterson JW, Trapp BD, Durham SK, Loy JK, Bravo R, Ransohoff RM, Lira SA. Neutrophil infiltration, glial reaction, and neurological disease in transgenic mice expressing the chemokine N5/KC in oligodendrocytes. *J Clin Invest* 1996; 98:529-539.
[91] Calabresi PA, Pelfrey CM, Tranquil LR, Maloni H, McFarland HF. VLA-4 expression on peripheral blood lymphocytes is down-regulated after treatment of multiple sclerosis with interferon beta. *Neurology* 1997;49:1111-1116.
[92] Calabresi PA, Tranquil LA, Dambrosia JM, Stone LA, Maloni H, Bash CN, Frank JA, McFarland HF. Increases in soluble VCAM-1 correlate with a decrease in multiple sclerosis treated with interferon β-1b. *Ann Neurol* 1997;4 :669-674.
[93] Elovaara I, Lällä M, Spåre E, Lehtimäki T, Dastidar P. Methylprednisolone reduces adhesion molecules in blood and cerebrospinal fluid in patients with MS. *Neurology* 1998;51:1703-1708.
[94] Kent SJ, Karlik SJ, Rice GPA, Horner HC. A monoclonal antibody to α-4 integrin reverses the MR-detectable signs of experimental allergic encephalomyelitis in the guinea pig. *JMRI* 1995;5:535-540.
[95] Rice GAP, Hartung HP, Calabresi PA. Anti-α4 integrin therapy for multiple sclerosis. Mechanisms and rationale. *Neurology* 2005;64:1336-1342.
[96] Yednock T, Cannon C, Fritz L, Sanchez-Madrid R, Steinman L, Karin N. Prevention of experimental autoimmune encephalomyelitis by antibodies against α4β1 integrin. *Nature* 1992;356:63-66.
[97] Shimizu Y, van Seventer GA, Horgan KJ, Shaw S. Costimulation of proliferative responses of resting CD4+ T cells by the interaction of VLA-4 and VLA-5 with fibronectin or VLA-6 with laminin. *J Immunol* 1990;145:59–67.
[98] Davis LS, Oppenheimer-Marks N, Bednarczyk JL, McIntyre BW, Lipsky PE. Fibronectin promotes proliferation of naive and memory T cells by signaling through both the VLA-4 and VLA-5 integrin molecules. *J Immunol* 1990;145:785–793.
[99] Bayless KJ, Meininger GA, Scholtz JM, Davis GE. Osteopontin is a ligand for the alpha4beta1 integrin. J Cell Sci 1998;111:1165–1174.
[100] Chan PY, Aruffo A. VLA-4 integrin mediates lymphocyte migration on the inducible endothelial cell ligand VCAM-1 and the extracellular matrix ligand fibronectin. *J Biol Chem* 1993;268:24655–24664.
[101] Ferguson TA, Mizutani H, Kupper TS. Two integrin-binding peptides abrogate T cell-mediated immune responses in vivo. *Proc Natl Acad Sci USA* 1991;88:8072–8076.
[102] Niino M, Bodner C, Simard ML, Alatab S, Gano D, Kim HJ, Trigueiro M, Racicot D, Guerrete C, Antel JP, Fournier A, Grand' Maison F, Bar-Or A. Natalizumab effects on immune cell response in multiple sclerosis. *Ann Neurol* 2006;59:748-754.

[103] Miller DH, Khan OA, Sheremata WA, Blumhardt LD, rice GP, Libonati MA, Willmer –Hulme AJ, Dalton CM, Miszkiel KA, O'Connor PW, International Natalizumab Multiple Sclerosis Group. A controlled trial of natalizumab for relapsing multiple sclerosis. *N Engl J Med* 2003;348:15-23.

[104] O'Connor PW, Goodman A, Wilmer-Hulme AJ, Libonati MA, Metz L, Murray RS, Sheremata WA, Vollmer TL, Stone LA, Natalizumab multiple Sclerosis Trial Group. Randomized multicenter trial of natalizumab in acute MS relapses. Clinical and MRI effects. *Neurology* 2004;62 :2038-2043.

[105] Polman CH, O´Connor PW, Havrdova E, Hutchinson M, Kappos L, Miller DH, Phillips JT, Lublin FD, Giovannoni G, Wajgt A, Toal M, Lynn F, Panzara M, Sandrock AW for the AFFIRM Investigators. A randomized, placebo-controlled trial of natalizumab for relapsing Multiple Sclerosis. *N Engl J Med* 2006;354:899-910.

[106] Rudick RA, Stuart WH, Calabresi PA, Confavreaux C, Galetta SL, Radue EW, Lublin FD, Weinstock-Guttman B, Wynn DR, Lynn F, Panzara M, Sandrock AW for the SENTINEL investigators. Natalizumab plus interferon beta 1-a for relapsing Multiple Sclerosis. *N Engl J Med* 2006;354:911-923.

[107] Kleinschmidt-De Masters BK, Tyler KL. Progressive multifocal leukoencephalopathy complicating treatment with natalizumab and interferon beta –1a for multiple sclerosis. *N Engl J Med* 2005;353:369-374.

[108] Langer-Gould A, Atlas SW, Bollen AW, Pelletier D. Progressive multifocal leukoencephalopathy in a patient treated with natalizumab. *N Engl J Med* 2005;353: 375-381.

[109] Van Assche G, Van Ranst M, Sciot R, Dubois B, Vermeire S, Noman M, Verbeeck J, Geboes K, Robberecht W, Rutgeerts P. Progressive multifocal leukoencephalopathy after natalizumab therapy for Crohn's disease. *N Engl J Med* 2005;353:362-368.

[110] Yousry TA, Major EO, Ryschkewitsch C, Fahle G, Fischer S, Hou J, Curfman B, Miszkiel K, Mueller-Lenke N, Sanchez E, Barkhof F, Radue EW, Jäger HR, Clifford DB. Evaluation of patients treated with natalizumab for progressive multifocal leukoencephalopathy. *N Engl J Med* 2006;354:924-933.

[111] Ransohoff RM. Natalizumab for Multiple Sclerosis. *N Engl J Med* 2007;356:2622-2629.

[112] Davenport RJ & Munday JR. Alpha4-integrin antagonism-an effective approach for the treatment of inflammatory diseases? *Drug Discov Today* 2007;12:569-576.

[113] Piraino PS, Yednock TA, Freedman SB, Messermith EK, Pleiss MA, Karlik SJ. Suppression of acute experimental allergic encephalomyelitis with a small molecule inhibitor of α4 integrin. *Mult Scler* 2005;11:683-690.

[114] Kwak B, Mulhaupt F, Myit S, Mach F. Statins as a newly recognized type of immunomodulator. *Nat Med* 2000;6:1399-1402.

[115] Greenwood J, Walters CE, Pryce G, Kanuga N, Beraud E, Baker D, Adamson P. Lovastatin inhibits brain endothelial cell Rho-mediated lymphocyte migration and attenuates experimental utoimmune encephalomyelitis. *FASEB J* 2003; 17:905-907.

[116] Menge T, Hartung HP, Stuve O. Statins cure all for the brain? *Nat Rev Neurosci* 2005; 6:325-331.

[117] Weber MS, Steinman L, Zamvil SS. Statins-treatment option for Central Nervous System autoimmune disease? *Neurotherapeutics* 2007;4:693-700.

[118] Zipp F, Waiczies S, Aktas O, Neuhaus O, Hemmer B, Schraven B, Nitsch R, Hartung HP. Impact of HMG-CoA reductase inhibition on brain pathology. *Trends Pharmacol Sci* 2007;28:342-349.

[119] Kobashigawa JA, Katznelson S, Laks H, Johson JA, Yeatman L, Wang XM, Chia D, Terasaki PI, Sabad A, Cogert GA, Trosian K, Hamilton MA, Moriguchi JD, Kawata N, Hage A, Drinkwater DC, Stevenson LW. Effect of pravastatin on outcomes after cardiac transplantation. *N Engl J Med* 1995;333:621-627.

[120] Botti RE, Triscari J, Pan HY, Zayat J. Concentrations of pravastatin and lovastatin in cerebrospinal fluid in healthy subjects. *Clin Neuropharmacol* 1991;14:256-261.

[121] Hamelin BA & Turgeon J. Hydrophilicity/lipophilicity: relevance for the pharmacology and clinical effects of HMG-CoA reductase inhibitors. *Trends Pharmacol Sci* 1998;19:26-37.

[122] Pahan K, Sheik FG, Namboodiri AM, Singh I. Lovastatin and phenylacetate inhibit the induction of nitric oxide synthase and cytokines in rat primary astrocyte, macroglia and macrophages. *J Clin Invest* 1997;100:2671-2679.

[123] Nishibori M, Takahashi HK, Mori S. The regulation of ICAM-1 and LFA-1 interaction by autacoids and statins: a novel strategy for controlling inflammation and immune responses. *J Pharmacol Sci* 2003;92:7-12.

[124] Sadeghi MM Tiglio A, Sadigh K, O'Donnell L, Collinge M, Pardi R, Bender J. Inhibition of interferon-gamma mediated microvascular endotelial cell major histocompatibility complex class II gene activation by HMG-CoA reductase inhibitors. *Transplantation* 2001;71:1262-1268.

[125] Yilmaz A, Reiss C, Tantawi O, Weng A, Srumpf C, Raaz D, Ludwig J, Berger T, Steinkasserer A, Daniel WG, Garlichs CD. HMG-CoA reductase inhibitors suppress maturation of human dendritic cells: new implications for atherosclerosis. *Atherosclerosis* 2004;172:85-93.

[126] Ifergan I, Wosik K, Cayrol R, Kebir H, Auger C, Bernard M, Bouthillier A, Moumdjian R, Duquette P, Prat A. Statins reduce human blood-brain barrier permeability and restrict leukocyte migration: Relevance to multiple sclerosis. *Ann Neurol* 2006;60:45-55.

[127] Weitz-Schmidt G, Welzenbach K, Brinkmann V, Kamata T, Kallen J, Bruns C, Cottens S, Takada Y, Hommel U. Statins selectively inhibit leukocyte function antigen-1 by binding to a novel regulatory integrin site. *Nat Med* 2001;7:687-692.

[128] Weber C, Erl W, Weber KS, Weber PC. HMG-CoA reductase inhibitors decrease CD11b expression and CD11b-dependent adhesion of monocytes to endothelium and reduce increased adhesiveness of monocytes isolated from patients with hypercholesterolemia. *J Am Coll Cardiol* 1997;30:1212-1217.

[129] Chung HK, lee IK, Kang H, Suh J, Kim H, Park KC, Kim DW, Kim YK, Ro HK, Shong M. Statins inhibits interferon-gamma induced expression of intracellular adhesion molecule-1 (ICAM-1) in vascular endothelial and smooth muscle cells. *Exp Mol Med* 2002;34:451-461.

[130] Doo YC, Han SJ, Han SW, Park WJ, Choi SH, Cho GY, Hong KS, Han KR, Lee NH, Oh DJ, Ryu KH, Rim CY, Lee KH, Lee Y. Effect of preexisting statin use on expression of C-reactive protein, adhesion molecules, interleukin-6 and antioxidized low density lipoprotein antibody in patients with unstable angina undergoing coronary stenting. *Clin Cardiol* 2005;28:72-76.

[131] Prasad R, Giri S, Nath N, Singh AK. Inhibition of phosphoinositide 3 kinase-Akt (protein kinase B)-nuclear-factor-kappa B pathway by lovastatin limits endothelial-monocyte cell interaction. *J Neurochem* 2005;94:204-214.

[132] Ganne F, Vasse M, Beaudeux JL, Peynet J, francois A, Mishal Z, Chartier A, Tobelem G, Vannier JP, Soria J, Soria C. Cerivastatin, an inhibitor of HMG-CoA reductase, inhibits urokinase/urokinase-receptor expression and MMP-9 secretion by peripheral blood monocytes-a possible protective mechanism against atherotrombosis. *Haemost* 2000;84:680-688.

[133] Bellosta S, Via D, Canavesi M, Pfister P, Fumagalli R, Paoletti R, Bernini F. HMG-CoA reductase inhibitors reduce MMP-9 secretion by macrophages. *Artherioscler Thromb Vasc Biol* 1998;18:1671-1678.

[134] Youssef S, Stüve O, Patarroyo JC, Ruiz PJ, Radosevich JL, Hur EM, Bravo M, Mitchell DJ, Sobel RA, Steinman L, Zanvil SS. The HMG-CoA reductasa inhibitor, atorvastatin, promotes a Th2 bias and reverses paralysis in central nervous system autoimmune disease. *Nature* 2002;420:78-84.

[135] Aktas O, Waiczies S, Smorodchenko A, Dorr J, Seeger B, Prozorovski T, Sallach S, Endres M, Brocke S, Nitsch R, Zipp F. Treatment of relapsing paralysis in experimental encephalomyelitis by targeting Th1 cells through atorvastatin. *J Exp Med* 2003;197:725-733.

[136] Paintlia AS, Paintlia MK, Khan M, Vollmer T, Singh AK, Singh I. HMG-CoA reductase inhibitor augments survival and differentiation of oligodendrocyte progenitors in animal model of multiple sclerosis. *FASEB J* 2005;19:1407-1421.

[137] Vollmer T, Key L, Durkalski V,Tyor W, Corboy J, Matlovic-Plese S, Preiningerova J, Rizzo M, Singh I. Oral simvastatin treatment in relapsing remitting multiple sclerosis. *Lancet* 2004;363:1607-1608.

[138] National Multiple Sclerosis Society. Clinical trials in multiple sclerosis: planned, in progress, recently completed [online]. Available from: URL: htpp://www.nationalmssociety.org/docs/HOM/clinicaltrials.pdf

[139] Stuve O, Youssef S, Weber MS, Nessler S, vonBüdingen HC, Hemmer B, Prod´homme T, Sobel RA, Sreinman L, Zanvil SS. Immunomodulatory synergy by combination of atorvastatin and glatiramer acetate in treatment of CNS autoimmunity. *J Clin Invest* 2006;116:1037-1044.

[140] Birnbaum GA & Altafullah I. A double blind, placebo controlled trial of atorvastatin in combination with subcutaneous interferon beta 1a in persons with multiple sclerosis. Neurology 2007;68(Suppl1):A206-A207.

[141] Kuruganti PA, Hinojoza JR, Eaton MJ, Ehmann UK, Sobel RA. Interferon-beta counteracts inflammatory mediator-induced effects on brain endothelial cells tight junctions molecules-implications for multiple sclerosis. *J Neuropathol Exp Neurol* 2002;61:710-724.

[142] Minagar A, Long A, Ma T, Jackson TH, Kelley RE, Ostanin DV, Sasaki M, Warren AC, Jawahar A, Cappell B, Alexander JS. Interferon (IFN)-beta 1a and IFN-beta 1b block IFN-gamma-induced desintegration of endothelial junction integrity and barrier. *Endothelium* 2003;10:299-307.

[143] Förster C, Silwedel C, Golenhofen N, Burek M Kietz S, Mankertz J Drenckhahn D. Occludin as direct target for glucocorticoid-induced improvement of blood-brain barrier properties in a murine in vitro system. *J Physiol* 2005;565:475-486.

[144] Förster C, Waschke J, Burek M, Leers J, Drenckhahn D. Glucocorticoid effects on microvascular endothelial barrier permeability as brain specific. *J Physiol* 2006;573:413-425.

[145] Szczucinski A & Losy J. Chemokines and chemokine receptors in multiple sclerosis. Potential targets for new therapies. *Acta Neurol Scand* 2007;115:137-146.

[146] Proudfoot AEI, Power CA, Rommel C, Wells TNC. Strategies for chemokine antagonists as therapeutics. *Sem Immunol* 2003;15:57-65.

[147] Lund BT, Ashikian N, Ta HQ,Charyian Y, Manoukian K, Groshen S, Gilmore W, Cheema GS, Stohl W, Burnett ME, Ko D, Kachuck NJ, Weiner LP. Increased CXCL8 (IL-8) expression in multiple sclerosis. *J Neuroimmunol* 2004;155:161-171.

[148] Sorensen TL & Sellebjerg F. Selective suppression of chemokine receptor CXCR3 expression by interferon-beta 1a in multiple sclerosis. *Mult Scler* 2002;8:104-107.

[149] Iarlori C, Reale A, Lugaresi GD. RANTES production and expression is reduced in relapsing-remitting multiple sclerosis patients treated with interferon-beta 1b. *J Neuroimmunol* 2000;107:100-107.

[150] Elovaara I, Kuusisto H, Paalavuo R, Särkijärvi S, Lehtimäki T, Huhtala H, Vilpo J. . Effect of high-dose methylprednisolone treatment on CCR5 expression on blood cells in MS exacerbation. *Acta Neurol Scand* 2006;113:163-166.

[151] Bartosik-Psujek H, Belniak E, Mitosek-Swewczyk K, Dobosz B, Stelmasiak Z. Interleukin-8 and RANTES levels in patients with relapsing-remitting multiple sclerosis (RR-MS) treated with cladribine. *Acta Neurol Scand* 2004;109:390-392.

[152] Johnson Z, Schwarz M, Power CA, Wells TNC, Proufoot AEI. Multi-faceted strategies to combat disease by interference with the chemokine system. *Trends Immunol* 2005;26:268-274.

[153] Haringman JJ, Kraan MC, Smeets TJ, Zwinderman KH, Tak PP. Chemokine blockade and chronic inflammatory disease:proof of concept in patients with rheumatoid arthritis. *Ann Rheum Dis* 2003;62:715-721.

[154] Schwarz MK & Wells TN. New therapeutics that modulate chemokine networks. *Nat Rev Drug Discov* 2002;1:347-358.

[155] Zipp F, Hartung HP, Hillert J, Schimrigk S, Trebst C, Stangel M, Infante-Duarte C, Jakobs P, Wolf C, Sandbrink R, Pohl C, Filippi M. Blockade of chemokine signaling in patients with multiple sclerosis. *Neurology* 2006;67:1880-1883.

[156] Brodmerkel CM, Huber R, Covington M, Diamond S, Hall L, Collins R, Leffet L, Gallagher K, Fledman P, Collier P, Stow M, Gu X, Baribaud F, Shin N, Thomas B, Burn T, Hollis G, Yeleswaram S, Solomon K, Friedman S, Wang A, Xue CB, Newton RC, Scherle P, Vaddi K . Discovery and pharmacological characterization of a novel rodent-active CCR2 antagonist INCB3344. *J Immunol* 2005;175:5370-5378.

[157] Gao P, Zhou XY, Yashiro-Ohtani Y, Yang YF, Sugimoto N, Ono S, Nakanishi T, Imanishi T, Egawa T, Nagasawa T, Fujiwara H, Hamaoka T. The unique target specificity of a nonpeptide chemokine receptor antagonist: selective blockade of two Th1 chemokine receptors CCR5 and CXCR3. *J Leukoc Biol* 2003;73:273-280.

[158] Blampain C, Buser R, Power CA, Edgerton M, Buchanan C, Mack M,Simmon G, Clapham PR, Parmentier M, Proudfoot AE. A chimeric MIP-1α/RANTES protein demonstrates the use of different regions of RANTES proteins to bind and activate its receptors. *J Leukoc Biol* 2001;69:977-985.

[159] Cox MA, Jenh CH, Gonsiorek W, Fine J, Narula SK, Zavodny PJ, Hipkin RW. Human Interferon-inducible 10-kDA protein and human interferon-inducible T cell alpha chemoattractant are allotropic ligands for CXCR3: differential binding to receptors states. *Mol Pharmacol* 2001;59:707-715.

[160] Liang M, Rosser M, Ng HP, May K, Bauman JG, Islam I, Ghannam A, Kretschmer PJ, PuH, Dunning L, Snider RM, Morrisey MM, Hesselgesser J, Perez HD, Horuk R. Species selectivity of a small molecule antagonist of CCR1chemokine receptor. *Eur J Pharmacol* 2000;389:41-49.

[161] Liang M, Mallari C, Rosser M, Ng HP, May K, Monahan S, Bauman JG, Islam I, Ghannam A, Buckman B, Shaw K, Wei GP, Xu W, Zhao Z, Ho E, Shen J, Oanh H, Subramanyan B, Vergona R, Taub D, Dunning L, Harvey S, Snider RM, Hesselgesser J, Morrisey MM, Perez HD. Identification and characterization of a potent, selective, and orally active antagonist of the CC chemokine receptor-1. *J Biol Chem* 2000;275:19000-19008.

[162] Karpus WJ, Lukacs NW, McRae BL, Strieter RM, Kunkel SL, Miller SD. An important role of the chemokine macrophage inflammatory protein-1 alpha in the pathogenesis of the T cell mediated autoimmune disease, experimental autoimmune encephalomyelitis. *J Immunol* 1995; 155:5003-5010.

[163] Gonzalo JA, Lloyd CM, Albar JP, Wen D, Wells TNC, Proudfoot A, Martinez-A C, Dorf M, Bjerke T, Coyle AJ, Gutierrez-Ramos JC. The coordinated action of CC chemokines in the lung orchestrates allergic inflammation and airway hyperresponsiveness. *J Exp Med* 1998;188:157-167.

[164] Gonzalo JA, Pan Y, Lloyd CM, Jia GQ, Yu G, Dussault B, Powers CA, Proudfoot AE, Coyle AJ, Gearing D, Gutierrez-Ramos JC. Mouse monocyte-derived chemokine is involved in airway hyperreactivity and lung inflammation. *J Immunol* 1999;163:403-411.

[165] Lloyd CM, Minto AM, Dorf ME, Proudfoot AEI, Wels TNC, Salant DJ, Gutierrez-Ramos JC. RANTES and monocyte chemoattractan protein-1 (MCP-1) play an important role in the inflammatory phase of crescentic nephritis but only MCP-1 is involved in crescent formation and intersticial fibrosis. *J Exp Med* 1997;185:1371-1380.

[166] Xie JH, Nomura N, Lu M, Chen SL, Koch GE, Weng Y, Rosa R, Di Salvo J, Mudgett J, Peterson LB, Wicker LS, Dimartino JA . Antibody-mediated blockade of the CXCR3 chemokine receptor results in diminished recruitment of T helper 1 cells into sites of inflammation. *J Leukoc Biol* 2003;73:771-780.

[167] Lazzeri E & Romagnani P. CXCR3-binding chemokines: novel multifunctional therapeutic targets. *Curr Drug Targets Immune Endocr Metabol Disord* 2005;5:109-118.

[168] Glass WG, Hickey MJ, Hardison JL, Liu MT, Manning JE, Lane TE. Antibody targeting of the CC chemokine ligand 5 results in diminished leukocyte infiltration into the central nervous system and reduced neurologic disease in a viral model of multiple sclerosis. *J Immunol* 2004;172:4018-4025.

[169] Gong JH, Ratkay LG, Waterfield JD, Clark LI. An antagonist of monocyte chemoattractant protein 1 (MCP-1) inhibits arthritis in the MRL-lpr mouse model. *J Exp Med* 1997;186:131-137.

[170] Plater-Zyberk C, Hoogewerf AJ, Proudfoot AEI, Power CA, Wells TNC. Effect of CC chemokine receptor antagonist on collagen-induced arthritis in DBA/l mice. *Immunol Lett* 1997;57:117-120.

[171] Ajuebor MN, Hogaboam CM, Kunkel SL, Proudfoot AE, Wallace JL. The chemokine RANTES is a crucial mediator of the progression from acute to chronic colitis in rat. *J Immunol* 2001;166:552-558.

[172] Mack M, Luckow B, Nelson PJ, Cihak J, Simmons G, Clapham PR, Signoret N, Marsh M, Stangassinger M, Borlat F, Wells TN, Schlöndorff D, Proudfoot AE. Amynooxypentane-RANTES induces CCR5 internalization but inhibits recycling: a novel inhibitory mechanism of HIV infectivity. *J Exp Med* 1998;187:1215-1224.

[173] Ozenci V, Kouwenhoven M, Teleshova N, Pashenkov M, Fredrikson S, Link H. Multiple sclerosis: pro and anti-inflammatory cytokines and metalloproteinases are affected differentially by treatment with IFN-beta. *J Neuroimmunol* 2000;108:236-243.

[174] Waubant E, Gee L, Miller K, Satbler G, Goodkin D. IFN-beta 1a may increase serum levels of TIMP-1 in patients with relapsing-remitting multiple sclerosis. *J Interferon Cytokine Res* 2001;21:181-185.

[175] Avolio C, Filippi M, Tortorella C, Rocca MA, Ruggieri M, Agosta F, Tomassini V, Pozzilli C, Stechhi S, Giaquinto P, Livrea P, Trojano M. Serum MMP-9/TIMP-1 and MMP-2/TIMP-2 ratios in multiple sclerosis: relationship with different magnetic resonance imaging measures of disease activity during IFN-beta-1a treatment *Mult Scl* 2005;11:441-446.

[176] Neuhaus O, Strasser-Fuchs S, Fasekas F, Kieseier BC, Niederwieser G, Hartung HP, Archelos JJ. Statins as immunomodulators. Comparison with interferon-β 1b in MS. *Neurology* 2002;59:990-997.

[177] Kopadze T, Dehmel T, Hartung HP, Stüve O, Kieseier BC. Inhibition of mitoxantrone of in vitro migration of immunocompetent cells. A possible mechanism of therapeutic efficacy in the treatment of multiples sclerosis. *Arch Neurol* 2006;63:1572-1578.

[178] Förster C, Kahles T, Kietz S, Drenckhahan. Dexametasone induces the expression of metalloproteinase inhibitor TIMP-1 in the murine cerebral vascular endothelial cell line cEND. *J Physiol* 2007;580:937-949.

[179] Rosenberg GA, Dencoff JE, Correa N, Reiners M, Ford CC. Effects of steroids on CSF matrix metalloproteinases in multiple sclerosis: relation to blood-brain barrier injury. *Neurology* 1996;46:1626-1632.

[180] Yong VW, Power C, Forsyth P, Edwards DR. Metalloproteinases biology and pathology of the nervous system. *Nat Rev Neurosci* 2001;2:502-511.

[181] Yong VW, Agrawal SM, Stirling DP. Targeting MMPs in acute and chronic neurological conditions. *Neurotherapeutics* 2007;4:580-589.

[182] Lapchack PA, Chapman DF, Zivin JA. Metalloproteinase inhibition reduces thrombolitic (Tissue-plasminogen activator)-induced hemorrhage after tromboembolic stroke. *Stroke* 2000;31:3034-3040

[183] Leib SL, Clements JM, Lindberg RL, Heimgartner C, Loeffler JM, Pfister LA, Tauber MG, Leppert D. Inhibition of matrix metalloproteinases and tumor necrosis factor alpha converting enzyme as adjuvant therapy in pneumococcal meningitis. *Brain* 2001;124:1734-1742.

[184] Leppert D. Lindberg RL, Kappos L, Leib SL. Matrix metalloproteinases : multifunctional effectors of inflammation in multiple sclerosis and bacterial meningitis. *Brain Res Brain Res Rev* 2001; 36:249-257.

[185] Wang J & Tsirka SE. Neuroprotection by inhibition of matrix metalloproteinases in a mouse model of intracerebral haemorrhage. *Brain* 2005; 128:1622-1633.

[186] Gijbels K, Galardy RE, Steinman L. Reversal of experimental allergic encephalomyelitis with a hydroxamate inhibitor of matrix metalloproteinases. *J Clin Invest* 1994;94:2177-2182.

[187] Toft-Hansen H, Babcock AA, Milward JM, Owens T. Downregulation of membrane type-matrix metalloproteinases in the inflamed or injured central nervous system. *J Neuroinflammation* 2007; doi:10.186/1742-2094-4-24

[188] Lee SR, Kim HY, Rogowaska J, Zhao BQ, Bhide P, Parent JM, Lo EH. Involvement of matrix metalloproteinase in neuroblast cell migration from the subventricular zone after stroke. *J Neurosci* 2006;26:3491-3495.

[189] Zhao BQ, wang S, Kim HY, Storrie H, Rosen BR, Mooney DJ, Wang X, Lo EH. Role of matrix metalloproteinases in delayed cortical responses after stroke. *Nat Med* 2006;12:441-445.

[190] Coussens L, Fingleton B, Matrisian LM, Matrix metalloproteinase inhibitors and cancer: trials and tribulations. *Science* 2002; 295:2387-2892.

[191] Yong VW. The potential use of MMP inhibitors to treat CNS diseases. *Expert Opin Investig Drugs* 1999;8:255-268.

[192] Stirling DP, Koochesfahani KM, Steeves JD, Tetzlaff W. Minocycline as a neuroprotective agent. *Neuroscientist* 2005;11:308-322.

[193] Yong VW, Wells J, Giuliani F, Casha S, Power C, Metz LM. The promise of minocycline in neurology. Lancet Neurol 2004;3:744-751.

[194] Yrjanheikki J, Tikka T, Keinamen R, Goldstein G, Cahn PH, Koistinaho J. A tetracycline derivative, minocycline, reduces inflammation and protect against focal cerebral ischemia with a wide therapeutic window. *Proc Natl Acad Sci USA* 1999;96:13496-13500.

[195] Chen M, Ona VO, Li M, Ferrante RJ, Fink KB, Zhu S, Bian J, Guo L, Farrel LA, Hersch SM, Hobbs W, Vonsattel JP, Cha JH, Friedlander RM. Minocycline inhibits caspase-1 and caspase-3 expression and delays mortality in a transgenic mouse model of Huntington disease. *Nat Med* 2000;6:797-801.

[196] Suk K. Minocycline suppresses hypoxic activation of rodent microglia in culture. *Neurosci Lett* 2004;366:167-171.

[197] Zabad RK, Metz LM, Todoruk TR, Zhang Y, Mitchell JR, Yeung M, Patry DG, Bell RB, Yong VW. The clinical response to minocycline in multiple sclerosis is accompanied by beneficial immune changes: a pilot study. *Mult Scl* 2007;13:517-526.

[198] Brundula V, Rewscale NB, Metz LM, Bernard CC, Yong VW . Targeting leukocyte MMPs and transmigration. Minocycline as a potential therapy for multiple sclerosis. *Brain* 2002;125:1297-1308.

[199] Bickett D, Green MD; Berman J, Dezube M, Howe AS, Brown PJ, Roth JT, McGeehan GM. A high throughput fluorogenic substrate for interstitial colleganese (MMP-1) and gelatinase (MMP-9). *Anal Biochem* 1993;212:58-64.

[200] Popovic N, Schubart A, Goetz BD, Zhang SC, Linington C, Duncan ID. Inhibition of autoimmune encephalomyelitis by a tetracycline. *Ann Neurol* 2002;51:215-223.

[201] Zabad RK, Metz LM, Todorouk TR, Zhang Y, Mitchell JR, Yeung M, Patry DG, Bell RB, Yong VW. The clinical response to minocycline in multiple sclerosis is accompanied by beneficial immune changes : a pilot study. *Mult Scl* 2007;13 :517-526.

[202] Persidsky Y, Ramirez SH, Haorah J, Kanmogne GD. Blood-brain barrier : structural components and function under physiologic and pathologic conditions. *J Neuroimmune Pharmacol* 2006;1:223-236.

[203] Pardridge WM. Blood-brain barrier delivery. *Drug Discov Today* 2007;12:54-61.

[204] Golden PL & Pardridge WM. P-glycoprotein on astrocyte foot processes of unfixed isolated human brain capillaries. *Brain Res* 1999;819:143-146.

[205] Begley DJ. Delivery of therapeutic agents to the central nervous system: the problems and the possibilities. *Pharmacol and Therap* 2004;104:29-45.

[206] Schinkel AH & Jonker JW. Mammalian drug efflux transporters of the ATP binding cassette (ABC) family: an overview. *Adv Drug Deliv Rev* 2003;55:3-29.

[207] Ford JM. Modulators of multidrug resistance. Preclinical studies. *Hematol Oncol Clin North Am* 1995;9:337-361.

[208] Borst P, evers R, Kool M, Winjnholds J. A family of drugs transporters: the multidrug resistance-associated proteins. *J Natl Cancer Inst* 2000;92:1295-1302.

[209] de Boer AG & Gaillard PJ. Strategies to improve drug delivery across the blood-brain barrier. *Clin Pharmocokinet* 2007;46:553-576.

[210] Zhang Y & Pardridge WM. Conjugation of brain derived neurotrophic factor to a blood-brain barrier drug targeting system enables neuroprotection in regional brain ischemia following intravenous injection of neurotrophin. *Brain Res* 2001;889:49-56.

[211] Smith MW & Gumbleton M. Endocytosis at the blood-brain barrier: from basic understanding to drug delivery strategies. *J Drug Target* 2006;14:191-214.

[212] Duffy KR & Pardridge WM. Blood-brain barrier transcytosis of insulin in developing rabbits. *Brain Res* 1987;420:32-38.

[213] Pardridge WM, Kang YS, Buciak JL, Yang J. Human insulin receptor monoclonal antibody undergoes high affinity binding to human brain capillaries in vitro and rapid transcytosis through the blood-brain barrier. *Pharm Res* 1995;12:807-816.

[214] Boado RJ, Zhang YF, Zhang Y, Pardridge WM. Humanization of anti-human insulin receptor antibody for drug targeting across the human blood-brain barrier. *Biotechnol Bioeng* 2007;96: 381-391.

[215] Smith MW & Gumbleton M. Endocytosis at the blood-brain barrier: from basic understanding to drug delivery strategies. *J Drug Target* 2006;14:191-214.

[216] Jones AR & Shusta EV. Blood-brain barrier transport and therapeutics via receptor mediation. *Pharmac Res* 2007;24:1759-1771.

[217] Cornford EM, Cornford ME. New systems for delivery of drugs to the brain in neurological diseases. *Lancet Neurol* 2002;1:306-315.

[218] Sindern E, Niederkinkhaus Y, Henschel M, Ossege LM, Patzold T, Malin JP. Differential release of beta-chemokines in serum and CSF of patients with relapsing-remitting multiple sclerosis. *Acta Neurol Scand* 2001;104:88-91.

[219] Gossen M, Freundlieb S, Bender G, Muller G, Hillen W, Bujard H. Transcriptional activation by tetracyclines in mammalian cells. *Science* 1995;268:1766-1769.

In: The Blood-Brain Barrier
Editor: Tomas R. Helio

ISBN 978-1-60456-894-3

Chapter 3

BLOOD–BRAIN BARRIER DISRUPTIONS IN STROKE: THE INFLUENCE OF AGING

R. L. Chen and J. E. Preston
Division of Pharmaceutical Research, King's College London, UK.

ABSTRACT

Cerebrovascular disease with inadequate blood supply to brain and ischemic stroke is largely a disease of later life and results in death or permanent disability in around 2/3rds of cases. An early event in stroke is damage to the brain microvasculature and disruption of the blood-brain barrier (BBB) which in itself can lead to neuronal damage since the BBB normally maintains homeostasis of the delicate brain environment. Current treatments for stroke focus on re-establishment of cerebral blood flow and on neuro-protection, however there is concern that blood reperfusion contributes to further BBB disruption with subsequent edema and the increased possibility of hemorrhage. There is increasing interest in the mechanisms underlying BBB disruption, both to further understanding of the pathogenesis of cerebral ischemia and to identify new therapeutic targets aiding vascular (and thus neuronal) integrity. The cause of BBB disruption is multi-factorial and may involve matrix metalloproteinases, reactive oxygen species, nitric oxide and inflammatory cytokines. A complicating factor is that, although stroke is more common in older population, many of the pre-clinical studies have used young adult animal models which do not adequately account for underlying age-related deficits in cerebral microvessels. This may contribute to the reasons why promising therapies at a pre-clinical stage later fail at clinical trial. Aging itself is associated with a host of changes in both BBB and brain, such as increased BBB permeability, reduced cerebral blood flow and neuronal atrophy and loss. These changes alone may not necessarily result in clinical symptoms, however they would render the old brain vulnerable to ischemic insult. Recent studies on stroke using aged animals indicate larger infarct volume, greater BBB permeability, more neuronal loss, less functional recovery and higher mortality compared to the young. Future pre-clinical research on stroke would benefit from attention to both BBB disruption and age-related tissue vulnerability to help development of targeted therapies of relevance to the clinical setting.

ABBREVIATIONS

AP,	alkaline phosphatase;
AQP,	aquaporin;
ATP,	adenosine triphosphate;
BCB,	blood-CSF barrier;
BBB,	blood–brain barrier;
BUI,	brain uptake index;
CBF,	cerebral blood flow;
CNS,	central nervous system;
CP,	choroid plexus;
CSF,	cerebrospinal fluid;
EB,	Evans Blue;
ECM,	extracellular matrix;
τ-GT,	τ– glutamyl transpeptidase;
HT,	hemorrhagic transformation;
ICAM,	immunoglobulin family of cellular adhesion molecule;
ICH,	intracerebral hemorrhage;
IL,	interleukin;
LDH,	lactate dehydrogenase;
MCAO,	middle cerebral artery occlusion;
MCP,	monocyte chemoattractant protein;
MMP,	matrix metalloproteinase;
MRI,	magnetic resonance imaging;
NMDA,	*N*-methyl-D-aspartate;
NO,	nitric oxide;
NOS,	nitric oxide synthase;
PA,	plasminogen activator;
PAF,	platelet activating factor;
RNS,	reactive nitrogen species;
ROS,	reactive oxygen species;
SOD,	superoxide dismutase;
TGF,	transforming growth factor;
TJ,	tight junctions;
TNF,	tumor necrosis factor;
tPA,	tissue-type PA;
uPA,	urokinase-type PA;
VEGF,	vascular endothelial growth factor;
ZO,	zonula occludens.

INTRODUCTION

Stroke is the third highest cause of mortality and the highest neurological cause of disability-adjusted life-years lost in major industrialized countries [1]. Stroke has recently been shown to cost the UK healthcare system £5.2 billion per year [2,3]. Over 80% of strokes are ischemic and result from vascular occlusion, most commonly by clot formation affecting the middle cerebral artery (MCA) [4], leading to reduced cerebral perfusion. Irreversible damage occurs in an 'ischemic core' of severe hypoperfusion [5], surrounding by the 'penumbra' and 'oligemia' [6]. Tissue within the penumbra may be salvageable [6] and is a key target for therapeutic intervention [7], while the oligemic compartment is not normally at risk of infarction [8] and is not therapeutically targeted [9]. Other forms of stroke are hemorrhagic, where a blood vessel bursts either in brain or on its surface. The proportion of this type of stroke is higher in Asian populations (China, Japan, Korea) compared to the Caucasian populations [10], probably due to environmental differences (e.g. lifestyles, diet) [10,11] and genetic predisposition to hypertension and ischemic stroke risk [12].

The fundamental approaches to acute stroke therapy are reperfusion and neuroprotection [13], with early reperfusion is the most effective therapy in humans [14]. Clinical outcome improves with early clot lysis 3 hours after stroke using intravenous recombinant tissue plasminogen activator (rtPA) [15]. This remains the only approved therapy for acute stroke [16], however, there are many limitations including the narrow time window, and few patients (1-3%) currently receive reperfusion therapies in actual practice [17]. In addition, if rtPA reaches the extracellular space of the central nervous system (CNS), it can induce neurotoxicity via proteolysis [18].

Neuroprotection strategies aim to protect neurons from ischemia-reperfusion injury and to amplify the time window for thrombolytic treatment [19]. Although more than 900 drugs have been investigated, only around 100 have reached clinical trials [20]. These include neurotransmitter agonists and antagonists (for GABA, 5HT, glycine), ion channel antagonists, Na^{+}/Ca^{2+} transport blockers and reactive oxygen species (ROS) scavengers [13]. Despite evidence of utility in animal models, none has been successful in humans [13]. One reason for this failure is that the primary focus of previous research has been on neurons, while brain microvessels have received relatively little attention [21]. Ischemia affects both neurons and microvessels rapidly [22], but the microvasculature generates free radicals earlier than neurons [23] and damaged microvasculature can then lead to neuronal injury [24]. The degree of blood brain barrier (BBB) breakdown is directly correlated with neurological deficit [25,26]. Drugs working on the neurovascular unit [27,28] are useful in protecting neurons following experimentally induced stroke [24], and will act as neuro-protective agents [13]. Cerebral vascular protection, which has not been well studied before, has the potential to be a new treatment for stroke [29]

An additional issue to take into account is that more than 80% of all strokes occur in people aged 64 or over, and the risk of stroke and likelihood of a poor outcome increases with age [30]. This may add to the reasons why neuroprotective drugs identified in preclinical studies on young animals fail at phase II-III clinical trials [31,32]. Ageing is associated with significant structural and functional alterations in BBB [33], and the response of the CNS to stroke differs as a function of age [32]. The Stroke Therapy Academic Industry Roundtable now recommends that aged animals be considered in preclinical studies [34]. There is an urgent need for research on the contribution of aged BBB to the pathophysiology of stroke [29].

This review is going to summarise BBB disruption in stroke, exploring the underlying mechanisms and the influence of ageing.

1. BBB Morphology and Function

Barriers between blood and brain comprise the blood-brain barrier (BBB), blood – cerebrospinal fluid (CSF) barrier (BCB) and the arachnoid membrane. The BBB is composed of endothelial cells that line the cerebral vasculature, their capillary basement membranes, the astrocyte end-feet, and pericytes [35]. Cerebral vascular endothelial cells differ from other endothelial cells in the body due to more extensive tight junctions (TJs) and relative lack of fenestrae and pinocytotic vesicles [36-38]. The highly developed TJs between adjacent endothelial cells are formed by a complex of integral membrane proteins [claudin (1, 5, and 12) [39], occludin [40,41], and junctional adhesion molecules [42], and a number of cytoplasmic accessory protein including zonula occludens proteins (ZO)[43-46], cingulin [47]. The end-feet of astrocytes contribute to the barrier permeability and almost completely cover the outer surface of the microvascular basement membranes [28]. Between the endothelium and astrocyte end-feet, is the extracellular matrix (ECM), which contains type IV collagen, laminin, and fibronectin. ECM supports the microvessels and regulates cell survival, growth, and differentiation [48]. At the BCB, TJs are formed between the epithelial cells rather than the endothelia, of the four choroid plexuses (CPs) in the cerebral ventricles. BCB epithelial TJs are different to those of BBB endothelial cells, containing claudin-2 rather than claudin-5 [49]. In addition, the ZOs are relatively short and concentrated close to the apical (CSF) side of the CP [50]. Functionally, the BCB is leakier to ions compared to BBB, as measured by the electrical resistance, which is 26 Ω cm^2 in the choroidal epithelium compared to 1462 Ω cm^2 in the cerebral endothelium [51,52]. Besides its barrier function, the CP avidly secretes CSF and synthesizes a number of proteins, many for secretion into CSF, e.g. transthyretin, insulin-like growth factor – II, vasopressin, transforming growth factor β [50].

The TJs normally prevent free exchange of solutes between blood and brain or CSF [53], except for small lipid-soluble molecules <400 Da which can cross the barriers unassisted via diffusion [54]. Hydrophilic molecules generally cross the endothelial wall via transcellular transport mechanisms, classified into five main categories: carrier-mediated transport, ion transport, active efflux transport, receptor-mediated transport, and caveolae-mediated transport [55].

2. BBB Disruption in Stroke: The Time Course

Following brain ischemia, there are a number of biochemical and molecular changes at the BBB, including glycolytic pathway stimulation, stress response, antioxidant defense, transport/transcytosis, inflammation, angiogenesis and ECM remodelling. BBB disruption occurs early after ischemia [56,57], although different models of cerebral ischemia show variability in the extent and time course [58-60]. BBB breakdown seems to be important during the initial stage of stroke [61], since the disruption is observed earlier than neuronal loss with opening of the BBB 6 h after the ischemia, while neuronal death becomes evident 1-3 days post ischemia [62,63].

Reperfusion leads to a characteristic "biphasic" opening of the BBB [64-69]. An immediate BBB opening was seen after reperfusion in the MAC occluded (MCAO) cat [64], and rat [56] using Evans blue (EB) extravasation or radioisotope measures, mainly in the caudate and cerebral cortex on the side of the MCAO. This was confirmed using magnetic resonance image (MRI), in which BBB damage was detected within minutes of recanulisation [57]. In humans, early BBB disruption (< 4 hours from onset) is seen in patients associated with acute thrombolytic therapy [61]. Several factors can contribute to this early BBB opening such as an increase in tissue water content [70,71], blood flow [72], oxygenation, ROS [73], and acute systemic hypertension [64]. After this initial opening, there is a "refractory" state, where no BBB disruption is observed [64-67]. The "refractory" time varies with different stroke models from a few hours [64] to several days [66,67]. Possible explanations are reduced hyperemia with re-establishment of vascular autoregulation, and inhibition of pinocytotic activity [64]. The second, more delayed BBB opening is associated with severe ischemic injury and infarction, with edema development. [74]. The mechanism for this opening is suggested to be associated with entry of inflammatory mediators and toxic substance from the blood to the brain [69]. It has been postulated that the secondary BBB opening is an integral part of inflammatory activation [75], with several cytokines implicated in the response [76].

Since the timing of BBB disruption is early in stroke, it is important to define the time course of BBB modifications following recanulisation, because: (a) with BBB disrupted, the brain is vulnerable to entry of potentially neurotoxic agents from blood, resulting in neuron death; (b) "BBB opening" may offer a therapeutic window for delivery of neuroprotective agents into brain, that would not normally cross the BBB [77,78]. In order to evaluate potential successful neuroprotective drugs, knowledge of how BBB changes as ischemic injury progresses is needed, especially in the elderly, and to bear in mind that drugs given acutely may need to function in energy-depleted conditions, (i.e. at the time of thrombolysis) [79].

3. Mechanisms of BBB Disruption in Stroke

The types of BBB disruption consistently seen in cerebral ischemia are widening of the endothelial TJ complexes [80-82] and enhancement of endothelial pinocytotic vesicular transport [83-86]. The mechanisms for the disruption are multi-factorial, and these factors can interact each other:

3.1. Matrix Metalloproteinases (MMPs)

MMPs are a family of zinc-dependent endopeptidases that can digest almost all ECM molecules [87]. MMP-9 and MMP-2 play key roles in the degradation of type IV collagen and laminin, which are major components of vascular basement membrane [88]. MMPs -2 is up-regulated by 1 hour after ischemia [89-92], and significant MMP-9 expression comes from microvessels and associated astrocytic end-feet [93], closely correlated with BBB disruption [92]. Increased MMP-9 in plasma of acute stroke patients demonstrates some correlation with clinical outcome, perhaps suggesting its use as a biomarker [94]. Inhibition of MMP 9 reduces infarct size and prevents ischemia-induced BBB breakdown and brain edema [95]. MMP inhibitors may be useful as adjunct therapies for combination with rtPA thrombolysis in acute ischemic stroke [96]. MMP might be helpful in later stages of stroke [97] for remodelling components of the ECM and participating in dendritic and axonal extension [98] as well as blood vessel formation [99].

3.2. Plasminogen Activators (PA)

Plasminogen activators such as tissue-type PA (tPA) and urokinase-type PA (uPA) convert inactive plasminogen to active plasmin, and are often used for clot lysis in the clinic as an exogenous source in the ischemic brain, however, in addition to clot lysis, PAs can degrade components of the basal lamina and participate in ECM remodelling [100,101]. A direct action of tPA on BBB opening is seen after tPA administration into CSF, which produces a rapid dose-dependent increase in vascular permeability [102]. Moreover, tPA may enhance BBB breakdown caused by MMPs [100,103], indeed inhibition of tPA activity in knockout mice or by inhibitors, blocks MMP-9 up-regulation after focal cerebral ischemia [104]. In clinical settings, the potential hazards of tPA may be offset by the benefits of clot lysis and reperfusion with subsequent clinical improvement [105].

3.3. Vascular Endothelial Growth Factor (VEGF)

VEGF is a vascular endothelial cell mitogen and a major inducer of angiogenesis. VEGF is expressed in the normal adult brain mainly by the CP epithelial cells but also by astrocytes and neurons [106,107]. It is expressed as early as 1-3 hours after focal cerebral ischemia in the rat and peaks after 24-48 h [108], localized primarily in the ischemic core where BBB leakage occurs [109]. VEGF exacerbates degradation of occludin and ZO-1 in vitro [110,111], and the loss of these two proteins increases BBB leakage in human brain [112]. However, delayed administration of VEGF on reperfusion days 1-3 promotes post-ischemic angiogensis and neurogenesis [113]. These diverse activities of VEGF on the nervous system present problems in applying the growth factor as a therapeutic agent for stroke treatment [114,115].

3.4. Ischemia-Reperfusion Injury

Cerebral ischemia treatments aim to re-establish brain perfusion, however this process can exacerbate damage to neurons and vasculture due to the oxygen "surge" and free radical production [116]. ROS are generated soon after vessel occlusion, as well as in later stages of ischemic reperfusion (e.g. by inflammatory cells), and are the fundamental mediators of reperfusion injury [105]. ROS cause cellular injury via peroxidation of cell membrane lipids

[117], and hydrolysis of phospholipids releases arachidonic acid, which causes non-specific opening of the BBB [118,119]. Indeed arachidonic acid alone increases the permeability of single cerebral microvessels [120], and suppression of arachidonic acid release by inhibition of phospholipase A2 decreases brain edema after ischemia [121]. Attenuation of ROS through over-expression of superoxide dismutase (SOD) -1, the major intracellular antioxidant enzyme, in transgenic mice, significantly reduces infarct volume after transient ischemia [122,123], whereas infarction is increased in SOD-1 knock-outs [124] suggesting that SOD plays a protective role [125,126].

3.5. Nitric Oxide (NO)

NO is a reactive nitrogen species (RNS) and ubiquitous intracellular signalling molecule, synthesized from the amino acid L-arginine by the enzyme NO synthase (NOS). NO has beneficial roles in increasing cerebral blood flow (CBF), decreasing platelet aggregation and leukocyte adhesion to the endothelium, and scavenging the free radicals [127]. Large amounts of NO are produced within minutes after MCAO [128]. At high concentration, NO reacts rapidly with superoxide free radical (O_2^-) to produce the cytotoxic oxidant peroxynitrite [129]. Peroxynitrite is thought to uncouple endothelial NOS which then produces further O_2^- [130] and also increases the expression of inflammatory cytokines interleukin 1β (IL-1β) and tumour necrosis factor α (TNF-α), is involved in TNF-α induced BBB opening [131]. In addition, NO mediates disruption of cerebral pial arteries via activation of guanylate cyclase [132], and also regulate MMPs -9 and -13 [133,134]. Nonselective NOS inhibitors reduce brain edema, BBB damage, and infarct size in experimental MCAO [135].

3.6. Inflammation

Inflammatory reaction is a common response of the cerebral parenchyma to various forms of insult. In stroke, the inflammatory reaction starts within hours and persist for days [136]. Ischemic injured tissue releases a number of inflammatory cytokines (e.g. IL-1,6,10, TNF-α, transforming growth factor (TGF)-β) and chemokines (e.g. CXC, CX3C, monocyte chemoattractant protein (MCP)-1), which cause, among other things, adhesion molecule upregulation in the cerebral vasculature and peripheral leukocyte recruitment [137]. Both P-selectin and E-selectin are rapidly secreted [138,139]. The expression of immunoglobulin family of cellular adhesion molecules (ICAM) -1 in ischemic brain increases within hours after stroke onset, peaking at about 12-24 h, and preceding leukocyte infiltration [140-142], which then migrate to the ischemic area [143]. Leukocyte adhesion to the endothelium triggers signal transduction cascades, leading to the loss of the TJ proteins occludin and ZO-1, directly causing BBB disruption [144], and reorganization of the actin cytoskeleton [145].

A number of inflammation mediators are upregulated after ischemic stroke and increase BBB permeability. Bradykinin promotes arteriolar dilatation, and increases endothelial permeability [146], by activating the B_2 receptor [147,148]. Selective inhibition of B_2 receptors significantly reduces post-ischemic brain edema and tissue damage in rats [149,150]. Histamine disrupts BBB and increases single cerebral microvessel permeability by increasing vesicular transport and by paracellular TJ opening [151,152]. Histamine antagonists reduce single cerebral microvessel permeability [153] and brain edema in MCAO rat [154]. In addition, activated neutrophils secrete MMP-9, superoxide, and platelet activating factor (PAF), which increase edema [155], and release glutamate, which may contribute to barrier opening via metabotropic glutamate receptors expressed by endothelial cells [156]. Interestingly, inflammatory responses in the later phases of cerebral ischemia are suggested to be beneficial in brain recovery and repair [137]. Whether inflammation is destructive or beneficial may depend on how severe the ischemia is and the stage of ischemia [137].

4. Brain Edema

The lack of adequate oxygen and energy supply during ischemia leads to depletion of adenosine triphosphate (ATP) and phosphocreatinine with subsequent reduction in ion transporter activity and fall in pH [157]. There is an increase in intracellular Na^+, Cl^-, and Ca^{2+} and a decrease in K^+ with membrane depolarisation (anoxic depolarisation), due to reduced Na^+,K^+-ATPase activity [158]. Increased intracellular Na^+ and Cl^- results in osmotic movement of water [157,159], and this translocation of interstitial water into the intracellular compartment causes cytotoxic edema. This change occurs early when BBB is still intact and does not contribute to a net increase in brain volume since it shifts water from extracellular to intracellular spaces [157]. Astrocyte end-feet swell within 5 minutes when brain cells are subjected to ischemia [160]. Neurons and oligodendrocytes seem to swell later but shrink earlier than astrocytes [161]. The water transporter, aquaporin (AQP) 4 is the most widely expressed aquaporin protein in the brain, predominantly found at the level of astrocytic foot processes adjacent to blood vessels, and has an important role in water transport and in the development of brain edema [162]. Increased AQP4 protein and mRNA expression in the peri-infarcted areas corresponds to the degree of brain edema [163]. In AQP4-deficient mice, there is reduced edema, improved neurological outcome, and decreased infarct size after experimental stroke [164].

Late restoration of blood flow may increase edematous damage by introducing different pathophysiological mechanisms (e.g., increase in ROS and excitatory amino acids, Ca^{++} influx), to further worsen edema [165]. Substances in blood such as ions and serum proteins will enter into the extracellular space of the brain, causing vasogenic edema [157], characterised by fluid movement from vascular to extravascular spaces [166]. Vasogenic edema occurs late while the BBB is disrupted [166] and leads to an expansion of brain volume with a crucial impact on mortality after stroke in that it increases intracranial pressure, favours herniations, and contributes to additional ischemic injuries [167]. Brain edema is a leading cause of death after stroke, especially within the first week after a stroke [168].

5. Intracerebral Hemorrhage (ICH) Conversion

Approximately one third of ischemic stroke will undergoes some degree of hemorrhagic conversion [169]. Brain hemorrhage following reperfusion is particular devastating, where

BBB alterations appear to precede the hemorrhage [170]. ICH expands brain edema and leads to displacement and disruption of brain structures, increases intracranial pressure, induces apoptotic neuronal and glial cell death [171], and is associated with extremely high rates of mortality. The main causes for the conversion are loss of microvascular integrity and disruption of neurovascular homeostasis [172], with MMP-9 mediated BBB disruption is implicated [173]. Hemorrhagic transformation (HT) after MCA occlusion/reperfusion in non-human primates is associated with significantly higher MMP-9 levels in the brain [89], and in stroke patients plasma MMP-9 levels are correlated with HT and with development of thrombolytic-induced hemorrhage [173,174]. ROS may also play a role in the pathogenesis since low plasma levels of the antioxidant ascorbic acid correlate with increased diameter of ICH and severity of clinical impairment [175]. ROS effects are likely to be exacerbated by release of heme iron, which is a neurotoxin at the concentrations observed in ICH [176]. Free iron mediates conversion of hydrogen peroxide to hydroxyl free radicals and lipid hydroperoxides to lipid alkoxyl radicals, so contributing to lipid peroxidation and further expand the radical chain reaction [177].

6. Age-Related BBB Changes

Age-related physiological and molecular degeneration is a consequence of multiple failures of homeostasis caused by complex dysfunction. The stochastic theories of ageing suggest that oxidative stress is an important component [178], affecting a number of vital organs, including the brain. There are several potential sources of ROS in brain, including monoamine oxidase, xanthine oxidase, mitochondrial oxidative phosphorylation, and enzymes involved in NO synthesis and arachidonic acid metabolism [179-181]. The cerebral endothelium in particular is rich in mitochondria [182], and during aging, there is a slow accumulation of mitochondrial DNA mutations [183], which beyond a certain threshold, are associated with decline in respiration and ATP–synthase activity [184,185]. Compared to young rats, the activities of antioxidants superoxide dismutase, glutathione peroxidase and catalase increase in aged rat brain microvessels [186]. In term of enzyme system, Mooradian and Scarpace [187] observed an age-related reduction in isoproterenol-stimulated adenylate cyclase activity of rat cerebral microvessels, however Agrawal et al [188] found either no change in lactate dehydrogenase (LDH) and acetylcholinesterase activities, or age-related increases of alkaline phosphatase (AP) and τ– glutamyl transpeptidase (τ-GT) of rat cerebral microvessels. Other age-related changes include altered lipid and protein composition in microvessel [189-191]. With a significant reduction in cerebral occludin protein but not ZO-1, at mRNA level occludin is not changed although ZO-1 increases, suggesting altered translation or post-translational processing of these products with age [192]. The most consistent changes recorded are thickening of the basement membrane, and thinning of the capillary endothelium [193]. This may be region specific since an endothelial barrier antigen in cerebral capillaries is significantly reduced in hippocampus, but not in the neocortex, of aged rats compared with the adults [194]. In humans, capillary walls, especially in the white matter became thinner with loss of endothelial cytoplasm and pericytes, indicating that the BBB is less able to compensate for transient leaks in elderly people [195]. In healthy ageing subjects, between the 6th and 7th decades, capillary surface area is decreased while capillary diameter, volume and total length increase [196], suggested to be induced by recurrent hypoxic episodes [197]. In aged rats, the response of cerebral arterioles to endogenous dilators such as acetylcholine and bradykinin [198], and β-adrenergic agonists [199] is impaired, resulting in less arteriole compliance. Such age–related degeneration of brain vasculture structure and function may lead to disruption of local perfusion. Modest, 20% reductions in CBF are associated with diminished cerebral protein synthesis [200]. More severe reductions in CBF result in shifts in intracellular pH and water, and accumulation of glutamate and lactate in brain interstitial fluid [201]. CBF reductions greater than 50% impair ATP synthesis and decrease the ability of neurons to fire action potentials [202]. Finally, the severe reductions in CBF (>80%), similar to ischemic stroke, lead to electrolyte imbalance and ischemic neuronal death [202]. Cerebral hypoperfusion may not necessarily cause an ischemic injury, as severe as stroke, but does lead to oligemia with subsequent disruption of the microcirculation, damage to the cerebral endothelium, and breach of BBB integrity [201].

Studies on whether there is gross age-related change in BBB permeability have generated conflicting results. The BBB permeability to the radiolabeled extracellular marker sucrose does not change with age in Fisher 344 rats up to 31 months of age, indicating BBB integrity is maintained with aging [203,204]. BBB permeability to larger molecules, horseradish peroxidase or albumin is not increased in senescent mice [205]. Farrall and Wardlaw [206] have recently systematically reviewed the literature on BBB integrity during ageing focusing on human studies where the CSF / plasma ratio is used as an index for BBB permeability. They found significant increase in the albumin ratio during normal ageing and concluded that BBB permeability increases with normal ageing. However, age-related increase of albumin in CSF may also be caused by age-related slow-down in CSF turn over. In young adult humans, CSF is replaced approximately four times each day [207] while with ageing or disease this may occur only one to two times a day [207,208]. CSF intracranial volume is also larger among elderly people [209], which would contribute to the slower replacement of CSF each day. Slower turn over will encourage build-up of molecules or metabolites that rely on CSF drainage for removal, some of which are of plasma origin such as albumin [210], and this needs to be quantified before CSF:plasma albumin ratio can be used to indicate barrier dysfunction for any individual. In addition, albumin is taken up via BBB receptor – mediated routes, such as TGF β receptor [211]. Since the density of endothelial vesicles and numbers of junctional gaps do not significantly change with age and there appears to be no morphological basis for general increased BBB permeability in ageing [193], and the BBB may remain functionally intact during aging under homeostatic conditions [33]. However, BBB may become more susceptible to disruption by external factors with increasing age [212], and indeed older rats show increased vulnerability to haloperidol-induced BBB disruption [213] and higher susceptibility to electroconvulsive shocks [214].

The effect of ageing on BBB transport process has been investigated in a number of studies. The uptake of glucose declines gradually [215], and the Vmax of the transporter is reduced with increasing age [216]. Similar declines are reported for choline [217], butyrate [218], triiodothyronine (T_3) [219], thyroxine (T_4) [220], Tyr-MIF and methionine-enkephalin peptides [221]. Studies on the effect of aging on amino acid transport kinetics are not so consistent. Brain Uptake Index (BUI) for methionine showed biphasic change with age in rats: adult animals had the highest BUI for methionine compared to the young and old animal groups [222], while neither lysine nor glutamic acid showed age-related difference [222]. There are age-related declines of BBB transport parameters for tryptophan in rats [223], and an exponential decline in valine and tyrosine brain uptakes in mice [224]. In humans, O'Tuama et al [225] reported [^{11}C]-L-methionine transport decreased with advancing age, however, Koeppe et al [226] using the synthetic amino acid [^{11}C]-aminocyclohexanecarboxylate demonstrated no significant change with age. Simlarly, Ito et al [227] using ^{18}F-Phe in a dynamic PET study and did not find any age-dependent changes in amino acid transport from the blood to the brain. In addition to carrier-mediated transport of small molecules, receptor-mediated transport of macromolecules into the brain from the blood during ageing has also been studied. There is no significant difference in the kinetics of insulin transport across BBB in senescent mice [228], nor is there any difference in IGF-II transport across BCB [229].

Brain cells, including neurons and glia constantly change to adapt to the environment even in ageing and the cerebral endothelium is no exception [230]. It is conceivable that the BBB may be able to accommodate subtle age-related damage such as degeneration of capillaries or reductions in resting blood flow, which do not obviously result in measurable functional changes under basal conditions. However, it has been suggested that these alterations reduce cerebrovascular reserves and increase the susceptibility of the brain to vascular insufficiency and ischemia injury [231] underlying the increased morbidity and mortality of ischemic stroke and vascular cognitive impairment affecting older individuals [232].

7. Stroke in Old Age

Although the importance of age during stroke is obvious, there are few studies on stroke using aged animals. Debow et al report that from 1990 to 2002, of 138 studies on stroke only two involved the study of older animals [233]. There are probably two main reasons for this; aged animals have higher mortality after brain ischemia and aged animals are more expensive than young. Since 2002 more research on older animals has been carried out to more accurately reflect the clinical situation [234] and several studies have been published evaluating the effect of aging in rodent models of ischemia [31,32,234,235]. A common finding is significantly increased infarction volume is in aged animals [31,234,236,237] increasing from around 135 mm^3 in young adult rats [236,238-241] to 156 mm^3 in 9-month-olds, and 232 mm^3 in the 18-month-olds [234]. The brain regions most significantly affected by animal age are in cortical and striatal areas [31].

Age-dependent impairment in tissue handling of ischemic stress is supported by various lines of evidence. The mean arterial blood pressure rises significantly during MCAO in the young rats, but there's a significant decrease in the aged rats which could contribute to larger infarct volume in the latter [234]. The aged brain is more susceptible to the excitotoxic damage, sensitive to excitotoxic amino acids [242,243], and the release of glutamate increases in the striatum and hippocampus in older rats [244]. Excessive release of glutamate is thought to play a major role in the susceptibility of neurons to ischemia [245] and extracellular concentrations of glutamate increase during ischemic challenge [244]. Interventions to reduce excitotoxic ischemic damage with NMDA receptor antagonists are effective in young-animal [246] but have reduced effect with increasing age [247].As the respiratory chain is impaired leading to increased production of ROS in ageing cells [248,249], impaired cellular energetics and increased availability of ROS might explain part of the link between impaired tolerance to ischemia and aging.

BBB permeability is also increased in old rats after MCAO. Old rats have two-fold greater BBB disruption, more neuronal loss and vacuolation following the disruption compared to young rats [31]. Given considerable cortical atrophy shown in human aging [250-252] as well as aged rats [253,254], this should impact recovery, morbidity and mortality. Aged rats exhibit severe hemiplegia, consistent circling, inability to feed, limb paresis, and poor performance in functional tests [31,234]. Although hemiparesis is also seen in young animals, the young rats are active after MCAO and continued to feed and groom as they had before the procedure [234]. Since aged rats are more severely affected and recovery diminished after cerebral ischemia [255], their functional status after MCAO is very similar to that seen clinically in older patients with stroke [31], who suffer from more permanently severe functional disabilities [256,257].

Mortality in aged animals after cerebral ischemia varies between 20-80% [31,234,236,237]. This reflects the larger biological variations in aged animal and differences between details of the experimental protocols (type of anaesthesia, surgery). Nevertheless, in all these studies the aged animals have higher mortality compared to the young, which is around 10% [31,234,236,237], and this is consistent with clinical observations. Survival and outcome after stroke are highly influenced by age in the clinic [258] with up to half of patients > 70 years old dying within the first 3 months after stroke [259]. The risk of symptomatic intracranial hemorrhage after thrombolysis is higher in patients with more severe stroke and with increased age [260]. The poorer outcome is contributed to by pre-stroke comorbidity, as well as higher stroke severity [234], due to alteration in pathophysiological responses of the aging CNS to severe trauma, rather than to increased incidence of non-neurological complications or subarachnoid hemorrhage [261].

Conclusions

The neurodegenerative responses of the CNS to stroke have been better understood over the last 10 years. Causative factors include a significant role for BBB disruption in the early stages of stroke, study of which could usefully provide new therapeutic targets. However, the reasons for increased vulnerability of the aged brain have only relatively recently been systematically investigated, as the prevalence of stroke in the elderly population has increased. The aim of future research should be to dissect the interaction between stroke and increased age-related CNS compromise to understand why old age imposes this great vulnerability, and allow development of more targeted therapies.

REFERENCES

[1] Seshadri S, Wolf PA: Lifetime risk of stroke and dementia: current concepts, and estimates from the Framingham Study. *Lancet Neurol* 2007, 6:1106-1114.

[2] Luengo-Fernandez R, Leal J, Gray A, Petersen S, Rayner M: Cost of cardiovascular diseases in the United Kingdom. *Heart* 2006, 92:1384-1389.

[3] Luengo-Fernandez R, Gray AM, Rothwell PM: Population-based study of determinants of initial secondary care costs of acute stroke in the United Kingdom. *Stroke* 2006, 37:2579-2587.

[4] Feigin V, Anderson N, Gunn A, Rodgers A, Anderson C: The emerging role of therapeutic hypothermia in acute stroke. *Lancet Neurol* 2003, 2:529.

[5] Astrup J, Siesjo BK, Symon L: Thresholds in cerebral ischemia - the ischemic penumbra. *Stroke* 1981, 12:723-725.

[6] Moustafa RR, Baron JC: Pathophysiology of ischaemic stroke: insights from imaging, and implications for therapy and drug discovery. *Br J Pharmacol* 2007.

[7] Baron JC, von Kummer R, del Zoppo GJ: Treatment of acute ischemic stroke. Challenging the concept of a rigid and universal time window. *Stroke* 1995, 26:2219-2221.

[8] Furlan M, Marchal G, Viader F, Derlon JM, Baron JC: Spontaneous neurological recovery after stroke and the fate of the ischemic penumbra. *Ann Neurol* 1996, 40:216-226.

[9] Baron JC: Perfusion thresholds in human cerebral ischemia: historical perspective and therapeutic implications. *Cerebrovasc Dis* 2001, 11 Suppl 1:2-8.

[10] Zhang LF, Yang J, Hong Z, Yuan GG, Zhou BF, Zhao LC, Huang YN, Chen J, Wu YF: Proportion of different subtypes of stroke in China. *Stroke* 2003, 34:2091-2096.

[11] Thrift AG, Dewey HM, Macdonell RA, McNeil JJ, Donnan GA: Incidence of the major stroke subtypes: initial findings from the North East Melbourne stroke incidence study (NEMESIS). *Stroke* 2001, 32:1732-1738.

[12] Nakase T, Mizuno T, Harada S, Yamada K, Nishimura T, Ozasa K, Watanabe Y, Nagata K: Angiotensinogen gene polymorphism as a risk factor for ischemic stroke. *J Clin Neurosci* 2007, 14:943-947.

[13] Green AR: Pharmacological approaches to acute ischaemic stroke: reperfusion certainly, neuroprotection possibly. *Br J Pharmacol* 2007.

[14] Martinez-Sanchez P, Diez-Tejedor E, Fuentes B, Ortega-Casarrubios MA, Hacke W: Systemic reperfusion therapy in acute ischemic stroke. *Cerebrovasc Dis* 2007, 24 Suppl 1:143-152.

[15] Kwiatkowski TG, Libman RB, Frankel M, Tilley BC, Morgenstern LB, Lu M, Broderick JP, Lewandowski CA, Marler JR, Levine SR, Brott T: Effects of tissue plasminogen activator for acute ischemic stroke at one year. National Institute of Neurological Disorders and Stroke Recombinant Tissue Plasminogen Activator Stroke Study Group. *N Engl J Med* 1999, 340:1781-1787.

[16] Grotta J, Marler J: Intravenous rt-PA: a tenth anniversary reflection. *Surg Neurol* 2007, 68 Suppl 1:S12-16.

[17] Molina CA, Saver JL: Extending reperfusion therapy for acute ischemic stroke: emerging pharmacological, mechanical, and imaging strategies. *Stroke* 2005, 36:2311-2320.

[18] Kaur J, Zhao Z, Klein GM, Lo EH, Buchan AM: The neurotoxicity of tissue plasminogen activator? *J Cereb Blood Flow Metab* 2004, 24:945-963.

[19] Perez de la Ossa N, Davalos A: Neuroprotection in cerebral infarction: the opportunity of new studies. *Cerebrovasc Dis* 2007, 24 Suppl 1:153-156.

[20] O'Collins VE, Macleod MR, Donnan GA, Horky LL, van der Worp BH, Howells DW: 1,026 experimental treatments in acute stroke. *Ann Neurol* 2006, 59:467-477.

[21] Keep RF, Ennis SR, Xiang JM: The Blood - CSF Barrier and Cerebral Ischemia. In *The Blood - Cerebrospinal Fluid Barrier. Volume* 13. Edited by Zheng W, Chodobski A. New York: Taylor and Francis Group; 2005: 345-360

[22] Mabuchi T, Lucero J, Feng A, Koziol JA, del Zoppo GJ: Focal cerebral ischemia preferentially affects neurons distant from their neighboring microvessels. *J Cereb Blood Flow Metab* 2005, 25:257-266.

[23] Kontos CD, Wei EP, Williams JI, Kontos HA, Povlishock JT: Cytochemical detection of superoxide in cerebral inflammation and ischemia in vivo. *Am J Physiol* 1992, 263:H1234-1242.

[24] del Zoppo GJ: Stroke and neurovascular protection. *N Engl J Med* 2006, 354:553-555.

[25] Lampl Y, Sadeh M, Lorberboym M: Prospective evaluation of malignant middle cerebral artery infarction with blood-brain barrier imaging using Tc-99m DTPA SPECT. *Brain Res* 2006, 1113:194-199.

[26] Lorberboym M, Blankenberg FG, Sadeh M, Lampl Y: In vivo imaging of apoptosis in patients with acute stroke: correlation with blood-brain barrier permeability. *Brain Res* 2006, 1103:13-19.

[27] Lo EH, Dalkara T, Moskowitz MA: Mechanisms, challenges and opportunities in stroke. *Nat Rev Neurosci* 2003, 4:399-415.

[28] Abbott NJ, Ronnback L, Hansson E: Astrocyte-endothelial interactions at the blood-brain barrier. *Nat Rev Neurosci* 2006, 7:41-53.

[29] Fagan SC, Hess DC, Hohnadel EJ, Pollock DM, Ergul A: Targets for vascular protection after acute ischemic stroke. *Stroke* 2004, 35:2220-2225.

[30] Tanne D, Yaari S, Goldbourt U: Risk profile and prediction of long-term ischemic stroke mortality: a 21-year follow-up in the Israeli Ischemic Heart Disease (IIHD) Project. *Circulation* 1998, 98:1365-1371.

[31] Dinapoli VA, Huber JD, Houser K, Li X, Rosen CL: Early disruptions of the blood-brain barrier may contribute to exacerbated neuronal damage and prolonged functional recovery following stroke in aged rats. *Neurobiol Aging* 2007.

[32] Jin K, Minami M, Xie L, Sun Y, Mao XO, Wang Y, Simon RP, Greenberg DA: Ischemia-induced neurogenesis is preserved but reduced in the aged rodent brain. *Aging Cell* 2004, 3:373-377.

[33] Mooradian AD: Effect of aging on the blood-brain barrier. *Neurobiol Aging* 1988, 9:31-39.

[34] Fisher M, Albers GW, Donnan GA, Furlan AJ, Grotta JC, Kidwell CS, Sacco RL, Wechsler LR: Enhancing the development and approval of acute stroke therapies: Stroke Therapy Academic Industry roundtable. *Stroke* 2005, 36:1808-1813.

[35] Dejana E: Endothelial cell-cell junctions: happy together. *Nat Rev Mol Cell Biol* 2004, 5:261-270.

[36] Wolburg H, Lippoldt A: Tight junctions of the blood-brain barrier: development, composition and regulation. *Vascul Pharmacol* 2002, 38:323-337.

[37] Hawkins BT, Davis TP: The blood-brain barrier/neurovascular unit in health and disease. *Pharmacol Rev* 2005, 57:173-185.

[38] Kniesel U, Wolburg H: Tight junctions of the blood-brain barrier. *Cell Mol Neurobiol* 2000, 20:57-76.

[39] Furuse M, Fujita K, Hiiragi T, Fujimoto K, Tsukita S: Claudin-1 and -2: novel integral membrane proteins localizing at tight junctions with no sequence similarity to occludin. *J Cell Biol* 1998, 141:1539-1550.

[40] Furuse M, Hirase T, Itoh M, Nagafuchi A, Yonemura S, Tsukita S, Tsukita S: Occludin: a novel integral membrane protein localizing at tight junctions. *J Cell Biol* 1993, 123:1777-1788.

[41] Ando-Akatsuka Y, Saitou M, Hirase T, Kishi M, Sakakibara A, Itoh M, Yonemura S, Furuse M, Tsukita S: Interspecies diversity of the occludin sequence: cDNA cloning of human, mouse, dog, and rat-kangaroo homologues. *J Cell Biol* 1996, 133:43-47.

[42] Martin-Padura I, Lostaglio S, Schneemann M, Williams L, Romano M, Fruscella P, Panzeri C, Stoppacciaro A, Ruco L, Villa A, et al: Junctional adhesion molecule, a novel member of the immunoglobulin superfamily that distributes at intercellular junctions and modulates monocyte transmigration. *J Cell Biol* 1998, 142:117-127.

[43] Stevenson BR, Siliciano JD, Mooseker MS, Goodenough DA: Identification of ZO-1: a high molecular weight polypeptide associated with the tight junction (zonula occludens) in a variety of epithelia. *J Cell Biol* 1986, 103:755-766.

[44] Haskins J, Gu L, Wittchen ES, Hibbard J, Stevenson BR: ZO-3, a novel member of the MAGUK protein family found at the tight junction, interacts with ZO-1 and occludin. *J Cell Biol* 1998, 141:199-208.

[45] Jesaitis LA, Goodenough DA: Molecular characterization and tissue distribution of ZO-2, a tight junction protein homologous to ZO-1 and the Drosophila discs-large tumor suppressor protein. *J Cell Biol* 1994, 124:949-961.

[46] Balda MS, Anderson JM: Two classes of tight junctions are revealed by ZO-1 isoforms. *Am J Physiol* 1993, 264:C918-924.

[47] Citi S, Sabanay H, Kendrick-Jones J, Geiger B: Cingulin: characterization and localization. *J Cell Sci* 1989, 93 (Pt 1):107-122.

[48] Begley DJ, Brightman MW: Structural and functional aspects of the blood-brain barrier. *Prog Drug Res* 2003, 61:39-78.

[49] Wolburg H, Wolburg-Buchholz K, Liebner S, Engelhardt B: Claudin-1, claudin-2 and claudin-11 are present in tight junctions of choroid plexus epithelium of the mouse. *Neurosci Lett* 2001, 307:77-80.

[50] Redzic ZB, Segal MB: The structure of the choroid plexus and the physiology of the choroid plexus epithelium. *Adv Drug Deliv Rev* 2004, 56:1695-1716.

[51] Zeuthen T, Wright EM: Epithelial potassium transport: tracer and electrophysiological studies in choroid plexus. *J Membr Biol* 1981, 60:105-128.

[52] Butt AM, Jones HC, Abbott NJ: Electrical resistance across the blood-brain barrier in anaesthetized rats: a developmental study. *J Physiol* 1990, 429:47-62.

[53] Ohtsuki S, Terasaki T: Contribution of carrier-mediated transport systems to the blood-brain barrier as a supporting and protecting interface for the brain; importance for CNS drug discovery and development. *Pharm Res* 2007, 24:1745-1758.

[54] Pardridge WM: Brain drug development and brain drug targeting. *Pharm Res* 2007, 24:1729-1732.

[55] Zlokovic BV: The blood-brain barrier in health and chronic neurodegenerative disorders. *Neuron* 2008, 57:178-201.

[56] Preston E, Webster J: Differential passage of [14C]sucrose and [3H]inulin across rat blood-brain barrier after cerebral ischemia. *Acta Neuropathol (Berl)* 2002, 103:237-242.

[57] Grillon E, Provent P, Montigon O, Segebarth C, Remy C, Barbier EL: Blood-brain barrier permeability to manganese and to Gd-DOTA in a rat model of transient cerebral ischaemia. *NMR Biomed* 2007.

[58] Gartshore G, Patterson J, Macrae IM: Influence of ischemia and reperfusion on the course of brain tissue swelling and blood-brain barrier permeability in a rodent model of transient focal cerebral ischemia. *Exp Neurol* 1997, 147:353-360.

[59] Harris NG, Gauden V, Fraser PA, Williams SR, Parker GJ: MRI measurement of blood-brain barrier permeability following spontaneous reperfusion in the starch microsphere model of ischemia. *Magn Reson Imaging* 2002, 20:221-230.

[60] Nagaraja TN, Karki K, Ewing JR, Croxen RL, Knight RA: Identification of variations in blood-brain barrier opening after cerebral ischemia by dual contrast-enhanced magnetic resonance imaging and T 1sat measurements. *Stroke* 2008, 39:427-432.

[61] Latour LL, Kang DW, Ezzeddine MA, Chalela JA, Warach S: Early blood-brain barrier disruption in human focal brain ischemia. *Ann Neurol* 2004, 56:468-477.

[62] Kirino T: Delayed neuronal death in the gerbil hippocampus following ischemia. *Brain Res* 1982, 239:57-69.

[63] Pulsinelli WA, Brierley JB, Plum F: Temporal profile of neuronal damage in a model of transient forebrain ischemia. *Ann Neurol* 1982, 11:491-498.

[64] Kuroiwa T, Ting P, Martinez H, Klatzo I: The biphasic opening of the blood-brain barrier to proteins following temporary middle cerebral artery occlusion. *Acta Neuropathol* 1985, 68:122-129.

[65] Preston E, Sutherland G, Finsten A: Three openings of the blood-brain barrier produced by forebrain ischemia in the rat. *Neurosci Lett* 1993, 149:75-78.

[66] Baskaya MK, Rao AM, Dogan A, Donaldson D, Dempsey RJ: The biphasic opening of the blood-brain barrier in the cortex and hippocampus after traumatic brain injury in rats. *Neurosci Lett* 1997, 226:33-36.

[67] Wu XD, Du LN, Wu GC, Cao XD: Effects of electroacupuncture on blood-brain barrier after cerebral ischemia-reperfusion in rat. *Acupunct Electrother Res* 2001, 26:1-9.

[68] Haqqani AS, Nesic M, Preston E, Baumann E, Kelly J, Stanimirovic D: Characterization of vascular protein expression patterns in cerebral

ischemia/reperfusion using laser capture microdissection and ICAT-nanoLC-MS/MS. *Faseb J* 2005, 19:1809-1821.
[69] Witt KA, Mark KS, Sandoval KE, Davis TP: Reoxygenation stress on blood-brain barrier paracellular permeability and edema in the rat. *Microvasc Res* 2008, 75:91-96.
[70] Kettunen MI, Grohn OH, Lukkarinen JA, Vainio P, Silvennoinen MJ, Kauppinen RA: Interrelations of T(1) and diffusion of water in acute cerebral ischemia of the rat. *Magn Reson Med* 2000, 44:833-839.
[71] Barbier EL, Liu L, Grillon E, Payen JF, Lebas JF, Segebarth C, Remy C: Focal brain ischemia in rat: acute changes in brain tissue T1 reflect acute increase in brain tissue water content. *NMR Biomed* 2005, 18:499-506.
[72] Calamante F, Thomas DL, Pell GS, Wiersma J, Turner R: Measuring cerebral blood flow using magnetic resonance imaging techniques. *J Cereb Blood Flow Metab* 1999, 19:701-735.
[73] Kettunen MI, Grohn OH, Silvennoinen MJ, Penttonen M, Kauppinen RA: Effects of intracellular pH, blood, and tissue oxygen tension on T1rho relaxation in rat brain. *Magn Reson Med* 2002, 48:470-477.
[74] Belayev L, Busto R, Zhao W, Ginsberg MD: Quantitative evaluation of blood-brain barrier permeability following middle cerebral artery occlusion in rats. *Brain Res* 1996, 739:88-96.
[75] Preston E, Webster J: A two-hour window for hypothermic modulation of early events that impact delayed opening of the rat blood-brain barrier after ischemia. *Acta Neuropathol* 2004, 108:406-412.
[76] Stamatovic SM, Dimitrijevic OB, Keep RF, Andjelkovic AV: Inflammation and brain edema: new insights into the role of chemokines and their receptors. *Acta Neurochir Suppl* 2006, 96:444-450.
[77] Abbott NJ: Evidence for bulk flow of brain interstitial fluid: significance for physiology and pathology. *Neurochem Int* 2004, 45:545-552.
[78] Krizanac-Bengez L, Mayberg MR, Janigro D: The cerebral vasculature as a therapeutic target for neurological disorders and the role of shear stress in vascular homeostatis and pathophysiology. *Neurol Res* 2004, 26:846-853.
[79] Pardridge WM: Blood-brain barrier drug targeting enables neuroprotection in brain ischemia following delayed intravenous administration of neurotrophins. *Adv Exp Med Biol* 2002, 513:397-430.
[80] Brown RC, Davis TP: Hypoxia/aglycemia alters expression of occludin and actin in brain endothelial cells. *Biochem Biophys Res Commun* 2005, 327:1114-1123.
[81] Brown RC, Davis TP: Calcium modulation of adherens and tight junction function: a potential mechanism for blood-brain barrier disruption after stroke. *Stroke* 2002, 33:1706-1711.
[82] Rosell A, Lo EH: Multiphasic roles for matrix metalloproteinases after stroke. *Curr Opin Pharmacol* 2008, 8:82-89.
[83] Preston E, Foster DO: Evidence for pore-like opening of the blood-brain barrier following forebrain ischemia in rats. *Brain Res* 1997, 761:4-10.

[84] Westergaard E, Go G, Klatzo I, Spatz M: Increased permeability of cerebral vessels to horseradish peroxidase induced by ischemia in Mongolian Gerbils. *Acta Neuropathol* 1976, 35:307-325.

[85] Plateel M, Teissier E, Cecchelli R: Hypoxia dramatically increases the nonspecific transport of blood-borne proteins to the brain. *J Neurochem* 1997, 68:874-877.

[86] Cipolla MJ, Crete R, Vitullo L, Rix RD: Transcellular transport as a mechanism of blood-brain barrier disruption during stroke. *Front Biosci* 2004, 9:777-785.

[87] Malemud CJ: Matrix metalloproteinases (MMPs) in health and disease: an overview. *Front Biosci* 2006, 11:1696-1701.

[88] Gasche Y, Soccal PM, Kanemitsu M, Copin JC: Matrix metalloproteinases and diseases of the central nervous system with a special emphasis on ischemic brain. *Front Biosci* 2006, 11:1289-1301.

[89] Heo JH, Lucero J, Abumiya T, Koziol JA, Copeland BR, del Zoppo GJ: Matrix metalloproteinases increase very early during experimental focal cerebral ischemia. *J Cereb Blood Flow Metab* 1999, 19:624-633.

[90] Chang DI, Hosomi N, Lucero J, Heo JH, Abumiya T, Mazar AP, del Zoppo GJ: Activation systems for latent matrix metalloproteinase-2 are upregulated immediately after focal cerebral ischemia. *J Cereb Blood Flow Metab* 2003, 23:1408-1419.

[91] Romanic AM, White RF, Arleth AJ, Ohlstein EH, Barone FC: Matrix metalloproteinase expression increases after cerebral focal ischemia in rats: inhibition of matrix metalloproteinase-9 reduces infarct size. *Stroke* 1998, 29:1020-1030.

[92] Fujimura M, Gasche Y, Morita-Fujimura Y, Massengale J, Kawase M, Chan PH: Early appearance of activated matrix metalloproteinase-9 and blood-brain barrier disruption in mice after focal cerebral ischemia and reperfusion. *Brain Res* 1999, 842:92-100.

[93] Asahi M, Wang X, Mori T, Sumii T, Jung JC, Moskowitz MA, Fini ME, Lo EH: Effects of matrix metalloproteinase-9 gene knock-out on the proteolysis of blood-brain barrier and white matter components after cerebral ischemia. *J Neurosci* 2001, 21:7724-7732.

[94] Montaner J, Rovira A, Molina CA, Arenillas JF, Ribo M, Chacon P, Monasterio J, Alvarez-Sabin J: Plasmatic level of neuroinflammatory markers predict the extent of diffusion-weighted image lesions in hyperacute stroke. *J Cereb Blood Flow Metab* 2003, 23:1403-1407.

[95] Asahi M, Asahi K, Jung JC, del Zoppo GJ, Fini ME, Lo EH: Role for matrix metalloproteinase 9 after focal cerebral ischemia: effects of gene knockout and enzyme inhibition with BB-94. *J Cereb Blood Flow Metab* 2000, 20:1681-1689.

[96] Rosenberg GA, Estrada EY, Mobashery S: Effect of synthetic matrix metalloproteinase inhibitors on lipopolysaccharide-induced blood-brain barrier opening in rodents: Differences in response based on strains and solvents. *Brain Res* 2007, 1133:186-192.

[97] Zhao BQ, Wang S, Kim HY, Storrie H, Rosen BR, Mooney DJ, Wang X, Lo EH: Role of matrix metalloproteinases in delayed cortical responses after stroke. *Nat Med* 2006, 12:441-445.

[98] Kaczmarek L, Lapinska-Dzwonek J, Szymczak S: Matrix metalloproteinases in the adult brain physiology: a link between c-Fos, AP-1 and remodeling of neuronal connections? *Embo J* 2002, 21:6643-6648.

[99] Pepper MS: Role of the matrix metalloproteinase and plasminogen activator-plasmin systems in angiogenesis. *Arterioscler Thromb Vasc Biol* 2001, 21:1104-1117.
[100] Lo EH, Broderick JP, Moskowitz MA: tPA and proteolysis in the neurovascular unit. *Stroke* 2004, 35:354-356.
[101] Wang J, Tsirka SE: Contribution of extracellular proteolysis and microglia to intracerebral hemorrhage. *Neurocrit Care* 2005, 3:77-85.
[102] Yepes M, Sandkvist M, Moore EG, Bugge TH, Strickland DK, Lawrence DA: Tissue-type plasminogen activator induces opening of the blood-brain barrier via the LDL receptor-related protein. *J Clin Invest* 2003, 112:1533-1540.
[103] Tsuji K, Aoki T, Tejima E, Arai K, Lee SR, Atochin DN, Huang PL, Wang X, Montaner J, Lo EH: Tissue plasminogen activator promotes matrix metalloproteinase-9 upregulation after focal cerebral ischemia. *Stroke* 2005, 36:1954-1959.
[104] Wang X, Lee SR, Arai K, Lee SR, Tsuji K, Rebeck GW, Lo EH: Lipoprotein receptor-mediated induction of matrix metalloproteinase by tissue plasminogen activator. *Nat Med* 2003, 9:1313-1317.
[105] Heo JH, Han SW, Lee SK: Free radicals as triggers of brain edema formation after stroke. *Free Radic Biol Med* 2005, 39:51-70.
[106] Monacci WT, Merrill MJ, Oldfield EH: Expression of vascular permeability factor/vascular endothelial growth factor in normal rat tissues. *Am J Physiol* 1993, 264:C995-1002.
[107] Marti HH, Risau W: Systemic hypoxia changes the organ-specific distribution of vascular endothelial growth factor and its receptors. *Proc Natl Acad Sci U S A* 1998, 95:15809-15814.
[108] Croll SD, Wiegand SJ: Vascular growth factors in cerebral ischemia. *Mol Neurobiol* 2001, 23:121-135.
[109] Zhang ZG, Zhang L, Tsang W, Soltanian-Zadeh H, Morris D, Zhang R, Goussev A, Powers C, Yeich T, Chopp M: Correlation of VEGF and angiopoietin expression with disruption of blood-brain barrier and angiogenesis after focal cerebral ischemia. *J Cereb Blood Flow Metab* 2002, 22:379-392.
[110] Antonetti DA, Barber AJ, Hollinger LA, Wolpert EB, Gardner TW: Vascular endothelial growth factor induces rapid phosphorylation of tight junction proteins occludin and zonula occluden 1. A potential mechanism for vascular permeability in diabetic retinopathy and tumors. *J Biol Chem* 1999, 274:23463-23467.
[111] Wang W, Dentler WL, Borchardt RT: VEGF increases BMEC monolayer permeability by affecting occludin expression and tight junction assembly. *Am J Physiol Heart Circ Physiol* 2001, 280:H434-440.
[112] Dallasta LM, Pisarov LA, Esplen JE, Werley JV, Moses AV, Nelson JA, Achim CL: Blood-brain barrier tight junction disruption in human immunodeficiency virus-1 encephalitis. *Am J Pathol* 1999, 155:1915-1927.
[113] Sun Y, Jin K, Xie L, Childs J, Mao XO, Logvinova A, Greenberg DA: VEGF-induced neuroprotection, neurogenesis, and angiogenesis after focal cerebral ischemia. *J Clin Invest* 2003, 111:1843-1851.
[114] Carmeliet P, Storkebaum E: Vascular and neuronal effects of VEGF in the nervous system: implications for neurological disorders. *Semin Cell Dev Biol* 2002, 13:39-53.

[115] Zhang Z, Chopp M: Vascular endothelial growth factor and angiopoietins in focal cerebral ischemia. *Trends Cardiovasc Med* 2002, 12:62-66.

[116] Aronowski J, Strong R, Grotta JC: Reperfusion injury: demonstration of brain damage produced by reperfusion after transient focal ischemia in rats. *J Cereb Blood Flow Metab* 1997, 17:1048-1056.

[117] Awasthi D, Church DF, Torbati D, Carey ME, Pryor WA: Oxidative stress following traumatic brain injury in rats. *Surg Neurol* 1997, 47:575-581; discussion 581-572.

[118] Bhakoo KK, Crockard HA, Lascelles PT: Regional studies of changes in brain fatty acids following experimental ischaemia and reperfusion in the gerbil. *J Neurochem* 1984, 43:1025-1031.

[119] Tomimoto H, Shibata M, Ihara M, Akiguchi I, Ohtani R, Budka H: A comparative study on the expression of cyclooxygenase and 5-lipoxygenase during cerebral ischemia in humans. *Acta Neuropathol* 2002, 104:601-607.

[120] Easton AS, Fraser PA: Arachidonic acid increases cerebral microvascular permeability by free radicals in single pial microvessels of the anaesthetized rat. *J Physiol* 1998, 507 (Pt 2):541-547.

[121] Dux E, Ismail M, Szerdahelyi P, Joo F, Dux L, Koltai M, Draskoczy M: Dexamethasone treatment attenuates the development of ischaemic brain oedema in gerbils. *Neuroscience* 1990, 34:203-207.

[122] Kinouchi H, Kamii H, Mikawa S, Epstein CJ, Yoshimoto T, Chan PH: Role of superoxide dismutase in ischemic brain injury: a study using SOD-1 transgenic mice. *Cell Mol Neurobiol* 1998, 18:609-620.

[123] Yang G, Chan PH, Chen J, Carlson E, Chen SF, Weinstein P, Epstein CJ, Kamii H: Human copper-zinc superoxide dismutase transgenic mice are highly resistant to reperfusion injury after focal cerebral ischemia. *Stroke* 1994, 25:165-170.

[124] Fujimura M, Morita-Fujimura Y, Kawase M, Copin JC, Calagui B, Epstein CJ, Chan PH: Manganese superoxide dismutase mediates the early release of mitochondrial cytochrome C and subsequent DNA fragmentation after permanent focal cerebral ischemia in mice. *J Neurosci* 1999, 19:3414-3422.

[125] Chan PH: Role of oxidants in ischemic brain damage. *Stroke* 1996, 27:1124-1129.

[126] Kondo T, Reaume AG, Huang TT, Murakami K, Carlson E, Chen S, Scott RW, Epstein CJ, Chan PH: Edema formation exacerbates neurological and histological outcomes after focal cerebral ischemia in CuZn-superoxide dismutase gene knockout mutant mice. *Acta Neurochir Suppl* 1997, 70:62-64.

[127] Zhang F, White JG, Iadecola C: Nitric oxide donors increase blood flow and reduce brain damage in focal ischemia: evidence that nitric oxide is beneficial in the early stages of cerebral ischemia. *J Cereb Blood Flow Metab* 1994, 14:217-226.

[128] Nagafuji T, Sugiyama M, Matsui T, Muto A, Naito S: Nitric oxide synthase in cerebral ischemia. Possible contribution of nitric oxide synthase activation in brain microvessels to cerebral ischemic injury. *Mol Chem Neuropathol* 1995, 26:107-157.

[129] Laffey JG, Boylan JF, Cheng DC: The systemic inflammatory response to cardiac surgery: implications for the anesthesiologist. *Anesthesiology* 2002, 97:215-252.

[130] Schulz E, Jansen T, Wenzel P, Daiber A, Munzel T: Nitric Oxide, Tetrahydrobiopterin, Oxidative Stress, and Endothelial Dysfunction in Hypertension. *Antioxid Redox Signal* 2008.

[131] Gursoy-Ozdemir Y, Can A, Dalkara T: Reperfusion-induced oxidative/nitrative injury to neurovascular unit after focal cerebral ischemia. *Stroke* 2004, 35:1449-1453.

[132] Chi OZ, Liu X, Weiss HR: Effects of cyclic GMP on microvascular permeability of the cerebral cortex. *Microvasc Res* 1999, 58:35-40.

[133] Marcet-Palacios M, Graham K, Cass C, Befus AD, Mayers I, Radomski MW: Nitric oxide and cyclic GMP increase the expression of matrix metalloproteinase-9 in vascular smooth muscle. *J Pharmacol Exp Ther* 2003, 307:429-436.

[134] Akool el S, Kleinert H, Hamada FM, Abdelwahab MH, Forstermann U, Pfeilschifter J, Eberhardt W: Nitric oxide increases the decay of matrix metalloproteinase 9 mRNA by inhibiting the expression of mRNA-stabilizing factor HuR. *Mol Cell Biol* 2003, 23:4901-4916.

[135] Nagafuji T, Matsui T, Koide T, Asano T: Blockade of nitric oxide formation by N omega-nitro-L-arginine mitigates ischemic brain edema and subsequent cerebral infarction in rats. *Neurosci Lett* 1992, 147:159-162.

[136] Barone FC, Feuerstein GZ: Inflammatory mediators and stroke: new opportunities for novel therapeutics. *J Cereb Blood Flow Metab* 1999, 19:819-834.

[137] Wang Q, Tang XN, Yenari MA: The inflammatory response in stroke. *J Neuroimmunol* 2007, 184:53-68.

[138] Kishimoto TK, Rothlein R: Integrins, ICAMs, and selectins: role and regulation of adhesion molecules in neutrophil recruitment to inflammatory sites. *Adv Pharmacol* 1994, 25:117-169.

[139] Carlos TM, Harlan JM: Leukocyte-endothelial adhesion molecules. *Blood* 1994, 84:2068-2101.

[140] Wang X, Siren AL, Liu Y, Yue TL, Barone FC, Feuerstein GZ: Upregulation of intercellular adhesion molecule 1 (ICAM-1) on brain microvascular endothelial cells in rat ischemic cortex. *Brain Res Mol Brain Res* 1994, 26:61-68.

[141] Wang X, Feuerstein GZ: Induced expression of adhesion molecules following focal brain ischemia. *J Neurotrauma* 1995, 12:825-832.

[142] Zhang RL, Chopp M, Zaloga C, Zhang ZG, Jiang N, Gautam SC, Tang WX, Tsang W, Anderson DC, Manning AM: The temporal profiles of ICAM-1 protein and mRNA expression after transient MCA occlusion in the rat. *Brain Res* 1995, 682:182-188.

[143] Beck J, Stummer W, Lehmberg J, Baethmann A, Uhl E: Activation of leukocyte-endothelial interactions and reduction of selective neuronal death after global cerebral ischemia. *Neurosci Lett* 2007, 414:159-164.

[144] Bolton SJ, Anthony DC, Perry VH: Loss of the tight junction proteins occludin and zonula occludens-1 from cerebral vascular endothelium during neutrophil-induced blood-brain barrier breakdown in vivo. *Neuroscience* 1998, 86:1245-1257.

[145] Couraud PO: Infiltration of inflammatory cells through brain endothelium. *Pathol Biol (Paris)* 1998, 46:176-180.

[146] Sarker MH, Hu DE, Fraser PA: Acute effects of bradykinin on cerebral microvascular permeability in the anaesthetized rat. *J Physiol* 2000, 528 Pt 1:177-187.

[147] Kamiya T, Katayama Y, Kashiwagi F, Terashi A: The role of bradykinin in mediating ischemic brain edema in rats. *Stroke* 1993, 24:571-575; discussion 575-576.

[148] Butt AM: Effect of inflammatory agents on electrical resistance across the blood-brain barrier in pial microvessels of anaesthetized rats. *Brain Res* 1995, 696:145-150.

[149] Zausinger S, Lumenta DB, Pruneau D, Schmid-Elsaesser R, Plesnila N, Baethmann A: Effects of LF 16-0687 Ms, a bradykinin B(2) receptor antagonist, on brain edema formation and tissue damage in a rat model of temporary focal cerebral ischemia. *Brain Res* 2002, 950:268-278.

[150] Ding-Zhou L, Margaill I, Palmier B, Pruneau D, Plotkine M, Marchand-Verrecchia C: LF 16-0687 Ms, a bradykinin B2 receptor antagonist, reduces ischemic brain injury in a murine model of transient focal cerebral ischemia. *Br J Pharmacol* 2003, 139:1539-1547.

[151] Dux E, Joo F: Effects of histamine on brain capillaries. Fine structural and immunohistochemical studies after intracarotid infusion. *Exp Brain Res* 1982, 47:252-258.

[152] Schilling L, Wahl M: Opening of the blood-brain barrier during cortical superfusion with histamine. *Brain Res* 1994, 653:289-296.

[153] Sarker MH, Easton AS, Fraser PA: Regulation of cerebral microvascular permeability by histamine in the anaesthetized rat. *J Physiol* 1998, 507 (Pt 3):909-918.

[154] Joo F, Kovacs J, Szerdahelyi P, Temesvari P, Tosaki A: The role of histamine in brain oedema formation. *Acta Neurochir Suppl (Wien)* 1994, 60:76-78.

[155] Maier CM, Hsieh L, Yu F, Bracci P, Chan PH: Matrix metalloproteinase-9 and myeloperoxidase expression: quantitative analysis by antigen immunohistochemistry in a model of transient focal cerebral ischemia. *Stroke* 2004, 35:1169-1174.

[156] Goda H, Ooboshi H, Nakane H, Ibayashi S, Sadoshima S, Fujishima M: Modulation of ischemia-evoked release of excitatory and inhibitory amino acids by adenosine A1 receptor agonist. *Eur J Pharmacol* 1998, 357:149-155.

[157] Simard JM, Kent TA, Chen M, Tarasov KV, Gerzanich V: Brain oedema in focal ischaemia: molecular pathophysiology and theoretical implications. *Lancet Neurol* 2007, 6:258-268.

[158] Lee JM, Grabb MC, Zipfel GJ, Choi DW: Brain tissue responses to ischemia. *J Clin Invest* 2000, 106:723-731.

[159] Ayata C, Ropper AH: Ischaemic brain oedema. *J Clin Neurosci* 2002, 9:113-124.

[160] Dodson RF, Chu LW, Welch KM, Achar VS: Acute tissue response to cerebral ischemia in the gerbil. An ultrastructural study. *J Neurol Sci* 1977, 33:161-170.

[161] Garcia JH, Liu KF, Ho KL: Neuronal necrosis after middle cerebral artery occlusion in Wistar rats progresses at different time intervals in the caudoputamen and the cortex. *Stroke* 1995, 26:636-642; discussion 643.

[162] Badaut J, Hirt L, Granziera C, Bogousslavsky J, Magistretti PJ, Regli L: Astrocyte-specific expression of aquaporin-9 in mouse brain is increased after transient focal cerebral ischemia. *J Cereb Blood Flow Metab* 2001, 21:477-482.

[163] Ribeiro Mde C, Hirt L, Bogousslavsky J, Regli L, Badaut J: Time course of aquaporin expression after transient focal cerebral ischemia in mice. *J Neurosci Res* 2006, 83:1231-1240.

[164] Manley GT, Fujimura M, Ma T, Noshita N, Filiz F, Bollen AW, Chan P, Verkman AS: Aquaporin-4 deletion in mice reduces brain edema after acute water intoxication and ischemic stroke. *Nat Med* 2000, 6:159-163.

[165] Schaller B, Graf R: Cerebral ischemia and reperfusion: the pathophysiologic concept as a basis for clinical therapy. *J Cereb Blood Flow Metab* 2004, 24:351-371.

[166] Rosenberg GA, Yang Y: Vasogenic edema due to tight junction disruption by matrix metalloproteinases in cerebral ischemia. *Neurosurg Focus* 2007, 22:E4.

[167] Klatzo I: Brain oedema following brain ischaemia and the influence of therapy. *Br J Anaesth* 1985, 57:18-22.

[168] Hacke W, Schwab S, Horn M, Spranger M, De Georgia M, von Kummer R: 'Malignant' middle cerebral artery territory infarction: clinical course and prognostic signs. *Arch Neurol* 1996, 53:309-315.

[169] Lyden PD, Zivin JA: Hemorrhagic transformation after cerebral ischemia: mechanisms and incidence. *Cerebrovasc Brain Metab Rev* 1993, 5:1-16.

[170] del Zoppo GJ, von Kummer R, Hamann GF: Ischaemic damage of brain microvessels: inherent risks for thrombolytic treatment in stroke. *J Neurol Neurosurg Psychiatry* 1998, 65:1-9.

[171] Felberg RA, Grotta JC, Shirzadi AL, Strong R, Narayana P, Hill-Felberg SJ, Aronowski J: Cell death in experimental intracerebral hemorrhage: the "black hole" model of hemorrhagic damage. *Ann Neurol* 2002, 51:517-524.

[172] Wang X, Lo EH: Triggers and mediators of hemorrhagic transformation in cerebral ischemia. *Mol Neurobiol* 2003, 28:229-244.

[173] Montaner J, Molina CA, Monasterio J, Abilleira S, Arenillas JF, Ribo M, Quintana M, Alvarez-Sabin J: Matrix metalloproteinase-9 pretreatment level predicts intracranial hemorrhagic complications after thrombolysis in human stroke. *Circulation* 2003, 107:598-603.

[174] Heo JH, Kim SH, Lee KY, Kim EH, Chu CK, Nam JM: Increase in plasma matrix metalloproteinase-9 in acute stroke patients with thrombolysis failure. *Stroke* 2003, 34:e48-50.

[175] Polidori MC, Mecocci P, Frei B: Plasma vitamin C levels are decreased and correlated with brain damage in patients with intracranial hemorrhage or head trauma. *Stroke* 2001, 32:898-902.

[176] Goldstein L, Teng ZP, Zeserson E, Patel M, Regan RF: Hemin induces an iron-dependent, oxidative injury to human neuron-like cells. *J Neurosci Res* 2003, 73:113-121.

[177] Braughler JM, Hall ED: Involvement of lipid peroxidation in CNS injury. *J Neurotrauma* 1992, 9 Suppl 1:S1-7.

[178] Bokov A, Chaudhuri A, Richardson A: The role of oxidative damage and stress in aging. *Mech Ageing Dev* 2004, 125:811-826.

[179] Droge W: Free radicals in the physiological control of cell function. *Physiol Rev* 2002, 82:47-95.

[180] Kishida KT, Klann E: Sources and targets of reactive oxygen species in synaptic plasticity and memory. *Antioxid Redox Signal* 2007, 9:233-244.

[181] Valko M, Leibfritz D, Moncol J, Cronin MT, Mazur M, Telser J: Free radicals and antioxidants in normal physiological functions and human disease. *Int J Biochem Cell Biol* 2007, 39:44-84.

[182] Oldendorf W: Other likely BBB functions possibly related to aging. *Neurobiol Aging* 1988, 9:52.

[183] Simonetti S, Chen X, DiMauro S, Schon EA: Accumulation of deletions in human mitochondrial DNA during normal aging: analysis by quantitative PCR. *Biochim Biophys Acta* 1992, 1180:113-122.

[184] Cardellach F, Galofre J, Cusso R, Urbano-Marquez A: Decline in skeletal muscle mitochondrial respiration chain function with ageing. *Lancet* 1989, 2:44-45.

[185] Guerrieri F, Capozza G, Kalous M, Papa S: Age-related changes of mitochondrial F0F1 ATP synthase. *Ann N Y Acad Sci* 1992, 671:395-402.

[186] Minn A, Ghersi-Egea JF, Perrin R, Leininger B, Siest G: Drug metabolizing enzymes in the brain and cerebral microvessels. *Brain Res Brain Res Rev* 1991, 16:65-82.

[187] Mooradian AD, Scarpace PJ: The response to isoproterenol-stimulated adenylate cyclase activity after administration of L-triiodothyronine is reduced in aged rats. *Horm Metab Res* 1989, 21:638-639.

[188] Agrawal A, Shukla R, Tripathi LM, Pandey VC, Srimal RC: Permeability function related to cerebral microvessel enzymes during ageing in rats. *Int J Dev Neurosci* 1996, 14:87-91.

[189] Mooradian AD, Meredith KE: The effect of age on protein composition of rat cerebral microvessels. *Neurochem Res* 1992, 17:665-670.

[190] Mooradian AD, Uko-eninn A: Age-related changes in the antioxidative potential of cerebral microvessels. *Brain Res* 1995, 671:159-163.

[191] Mooradian AD, Smith TL: The effect of experimentally induced diabetes mellitus on the lipid order and composition of rat cerebral microvessels. *Neurosci Lett* 1992, 145:145-148.

[192] Mooradian AD, Haas MJ, Chehade JM: Age-related changes in rat cerebral occludin and zonula occludens-1 (ZO-1). *Mech Ageing Dev* 2003, 124:143-146.

[193] Kalaria RN: Cerebral vessels in ageing and Alzheimer's disease. *Pharmacol Ther* 1996, 72:193-214.

[194] Mooradian AD, Grabau G, Uko-eninn A: In situ quantitative estimates of the age-related and diabetes-related changes in cerebral endothelial barrier antigen. *Brain Res* 1993, 609:41-44.

[195] Stewart PA, Hayakawa K, Farrell CL, Del Maestro RF: Quantitative study of microvessel ultrastructure in human peritumoral brain tissue. Evidence for a blood-brain barrier defect. *J Neurosurg* 1987, 67:697-705.

[196] Hunziker O, Abdel'Al S, Schulz U: The aging human cerebral cortex: a stereological characterization of changes in the capillary net. *J Gerontol* 1979, 34:345-350.

[197] Cervos-Navarro J, Gertz HJ, Frydl V: Cerebral blood vessel changes in old people. *Mech Ageing Dev* 1987, 39:223-231.

[198] Mayhan WG, Faraci FM, Baumbach GL, Heistad DD: Effects of aging on responses of cerebral arterioles. *Am J Physiol* 1990, 258:H1138-1143.

[199] Mooradian AD: Potential mechanisms of the age-related changes in the blood-brain barrier. *Neurobiol Aging* 1994, 15:751-755; discussion 761-752, 767.

[200] Hossmann KA: Viability thresholds and the penumbra of focal ischemia. *Ann Neurol* 1994, 36:557-565.

[201] Drake CT, Iadecola C: The role of neuronal signaling in controlling cerebral blood flow. *Brain Lang* 2007, 102:141-152.

[202] Stoquart-ElSankari S, Baledent O, Gondry-Jouet C, Makki M, Godefroy O, Meyer ME: Aging effects on cerebral blood and cerebrospinal fluid flows. *J Cereb Blood Flow Metab* 2007, 27:1563-1572.

[203] Rapoport SI, Ohno K, Pettigrew KD: Blood-brain barrier permeability in senescent rats. *J Gerontol* 1979, 34:162-169.

[204] Wadhwani KC, Koistinaho J, Balbo A, Rapoport SI: Blood-nerve and blood-brain barrier permeabilities and nerve vascular space in Fischer-344 rats of different ages. *Mech Ageing Dev* 1991, 58:177-190.

[205] Rudick RA, Buell SJ: Integrity of blood-brain barrier to peroxidase in senescent mice. *Neurobiol Aging* 1983, 4:283-287.

[206] Farrall AJ, Wardlaw JM: Blood-brain barrier: Ageing and microvascular disease - systematic review and meta-analysis. *Neurobiol Aging* 2007.

[207] Silverberg GD, Mayo M, Saul T, Rubenstein E, McGuire D: Alzheimer's disease, normal-pressure hydrocephalus, and senescent changes in CSF circulatory physiology: a hypothesis. *Lancet Neurol* 2003, 2:506-511.

[208] Rubenstein E: Relationship of senescence of cerebrospinal fluid circulatory system to dementias of the aged. *Lancet* 1998, 351:283-285.

[209] Courchesne E, Chisum HJ, Townsend J, Cowles A, Covington J, Egaas B, Harwood M, Hinds S, Press GA: Normal brain development and aging: quantitative analysis at in vivo MR imaging in healthy volunteers. *Radiology* 2000, 216:672-682.

[210] Preston J, Wilson M, Chen R: Aging of the choroid plexus and CSF system: implications for neurodegeneration. In *The blood-cerebrospinal fluid barrier. Volume* 14. Edited by Zheng W, Chodobski A. New York: Taylor and Francis Group; 2005: 361-376

[211] Ivens S, Kaufer D, Flores LP, Bechmann I, Zumsteg D, Tomkins O, Seiffert E, Heinemann U, Friedman A: TGF-beta receptor-mediated albumin uptake into astrocytes is involved in neocortical epileptogenesis. *Brain* 2007, 130:535-547.

[212] Shah GN, Mooradian AD: Age-related changes in the blood-brain barrier. *Exp Gerontol* 1997, 32:501-519.

[213] Saija A, Princi P, Imperatore C, De Pasquale R, Costa G: Ageing influences haloperidol-induced changes in the permeability of the blood-brain barrier in the rat. *J Pharm Pharmacol* 1992, 44:450-452.

[214] Oztas B, Kaya M, Camurcu S: Age related changes in the effect of electroconvulsive shock on the blood brain barrier permeability in rats. *Mech Ageing Dev* 1990, 51:149-155.

[215] Daniel PM, Love ER, Pratt OE: The effect of age upon the influx of glucose into the brain. *J Physiol* 1978, 274:141-148.

[216] Mooradian AD, Morin AM, Cipp LJ, Haspel HC: Glucose transport is reduced in the blood-brain barrier of aged rats. *Brain Res* 1991, 551:145-149.
[217] Mooradian AD: Blood-brain barrier transport of choline is reduced in the aged rat. *Brain Res* 1988, 440:328-332.
[218] Mooradian AD: Metabolic fuel and amino acid transport into the brain in experimental hypothyroidism. *Acta Endocrinol (Copenh)* 1990, 122:156-162.
[219] Mooradian AD: Blood-brain transport of triiodothyronine is reduced in aged rats. *Mech Ageing Dev* 1990, 52:141-147.
[220] Chen RL, Athauda SB, Kassem NA, Zhang Y, Segal MB, Preston JE: Decrease of transthyretin synthesis at the blood-cerebrospinal fluid barrier of old sheep. *J Gerontol A Biol Sci Med Sci* 2005, 60:852-858.
[221] Banks WA, Kastin AJ: Aging and the blood-brain barrier: changes in the carrier-mediated transport of peptides in rats. *Neurosci Lett* 1985, 61:171-175.
[222] Bubna-Littitz H: [Age-related changes in the blood-brain barrier in the rat with reference to methionine, lysine, glutamic acid and N-methyl-N-nitrosourea]. *Z Gerontol* 1988, 21:93-101.
[223] Tang JP, Melethil S: Effect of aging on the kinetics of blood-brain barrier uptake of tryptophan in rats. *Pharm Res* 1995, 12:1085-1091.
[224] Samuels S, Fish I, Schwartz SA, Hochgeschwender U: Age related changes in blood-to-brain amino acid transport and incorporation into brain protein. *Neurochem Res* 1983, 8:167-177.
[225] O'Tuama LA, Phillips PC, Smith QR, Uno Y, Dannals RF, Wilson AA, Ravert HT, Loats S, Loats HA, Wagner HN, Jr.: L-methionine uptake by human cerebral cortex: maturation from infancy to old age. *J Nucl Med* 1991, 32:16-22.
[226] Koeppe RA, Mangner T, Betz AL, Shulkin BL, Allen R, Kollros P, Kuhl DE, Agranoff BW: Use of [11C]aminocyclohexanecarboxylate for the measurement of amino acid uptake and distribution volume in human brain. *J Cereb Blood Flow Metab* 1990, 10:727-739.
[227] Ito H, Hatazawa J, Murakami M, Miura S, Iida H, Bloomfield PM, Kanno I, Fukuda H, Uemura K: Aging effect on neutral amino acid transport at the blood-brain barrier measured with L-[2-18F]-fluorophenylalanine and PET. *J Nucl Med* 1995, 36:1232-1237.
[228] Banks WA, Farr SA, Morley JE: Permeability of the blood-brain barrier to albumin and insulin in the young and aged SAMP8 mouse. *J Gerontol A Biol Sci Med Sci* 2000, 55:B601-606.
[229] Chen RL, Kassem NA, Sadeghi M, Preston JE: Insulin-like growth factor-II uptake into choroid plexus and brain of young and old sheep. *J Gerontol A Biol Sci Med Sci* 2008, 63A:141-148.
[230] Black JE, Polinsky M, Greenough WT: Progressive failure of cerebral angiogenesis supporting neural plasticity in aging rats. *Neurobiol Aging* 1989, 10:353-358.
[231] Farkas E, Luiten PG: Cerebral microvascular pathology in aging and Alzheimer's disease. *Prog Neurobiol* 2001, 64:575-611.
[232] Rothwell PM: Is there a link between carotid artery stiffness and risk of cerebrovascular events? *Nat Clin Pract Cardiovasc Med* 2005, 2:78-79.

[233] DeBow SB, Clark DL, MacLellan CL, Colbourne F: Incomplete assessment of experimental cytoprotectants in rodent ischemia studies. *Can J Neurol Sci* 2003, 30:368-374.

[234] Rosen CL, Dinapoli VA, Nagamine T, Crocco T: Influence of age on stroke outcome following transient focal ischemia. *J Neurosurg* 2005, 103:687-694.

[235] Shapira S, Sapir M, Wengier A, Grauer E, Kadar T: Aging has a complex effect on a rat model of ischemic stroke. *Brain Res* 2002, 925:148-158.

[236] Sutherland GR, Dix GA, Auer RN: Effect of age in rodent models of focal and forebrain ischemia. *Stroke* 1996, 27:1663-1667; discussion 1668.

[237] Kharlamov A, Kharlamov E, Armstrong DM: Age-dependent increase in infarct volume following photochemically induced cerebral infarction: putative role of astroglia. *J Gerontol A Biol Sci Med Sci* 2000, 55:B135-141; discussion B142-133.

[238] McCullough LD, Blizzard K, Simpson ER, Oz OK, Hurn PD: Aromatase cytochrome P450 and extragonadal estrogen play a role in ischemic neuroprotection. *J Neurosci* 2003, 23:8701-8705.

[239] Alkayed NJ, Harukuni I, Kimes AS, London ED, Traystman RJ, Hurn PD: Gender-linked brain injury in experimental stroke. *Stroke* 1998, 29:159-165; discussion 166.

[240] Yang YL, Pan WH, Chiu TH, Lin MT: Striatal glutamate release is important for development of ischemic damage to striatal neurons during rat heatstroke. *Brain Res* 1998, 795:121-127.

[241] Wang LC, Futrell N, Wang DZ, Chen FJ, Zhai QH, Schultz LR: A reproducible model of middle cerebral infarcts, compatible with long-term survival, in aged rats. *Stroke* 1995, 26:2087-2090.

[242] Wozniak DF, Stewart GR, Miller JP, Olney JW: Age-related sensitivity to kainate neurotoxicity. *Exp Neurol* 1991, 114:250-253.

[243] Wheeler DD, Ondo JG: Time course of the aging of the high affinity L-glutamate transporter in rat cortical synaptosomes. *Exp Gerontol* 1986, 21:159-168.

[244] Dawson R, Jr., Wallace DR, Meldrum MJ: Endogenous glutamate release from frontal cortex of adult and aged rats. *Neurobiol Aging* 1989, 10:665-668.

[245] Rothman S: Synaptic release of excitatory amino acid neurotransmitter mediates anoxic neuronal death. *J Neurosci* 1984, 4:1884-1891.

[246] Bullock R, McCulloch J, Graham DI, Lowe D, Chen MH, Teasdale GM: Focal ischemic damage is reduced by CPP-ene studies in two animal models. *Stroke* 1990, 21:III32-36.

[247] Gonzales RA, Brown LM, Jones TW, Trent RD, Westbrook SL, Leslie SW: N-methyl-D-aspartate mediated responses decrease with age in Fischer 344 rat brain. *Neurobiol Aging* 1991, 12:219-225.

[248] Loschen G, Azzi A: On the formation of hydrogen peroxide and oxygen radicals in heart mitochondria. *Recent Adv Stud Cardiac Struct Metab* 1975, 7:3-12.

[249] Ungvari ZI, Labinskyy N, Gupte SA, Chander PN, Edwards JG, Csiszar A: Dysregulation of mitochondrial biogenesis in vascular endothelial and smooth muscle cells of aged rats. *Am J Physiol Heart Circ Physiol* 2008.

[250] Miller AK, Alston RL, Mountjoy CQ, Corsellis JA: Automated differential cell counting on a sector of the normal human hippocampus: the influence of age. *Neuropathol Appl Neurobiol* 1984, 10:123-141.

[251] Buckner RL: Memory and executive function in aging and AD: multiple factors that cause decline and reserve factors that compensate. *Neuron* 2004, 44:195-208.

[252] Anderson JM, Hubbard BM, Coghill GR, Slidders W: The effect of advanced old age on the neurone content of the cerebral cortex. Observations with an automatic image analyser point counting method. *J Neurol Sci* 1983, 58:235-246.

[253] Knox CA: Effects of aging and chronic arterial hypertension on the cell populations in the neocortex and archicortex of the rat. *Acta Neuropathol* 1982, 56:139-145.

[254] Landfield PW, Braun LD, Pitler TA, Lindsey JD, Lynch G: Hippocampal aging in rats: a morphometric study of multiple variables in semithin sections. *Neurobiol Aging* 1981, 2:265-275.

[255] Andersen MB, Zimmer J, Sams-Dodd F: Specific behavioral effects related to age and cerebral ischemia in rats. *Pharmacol Biochem Behav* 1999, 62:673-682.

[256] Olindo S, Cabre P, Deschamps R, Chatot-Henry C, Rene-Corail P, Fournerie P, Saint-Vil M, May F, Smadja D: Acute stroke in the very elderly: epidemiological features, stroke subtypes, management, and outcome in Martinique, French West Indies. *Stroke* 2003, 34:1593-1597.

[257] Sharma JC, Fletcher S, Vassallo M: Strokes in the elderly - higher acute and 3-month mortality - an explanation. *Cerebrovasc Dis* 1999, 9:2-9.

[258] Di Carlo A, Lamassa M, Pracucci G, Basile AM, Trefoloni G, Vanni P, Wolfe CD, Tilling K, Ebrahim S, Inzitari D: Stroke in the very old : clinical presentation and determinants of 3-month functional outcome: A European perspective. European BIOMED Study of Stroke Care Group. *Stroke* 1999, 30:2313-2319.

[259] Dennis MS, Burn JP, Sandercock PA, Bamford JM, Wade DT, Warlow CP: Long-term survival after first-ever stroke: the Oxfordshire Community Stroke Project. *Stroke* 1993, 24:796-800.

[260] Khatri P, Wechsler LR, Broderick JP: Intracranial hemorrhage associated with revascularization therapies. *Stroke* 2007, 38:431-440.

[261] Vollmer DG, Tormer JC, Jane JA, Sadovnic B, Charlebois D, Eisenberg HM, et a: Age and outcome following traumatic coma: why do older patients fare worse? *J Neurosurg* 1991, 75:S37-S49.

In: The Blood-Brain Barrier
Editor: Tomas R. Helio

ISBN 978-1-60456-894-3

Chapter 4

Blood-Brain Barrier in Ischemic Stroke: A Review

Yair Lampl[1,*] and Mordechai Lorberboym[2]

Departments of [1]Neurology, [2]Nuclear Medicine, Edith Wolfson Medical Center, Holon and Sackler Faculty of Medicine, Tel Aviv University, Israel.

Abstract

Blood-brain barrier (BBB) is a dynamic regulated system which is responsible for selective filtering of substances to and from the brain. This action has important significance in various pathophysiological processes of the central nervous system, including anoxia and stroke. Different animal model studies have demonstrated early disruption of the BBB ischemic cascade onset. Matrix metalloproteinase (MMP), serum proteinase (SP) and free radicals were found to have key roles in the breakdown of the BBB during stroke. It has been shown that MMP and SP have an affect on the early ischemic process of the extracellular matrix around the cerebral vessels and neurons. The reactive oxygen activated the signaling pathways influencing specific enzymes which lead to an ongoing disruption of the BBB during ischemia and anoxia. It has also been shown that VEGI and the proinflammatory cytokines, especially IL1β, TNFα, MCPI and E-selectin are actively involved in the post stroke BBB disruption. Probably neutrophil recruitment, damage of the tight junction system and adherens junction and loss of vital proteins - occludin and zonula occludens and vinculum - act also on this process. Molecular changes in the BBB during ischemia have been researched by application of the genomic and proteomic techniques.

The role of BBB disruption during stroke was less intensely evaluated in humans in vivo. Two main methods, MRI with contrast agent gadolinium-diethylene-triamine-pentaactic acid (Gd-DTPA) and DTPA single protein CT (SPECT), are used for demonstration of the BBB during stroke in patients. The cardinal role of BBB disruption

* Correspondence concerning this article should be addressed to: Yair Lampl, MD, Department of Neurology Edith Wolfson Medical Center, Holon 58100, Israel. Tel: 972 – 3 – 502-8512; Fax: 972 – 3 – 502-8681; Email: y_lampl@hotmail.com.

in humans during stroke has been hypothesized, but not proven. Its role has also been discussed involving small lacunar infarctions, ischemic damage of the white matter and diabetes mellitus patients. Little information is known about the etiology and clinical applications for BBB in the subchronic and chronic stages after stroke. The review will discuss these issues.

INTRODUCTION

Anatomy and Structure

The blood-brain barrier (BBB) is a dynamically regulated diffusion barrier system of the brain. The physiologic and metabolic goal is to regulate the exchange of nutrients, plus both the hydrophilic and lipophilic molecules, and to protect the microenvironment of the barrier from neurotoxic substances. The existence of a barrier between the systemic blood system and the brain had already been noted by Paul Erlich in the early 1900's [1,2]. The finding of the BBB, in relative primitive non-vertebrate life forms, underlies the importance of this system [3,4].

Characteristics of the BBB are its high transendothelial electrical resistance (1500-2000 Ωm^2), which is usually found in the epithelial cells, and the low paracellular permeability [5]. The cerebral vasculature is surrounded by tissue consisting of astrocytes, which have the BBB phenotype [6-8]. The intense interaction between the endothelial cells, other cell types and the extracellular matrix of the brain create one active neurovascular unit system. The endothelial cells of the BBB differ from other endothelial cells by the extensive presence of tight junctions (TJ), in addition to adherens junctions (AJ), and the fenestration of the cells and the presence of the active transport model of a pinocytic vascular system. The narrowness of the time barrier of the paracellular diffusion is dependent upon the amount and characteristics of the TJs. Even though this barrier is constructed as a continuous network, it acts virtually as a series of multiple ones [9,10]. The transport mechanisms include the diffusion-gradient dependent and energy independent systems for small water molecules and lipophilic solutes, the energy-dependent carrier mediated system for glucose and amino acids and the receptor-mediated endocytosis system for large molecules, such as insulin or transferrin [11-15].

The TJ complex is located in a region along the plasma membrane, which contains a high percentage of cholesterol. It included claudin as a major component of its membrane protein. Claudin is made up of at least 24 sub-members [16,17]. The other membrane proteins are occludin [18,19], the junction adhesion molecules (JAM) (which belong to the immunoglobulin subfamily) [20], the cytoplasmic accessory protein, including zonula occludens proteins (Z01, Z02, and Z03), and membrane-associated guanylate kinase-like protein (MAGUK's), AF6 and ZH6 [21]. The plasma membrane is associated with caveolin 1 which is responsible for the regulation of several signal transducing pathways. The adherens junctions are formed by the cadherin proteins and the interconnective protein, catenin.

Signaling Molecules

The signaling pathways may be activated by various systems. Ca^{+2} acts extracellulary and intracellulary to regulate TJ activity. The effect is based on a concurrent decrease of the membranal electrical resistance [22]. Another method of signal transducing is based on the phosphorylation of the transmembranal accessory proteins. The phosphorylation of serine, thyroxine and tyrosine happens on occludin and Z01 [23]. The tyrosine phosphorylation of the protein is done by cell to cell contact [24]. An additional pathway is based on the high sensitivity of the central nervous system (CNS) endothelials to changes in the cAMP level. The major regulating factor of TJ activity is the PKC, including both its isoenzymes - PKCα, and especially, the PKCξ, agouti signaling protein (ASIP) and the G protein group [25]. The PKC is virtually responsible for the physiological maintenance of the TJs. The PKC also regulates cytokines, such as the tumor necrosis factor α (TNFα) and the intercellular adhesion molecule (ICAM-1) via $_{k}$B activity [26]. The G protein fabricates the TJ and regulates its action by GTP-binding protein, especially the Rho subfamily members. The GTP-binding protein itself regulates the paracellular diffusion [27].

Transport of Polypeptides

The physiological patter of transport of poly peptides is a source of significant regarding the changes of BBB in many diverse neurological diseases. The main ways of transport for delivery of poly peptides across the BBB can be isolated and defined. There is the passive-diffuse, the absorptive transcytosis, the receptor-mediated and the carrier-mediated transports. Not all polypeptides have the same ways of delivery. Whereas, the nerve growth factor (NGF), neurotrophins 3 and 4/5 and brain derived neurotrophins (BDNF) have selective transport, mostly by receptor-mediated transcytosis, glial cell-derived neurotrophic factor (GDGF) has no capacity to cross the BBB at all. Other neurotrophic peptides have different ways of behavior. The transport may consist of a saturated solution type of system or even complete blockage of the crossing, as seen with the TGFα or TGFβ_1 type [28-31]. Among the cytokines, the concept of an individual form for each of the peptides is real as well; whereas, interleukin 1 (IL) 1α, IL 1β, and TNF α cross by a saturable transport system. IL 2 delivery is based on a diffuse mechanism, and IL 10 has no specific mechanism to cross the BBB [32,33]. The presence of brain edema dependence on the BBB disruption brings up the question of the role of aquaporin 4 which is responsible for water hemostasis in BBB. While using male stroke prone spontaneous hypertensive rats, a high aquaporin 4 level was found in the astrocytes cells which are located in brain microvessels [34].

Genomic and Proteomic Analyses

The genomic/proteomic laboratory technique included gene microarray, serial analysis of gene (SAGE), and suppression subtraction by hybridization (SSH) methods. This gene expression study method is based on isolation of cerebral microvessel from brain tissue surrounding the vessels. The practical means of demonstration of the microvessels is mostly by mechanical isolation of the capillaries from the brain tissue, although other methods, such as laser capture microdissection and preparation of cultured brain endothelial cells, are also in use. In comparing gene upregulating of the BBB and the SAGE catalization in the animal model and human BBB, some of the proteins were found to some extent in both these models. While other proteins, RGS5 in the signal transduction group, BBB specific anion transporter type 1 (BSAT1) and organic anion transporter polypeptide type 2 (OATP2) in the transport and myelin basic protein group and fms-like tyrosine kinase 1 (FLT1) in the vascular remodeling group, were found in all animal model studies, but not in human SSH analysis. Just the opposite of this was the demonstration of other genes and proteins in humans, but not in rats. To this category belong fibrinogen gamma (FGG1), insulin-like growth factor binding protein 3 (IGFBP3) and tomoregulin as growth factors, and HERC2 and Grb2-associated binder 2 (GAB2) as signal transducers and serglycin as TJ and matrix factors and paraoxonase as a lipid [35].

Using the SSH method, stroke was studied in stroke prone spontaneously hypertensive rats (SHRSP). Downregulation of the G protein signaling regulator and upregulation of sulfonylurea receptor 2B was demonstrated. In an analysis of whole brain stroke tissue by the SSH and KAT methods, 76 overexpressed genes were detected [36]. Other studies showed another profile of upregulation and downregulation of 57 genes [37].

Hypoxia-Reoxygenation (HR)

The hypoxia-reoxygenation stress model is an experimental in vitro yardstick for hypoxic damage and imitates some of the steps in the stroke cascade. The most common tissue model is bovine brain endothelial cells (BBMEC). Human models are based commonly on human fetal tissue. The hypoxia is known to lead to disruption of the TJ and to increase of BBB permeability. Marks et al [38] showed on BBMEC a 2.6-fold increase of sucrose level, a marker of paracellular permeability, after induction of hypoxia, and a dramatic decrease of this effect, up to 50%, in the reoxygenation phase. The actin expression increased up to 2.3-fold. The TJ proteins, occludin, Z01 and Z02 showed a lesser and more ambiguous effect, which disappeared after reoxygenation. The same research group [39] demonstrated also that specific protective media (C6 glioma conditioned media) inhibits the increased expression of claudin1 and actin associated with increase of basic fibroblast growth factor (bFGF) and vascular endothelial growth factor (VEGF). This effect is assumed to be mediated by the transcription factor NF-Kappa B. The effect of NF-Kappa B on the BBB in the H/R model is associated with increased expression of hypoxia inducible factor (HIF) 1α and HIB-1β in the cytoplasm and the nucleus. The location of the increased NF Kappa B p65 expression is in the nucleus and cytoplasm. The expression of NF Kappa B p50 is found only in the nucleus itself [40]. The main mediated substances on the TJ's disruption of the BBB increased permeability by hypoxia are the cytokines, VEGF and nitro oxide (NO). The hypoxic-induced permeability on the BBMEC is diminished by inhibition of the NO synthesis and lowering of NO metabolic levels [41]. The prevention of permeability increase by NO was confirmed by the inhibition effect of NO inhibitor NE monomethyl L arginine [5] and also in relation to endothelial growth factor [42].

Vascular Endothelial Growth Factor (VEGF)

The rationale for the role of VEGF in regulation of BBB permeability was reinforced in various research works. The time-dependent manner effect, as well as the one that induces the VEGF mRNA expression, most probably has protein kinase C (PKC) dependent and independent pathways. These would involve the pathway of phospholipase C gamma, phosphatidylinositol 3-kinase /AKT (PI3/AKT), protein kinase G (PKG) [43] and involving adenosine [44]. The effect of VEGF can be abolished by hypothermia [45] and decreased by steroids [46] and barbiturates [47].

Cytokines

The key effect of cytokines has been well documented as well. In humans, cerebrovmicrovascular endothelial cell tissue after inducing of the HR effect leads to upregulation of IL 1β and to increases of the IL 1β level 2-3 fold [48]. The upregulation of IL 1β is a transient phenomenon which takes a H/R experiment 4-18 hours post reoxygenation. On the same human cells, as well as on human fetal astrocytes, in addition to IL 1β, an increase of IL 8, MCP 1 and upregulation of their mRNA was demonstrated [49]. TNFα, E selectin and ICAM are also upregulated [1], as well as activation of metalloproteinase (MMP) and decrease of tissue inhibitors, TIMP 1 and 2 [50]. Chemokines, especially CCL2, has also been found to have an effect on the permeability of H/R BBB tissue [51].

Evidence of the role of intracellular calcium cascade was shown on the BBMEC tissue model. This effect was visible only after drug treatment and hypoxia and was reversible after treatment with Ca^{+2} channel blockers [52]. The intracellular release of Ca^{+2} followed by activation of the p44/42 MAP kinase was induced also by H_2O_2 [53]. The time profile of BBB disruption and induction of edema seems to be biphasic, reaching its peak 10 min post reoxygenation and 6-18 hours later [54].

BBB in Stroke on the Animal Model

The profile of time dependency of the BBB disruption is dependent upon the animal and the experiment for of the stroke. Most studies were constructed on the transient focal ischemia model with reperfusion. The importance of these studies is based on the impact of the high relevance for an eventual treatment usage in humans, and especially, for finding the optimal therapeutic window which includes thrombolytic treatment.

The ultimate method of demonstration may be histopathological, using mostly horseradish peroxidase (HRP) and Evans blue, in addition to the non-invasive method employing MRI in the various sequences (diffusion-weighted and T1 sequence) with Gd-DTPA as the contrast medium. It has been shown that both methods (HRP and Gd-DTPA MRI) do not reproduce the same results and was hypothesized that the incongruity is based on a difference in the molecule size of the functional tracers [55]. The method of quantitative measurement of the BBB disruption in ischemic animal models is mostly by using the MRI technique and calculating the blood to brain transfer constant (Kic) [56].

The fine points of the conclusions reached regarding the onset of BBB breakdown after initiation of stroke are controversial and might be dependent upon the animal model used.

Since the 1960s and 1970s, the basic assumption already has been that the BBB does not become disturbed directly after ischemia begins. However, in a rat model of transient unilateral carotid occlusion and systemic hypoxia, Petito found an immediate permeability to HRP after one minute, as well as after 30 minutes [57].

BBB and Matrix Metalloproteinases (MMPs)

Pathology of the BBB and Matrix Metalloproteinases (MMPs) in Animal Models

MMPs belong to the gene family of proteolytic enzymes responsible for the breakdown of the extracellular matrix around the cerebral vessels. This essential effect is concentrated on the basement membrane of the brain vasculature. The effect of MMP about its role in the process of BBB disruption was best researched in studies on the BBB, especially those concerning stroke leading to vasogenic edema and hemorrhage.

MMPs are divided into two families - the regular MMPs of which up to 25 members have been discovered and the disintegin metalloproteinases (ADAMs), which have a very significant enzymatic effect. The structure is characterized by a zinc atom which is located on its catalytic site. The MMPs are further categorized into four major subfamilies: (1) MMP1 and MMP8 (collegenases); (2) MMP3, MMP10 and MMP7 (stromelysins and matrilysin); (3) MMP 2 and 72kDa and 92kDa type IV collegenase; and (4) MMP14, MMP26 and other MMPs (membrane type metalloproteinases). MMPs are blocked by four endogenous inhibitors [58,59]. TIMP forms the main complex of the MMP and inhibits the apoptotic pathways. TIMP2 has a biphasic effect on MMP2 – activation at low concentrations and inhibition at higher concentrations. TIMP3 inhibits MMP and MMP7 by inducing cell death by acting on all levels of the cell surfaces' death.TIMP3 acts also by the blockage of the VEGF receptor 2 and the inhibition of angiogenesis [60,61].

Some data is well known about MMPs: (1) each brain cell produces one type of MMP (e.g., astrocytes produce MMP2 and microglias produce MMP9); (2) inflammatory reaction induces the secretion of MMPs; (3) cytokines are involved in the activation of MMP (e.g., NO activates MMP9); and (4) one MMP can activate the other MMPs along the MMP pathways MMP (e.g., MMP3 activates MMP9) [62-65]. The post ischemic breakdown of the BBB by the occlusion/reperfusion mechanism is characterized in a biphasic. The early phase is reversible, mostly associated with MMP2, production of mRNA and increased level of the astrocytic foot process [66,67]. The second late phase, which provides the most severe and long lasting disruption of the BBB, is related to increase of the MMP9. Induction of MMP3 was shown in microglia and neuron mechanisms [68]. MMP is probably associated with induction of the apoptotic pathway [69]. Induction of apoptosis, not in the central nervous system tissue, was shown also in melanoma cells by TIMP 3 [70]. There is also interaction between MMPs and free radicals which activate the MMP thru proMMPs in a direct pathway by its oxidation or nitrosylation [71] and by an indirect pathway via effecting transcription factors. Most of them involved are the $NF_{K}B$ and activator protein 1 (APA) [72,73].

In spontaneously hypertensive rats, the realtime PCR of mRNS was measured for MMP2, MMP9, furin, occludin and claudin 5 – proteins of the TJ. The measurements were performed on the occlusion/reperfusion model of 90 mins / 2, 3, 24 hours. After two hours, there was a decrease of occludin and claudin 5 mRNA expression, after three hours degradation of the TJ proteins, and after 24 hours, increase of the MMT9 level. It seemed that the MMPs act at least partially direct on the TJ by fragmentation of its proteins [74].

BBB and MMPs in Permanent MCA Occlusion Model

In permanent MCA occlusion rat model, the MMP9 expression was observed after 12 hours and reached it maximal level after 24 hours, persisting for 5 days. MMP appeared to be stained with endothelial cells around the infarct core within 24 hours, and after 5 days in the macrophages within the infarction areas. MMP1 and MMP3 were not active [75]. In a mice model, the pro MMP9 expression was found in the infracted area after 2 hours and up to 24 hours. The MMP9 was demonstrated after four hours with a correlative association with degree of the BBB disruption [76].

BBB and MMPs in the Transient Focal Cerebral Ischemic Model/ Ischemic Reperfusion Model

Reperfusion injury is characterized by the presence of biphasic breakdown phases of the BBB. The first phase period is between 2-4 hours in a first stroke, followed by a more extensive disruption period after 24-48 hours. However, there are differences in the profile of the BBB disruption and the MMP9 expression between the mechanical ischemic reperfusion model and the embolic model. In the spontaneous hypertensive rat model, the intensity of MMP9 upregulation and the degree of BBB disruption was much higher after embolic focal ischemia [77]. In the Knockout (KO) mice model of SOD2-KO (manganese superoxide dismutase), a mice model having a high sensitivity to stroke, the MMP9 expression was increased after 6-12 hours, reaching its maximal level after 48-72 hours. The activity was in direct correlation to the BBB breakdown, as demonstrated as by histochemical methods (Evans blue extravasation) [78]. In adult rats after two hours of MCA occlusion and two hours of reperfusion, the first phase of opening was associated with maximal increase of MMP9 and tissue inhibitors to metalloproteinase (TIMI)1. Increase of MMP9 was maximally detected on day 5. After 48 hours, the TIMI level returned to normal [79]. In other studies, MMP9 was detected after four hours and up to four days. It was associated with mild increase of MMP2, at the beginning and maximal activation on day 4 [80]. The role of the protective effect on MMP9 KO mice after transient focal ischemia is probably mediated by the reduction of proteolytic cleavage of BBB and of reduction degradation of the MMP9 substate myelin basic protein (MBP) in the brain white matter [81]. In other SOD2-KO studies, MMP9 expression was also biphasic, with significant high levels 6-12 hours and 48-72 hours post stroke. Dependent upon additional results of the study, the conclusion was that neutrophils are not the primary source of MMP9 proteins [78].

MMP and NO, Cytokines and VEGF

There is no doubt that abnormal expression of MMP has a direct effect on the pathophysiology of the neuroinflammatory processes. In a rate model of two hours occlusion and two hours reperfusion, an increased expression of activity of MMP2 and MMP9 were in association with increase up to 166% of interleukin (IL 1β) [82]. The role of VEGF was emphasized in local cerebral ischemia in rats. The interactive influence of MMP and VEGF was hypothesized by the fact that MMPs reduced endogenous VEGF signal [83]. In a two hour occlusion and three to five hour reperfusion mice model, the role of superoxide, nitrooxide and peroxynitrite was demonstrated. It was found that the location of oxidative stress substances on the microvessel were identical with those of the MMP9 expression [84]. An effect of MMPs was also identified in association with estrogens. In an ischemia-reperfusion model, the effect of 30%-50% reduction of the BBB breakdown was directly in correlation with the expression of MMP2 and MMP9 [85]. The association between MMP9 and leukocytes is controversial. Whereas, some studies on mice implied that neutrophils are most probably not the source of MMP9; other researchers disagreed with this assumption [86].

Protective Preconditioning

Various techniques of conditioning and treatment have been published as protective methods used to reduce the BBB post stroke injury and blockage of MMP9 production. Minocycline [87,88] BB 1101 [87], BB 3103 [89], GM 6001 [82] and hyperbaric oxygen [90] in Wistar Koyoto rats and cyclooxygenase inhibitors 1 and 2 [91], preischemic exercise [92] and treatment of hyperglycemia [93] in Sprague-Dawley rats were shown to have BBB protective effects by inhibition of MMP9. An inhibition of the upregulation of MMP9 and neuroprotective effect has also been shown in calpain and cathepsin inhibitors [94]. This is also been found in inhibitors of tumor necrosis-like weak inducer of apoptosis (TWEAK) [95], extracellular MMP inducers (EMMPRIN) in a permanent stroke model [96] and nimesulid, a NSAIDS, in embolic focal cerebral ischemia [97].

In a study of MM9KO and wild type hypoxic-ischemic mice model, the apoptotic process included the caspase3-dependent and caspase3-independent pathways were examined. Apoptosis did not appear to have a main role in part of the protective effect of the BBB breakdown [98]. However, another study showed that MMP3 and TIMP3 regulated the sensitivity of the BBB to the apoptotic process induced by doxorubicin. The effectiveness of this mechanism is due to the inactivation of Fas, an apoptotic receptor on the cell surface [69].

MMP and Thrombolysis

Thrombolytic therapy using recombinant tissue plasminogen activator (r-tPA) is standard treatment in a time period of three hours for acute stroke. The most common complication is hemorrhagic transformation of the infarction. An association between MMP and the hemorrhagic transformation has been shown. In spontaneously hypertensive rats after induced embolic focal stroke receiving 10mg/Kg r-tPA for six hours and a group receiving MMP inhibitor BB94, an increase of MMP9 level in the treated group was detected. The MMP9 increase was involved in the mechanisms of secondary bleeding [99]. The upregulation of MMP9 is significantly higher in the rat model after the thrombolytic procedure rather than after mechanically induced ischemic injury. The effect of BBB protection breakdown and reduction of the mortality in the male Wistar rats is suggested to be generally induced by MMP's changes [100]. The promoting of MMP9 after focal cerebral infarction followed by r-tPA (10mg/Kg) usage became apparent in comparison between the wild type and tPA Knockout mice [101]. The level of MMP9 is not only directly correlated to the r-tPA treatment dosage, but also to the hemoglobin content [102]. The pathophysiology of the BBB destruction by r-tPA via MMP is at least partially dependent on direct and indirect mechanisms leading to the breakup of the basal membrane in the cerebral microvasculature [103]. The temporal profile of MMP9 activation following treatment with r-tPA was determined in Sprague Dawley focal embolic ischemic model rats. r-tPA was associated with activation of MMP9 at 6,12 and 24 hours following the ischemic procedure. A similar profile of activation was not found in MMP2 [104].

BBB, Nitric Oxide (NO) and Reactive Oxygen Species (ROS)

There is evidence that nitric oxide has a direct effect on the BBB in vivo. An important role of NO is the ability to activate a regeneration process of the BBB in the reperfusion stage via peroxynitrite [105]. Inhibition of the inducible NOS (iNOS) protects the post stroke BBB and minimizes the BBB damage. Administration of selective NOS inhibitors, such as ARL 17477, provide neuroprotective effects in animal global and focal brain ischemia via stabilization of the BBB [106]. This effect also seems to be characteristic of curcumin [107] and scutellarin [108]. In the filament occlusion technique of the MCA in NADPH oxidase KO and in wild-type mice for two hours following reperfusion, breakdown of the BBB was mediated by activation of Rac1 and gp91 phox containing NADPH oxidase. The disturbance of the BBB was caused via formation of reactive oxygen species and Rho kinase-induced cell contraction [109].

BBB and VEGF

Increase of VEGF expression has been shown to have a negative effect on the integrity of the BBB. In transient MCA occlusion in mice, VEGF overexpression improved neurological deficits and reduced caspase 3 activity. On the other hand, VEGF overexpression induced blood-brain barrier leakage, mostly not associated with brain swelling vivo [110]. the VEGF effect on the integrity of the BBB may be blocked not only by direct inhibition of VEGF, but also indirectly, i.e., by inhibition of the integrin alfa beta 3 [111,112]. In an embolic stroke rat model two to four hours post occlusion, an increase of VEGF mRNA and decrease of angiopoietin 1 (Ang1), in the core of the stroke, and VEGF/VEGF-receptor and Ang/Tie 2 increase, in the surrounding peripheral infarct, was documented. The VEGF and Ang1 had direct influence on the breakdown of the BBB in the various infarct regimens [113]. The expression of VEGF receptor 2 is significantly reduced three days after erythropoientin treatment. The protective impact of erythropoientin and the promotion of angiogenesis, vascular stabilization and decrease of the BBB leakage seems, at least, partially dependent upon down regulation of fetal liver kinase receptor=VEGFR2 (Flk1) and VEGF down regulation of Flk1 expression and response to VEGF signaling [114]. Reduction of the BBB leakage after stroke was seen to be induced by Ang1 in the mice occlusion and to be associated with the final infarct's volume [115]. The impact of Ang1, Tie1, VEGF and FLK1 in stabilization of the damaged BBB was demonstrated also after the treatment with marrow stromal cells in male Wistar rats [116].

BBB and Endothelin1 (ET-1)

In the administration of Endothelin1 (ET-1) in various dosages 40 minutes after 40 minutes of MCA occlusion in the rat, the transfer coefficient of BBB after infarction was reduced. The effect is dose dependent [117].

BBB and Brain Derived Neurotrophic Factor (BDNF)

Studies on animal models showed that BDNF has a protective effect on the BBB post stroke lasting for at least seven days [118].

Acute Stroke in Humans

The presence of BBB disturbance during acute stroke was demonstrated by calculation of the results of total CSF protein and CSF/serum albumin ratio. Based on these laboratory methods, it was shown that 50% of the ischemic cerebral patients had a barrier disturbance, but without correlation to the enhancement on computed tomography (CT scan). [119,120]. Another study from the same research group found on a supratentorial stroke patient group that a late CT enhancement after two-three weeks was unrelated to infarction volume or to the BBB breakdown. CT enhancement in the first week was associated with large infarction and severe BBB disturbance. The peak time was the third day, and it persisted for several weeks [121]. Using the contrast infusion of meglumine amidotrizoate, CT scan demonstrated a breakdown of the BBB as an early event after stroke, even after only three hours [122]. A non-invasive marker of BBB function, including during ischemic stroke, is the serum S100B [123-125]. It is also used as a parameter for the damage of cerebral tissue, including after thrombolytic therapy [126]. Its usefulness is due to the release of astroglial proteins into the CSF, dependent upon the amount of BBB disruption. In the later stroke stages, it reflects the damage of astroglial cells in the penumbra area. Another parameter for BBB disruption in stroke is the β trace protein level [127]. The efficacy of MRI for evaluation of BBB disruption is dependent upon the technique of imaging [128-131]. Single photon emission computed tomography (SPECT) with (99m)Tc-diethylenetriaminepentaacetic acid (99m)Tc-DTPA showed a correlation between degree of blood brain disruption and clinical outcome with a cutoff threshold (2.5) reflecting a non linear correlation between degree of BBB breakdown and clinical outcome [132]. Using radiolabeled annexin V in the comparison between apoptotic brain lesion and BBB breakdown in acute stroke, no correlation regarding location was found [133].

Subacute and Chronic Stroke in Humans

Less is know about the behavior of BBB in human stroke in the subacute (hours to days) and chronic stroke (days to months), especially regarding condition of the BBB in the very late period post stroke. Cordes et al used single photon emission computed tomography (SPECT) for regional cerebral blood flow (rCBF) and regional cerebral blood volume (rCBV) examination. Using 23 patients – 19 with subacute and 7 with chronic infarction. The data was compared with MR findings. In the subacute stage, there was increased rCBV with either increased or decreased rCBF. In the chronic cases, rCBV and rCBF were decreased without contrast lubricant or MR [134]. Marks et al [135] investigated spin-echo (SE) motion correction sequence using diffusion-weighted (DW) MR in 29 patients. They found that the apparent diffusion coefficients (ADC) which were low among the acute stroke victims were supranormal in the chronic stroke ones in comparison with normal controls. Lorberboym et al found that the degree of BBB breakdown in the acute stage may suggest the clinical outcome in the late phase [132]. However, there is no data about the exact changes of the BBB with time in the chronic phase or information regarding individual characteristics and factors which may influence them. There is data which shows that in lacunar infarction and in persistence of white matter damage (ischemic leukoaraiosis), there are chronic endothelial and BBB dysfunctions. Correlation with dementia and age was assumed. The results of studies on this subject were mostly based on cerebrospinal fluid analysis of the albumin, IgG ratio and IgG index parameters compatible with intact function of the BBB [136-138].

BBB and Stroke Hemorrhage Transformation

Hemorrhagic transformation (HT) is a common complication following insults on the BBB. It is more frequent in embolic stroke and is mostly identified two to seven days (commonly three to five days) after stroke. Its critical importance is in its ability to limit revascularization therapy. Most studies underlie the fact that early breakdown of BBB is immeasurably associated with HT. Separate experimental rat and mouse models showed the relationship between early BBB disruption and HT, plus the association with diabetes mellitus [139]. Human data confirmed this conclusion by using diffusion-weighted imaging, T2 permeability magnetic resonance and another novel MRI imaging marker permeability technique [140-143], as well as with the computed tomography technique [144]. Various drugs, such as melatonin, inhibit the early effects of BBB disruption and protect against HT [145].

A highly clinical relevance of the early detection of BBB for forewarning from HT is present when tPA is used for early recanalization of the occluded artery. The rationale for the HT effect on the BBB can be due to its role as an extracellular protease and signaling substance in the brain, plus its mediation of matrix remodeling. The effects are unrelated to the therapeutic clot lysis mechanism, and further rationale for this can be due to interaction with the NMDA receptor, increase of calcium content, activation of the apoptotic pathway and direction action on the MMP.

The relationship of HT in rtPA and BBB was studied in the embolic rat model, as well as in the non embolic stroke model. In the embolic model, not only was an association between BBB and HT seen [146], but it was shown that on MRI Gd DTPA imaging, the breakdown of the BBB was the only MR parameter to anticipate HT [147]. With the use of monocrystalline iron oxide nanocolloids (MION) in a novel MRI method, which reflects the functioning of the BBB, it was shown that the thrombolytic treatment does not improve perfusion in the HT area [148]. However, other studies showed no direct correlation between HT and time, intensity and region of infarction [149]. MMP, especially MMP9, may play a key role in the association between tPA treatment and HT BBB breakdown [150]. The correlation between BBB disturbance, HT and clinical outcome was documented also on humans with and without association with the MMP using the MRI imaging technique [151-152].

BBB and Vascular Risk Factors

Diabetes Mellitus, BBB and Stroke

Diabetes mellitus (DM) is a risk factor for disturbance of the normal function of the BBB [153,154]. In a recent study, streptozotocin-induced DM rats have an increased permeability to small molecules and decreased occludin and Z01 content during the 14 days of the study [155,156]. Insulin treatment seems not to be effective enough to counteract this phenomenon [157]. The alteration of the BBB due to DM is shown by increase of insulin [158] and decrease of cholin transports [159]. It is also known that DM is associated with multidrug resistance-associated protein (MRP) upregulation in the BBB and increase of protein expression in the brain microvessels. These findings are associated with decrease of BBB permeability to fluorescein [160]. In the induced stroke rats when comparing hyperglycemic and non hyperglycemic rats, the BBB transport among the hyperglycemic animal was significantly reduced, in association with decrease of the cerebral blood flow [161]. In both permanent and transient type stroke models, BBB breakdown could be demonstrated soon after the occlusion; whereas, with an increase of glucose in the late post stroke stage (90 minutes into the stroke), the impact of the hyperglycemia was only limited. It was concluded that the correction of diabetes in stroke must be undertaken as soon as possible [162]. The devastating effect of hyperglycemia in stroke was shown also in occlusion of 3 hours to reperfusion at 21 hours in the diabetic Goto-Kakizaki rat model. The reasons for the significant larger infarct area demonstrated and the poor outcome was explained, at least partially, by the effect of the BBB disruption [139].

BBB and Hypertension

A dramatic increase of blood pressure, as well as chronic persistence of high levels may induce the breakdown of the BBB. The increased stress on the endothelium may exacerbate the leakage of the BBB. The vulnerability of the BBB to increased blood pressure was shown especially on spontaneously hypertensive rats [163]. In spontaneously hypertensive stroke rats (SHRSP) with increase of the blood pressure up to values of 250-270 mmHg, multilocation of BBB breakdown with leakage of plasma had already been noted at values of 210-220 mmHg of systolic pressure [164]. A similar finding has been found also in cats after increase of their blood pressure in 30%-40% [165]. Using the MRI technique, obligatory brain lesions were found in rats after increase of the systolic blood pressure up to 276 mmHg. In values of 210 mmHg, no lesions were noted [166]. Lacunar infarction was very commonly associated with damage of white matter and BBB disruption [167]. The cause of the BBB leakage in hypertension is due to changes in the TJ structure affecting the endothelial cell polarity of the BBB and alterations in the percentage relation of the 1 exocytoplastic leaflet (E face) to protoplastic leaflet (P face) [168], decrease of the TJ protein Z02 and increase of the ion transporter Na^+/H^+ exchanges 1 [169]. The characteristics of the BBB hypertension in correlation with ischemia were confirmed by studies showing the effect of antihypertensive drugs of the calcium antagonist family [170,171].

BBB and Lipids

There is some evidence that triglycerides and cholesterol play a role in the steady state of the BBB. Induction of leptin resistance of the BBB by triglycerides was shown by feeding milk with 98% triglycerides of fat [172]. It is interesting to note that the well-documented tPA activity of opening the BBB is at least partially affected via the LDL receptor related protein [173]. An important issue is the role of statin, especially, the atorvastatin in the downregulation of tPA by aggravating genes mediating coagulation and BBB permeability [174]. It also prevents the inflammation-dependent BBB disruption in humans [175].

CONCLUSION

The breakdown of the BBB seems to play a key role in the outcome of acute stroke. It may have also cardinal importance for the intracerebral bleeding, later rehabilitation potential and recurrency of stroke. Whereas, the pathophysiology and time behavior has been well studied, especially in animal models, very little is know about the behavior of the BBB during the late stage of stroke, as well as its variability between individuals.

The ability to influence the opening or closure of the BBB with medication made it possible to impact the functioning of the stroke outcome. Various medications have been tested, none of them are yet relevant. The forthcoming knowledge of the physiology and biology of the BBB and the present vast data of the behavior of the BBB post stroke in animal models and the novel techniques of demonstrating the degree of BBB breakdown, especially with MRI and SPECT-DTPA, make it easier to investigate and establish the behavior of the BBB at any stage of stroke.

References

[1] Ehrlick P. Das Sauerstoff-beduerfnis des organisjmus: eine farben analytische studie. Habilitation thesis, *Hirschwald*, 1885.

[2] Ehrlich P. Uber die beziehungen von chemischer constitution, vertheilung, und pharmakologischen wirkung. In: *Collected Studies on Immunity*. John Wiley and Sons; 1906;404-42.

[3] Carlson SD; Juang JL; Hilgers SL; Garment MB. Blood barriers of the insect. *Annu Rev Entomol.* 2000;45:151-74.

[4] Carlson SD; Hilgers SL; Juang JL. Ultrastructure and blood-nerve barrier of chordotonal organs in the *Drosophila* embryo. *J Neurocytol.* 1997;26(6):377-88.

[5] Butt AM; Jones HC; Abbott NJ. Electrical resistance across the blood-brain barrier in anaesthetized rats: a developmental study. *J Physiol.* 1990;429:47-62.

[6] Sobue K; Yamamoto N; Yoneda K; Hodgson ME; Yamashiro K; Tsuruoka N; et al. Induction of blood-brain barrier properties in immortalized bovine brain endothelial cells by astrocytic factors. *Neurosci Res.* 1999;35(2):155-64.

[7] Stewart PA; Hayakawa K. Early ultrastructural changes in blood-brain barrier vessels of the rat embryo. *Brain Res Dev Brain Res.* 1994;78(1):25-34.

[8] Rubin LL; Barbu K; Bard F; Cannon C; Hall DE; Horner H; et al. Differentiation of brain endothelial cells in cell culture. *A NY Acad Sci.* 1991;633:420-5.

[9] Schneeberger EE; Walters DV; Oliver RE. Development of intercellular junctions in the pulmonary epithelium of the fetal lamb. *J Cell Sci.* 1978;32:307-24.

[10] Claude P. morphological factors influencing transepithelial permeability: a model for the resistance of the zonula occludens. *J Membr Biol.* 1978;39(2-3):219-32.

[11] Grieb P; Forster RE; Strome D; Goodwin CW; Pape PC. O2 exchange between blood and brin tissues studied with18 O2 indicator-dilution technique. *J Appl Physiol.* 1985;58(6):1929-41.

[12] Pardridge WM; Eisenberg J; Yang J. Human blood-brain barrier insulin receptor. *J Neurochem.*1985;44(6):1771-8.

[13] Zhang Y; Pardridge WM. Rapid transferring efflux from brain to blood across the blood-brain barrier. *J Neurochem.* 2001;76(5):1597-1600.

[14] Smith MW; Gumbleton M. Endocytosis at the blood-brain barrier: from basic understanding to drug delivery strategies. *J Drug Target.* 2006;14(4):191-214.

[15] Hawkins RA; O'Kane RL; Simpson IA; Vina JR. Structure of the blood-brain barrier and its role in the transport of amino acids. *J Nutr.* 2006;136:218S-226S.

[16] Furuse M; Fujita K; Hiiragi T; Fujimoto K; Tsukita S. Claudin-1 and -2: novel integral membrane proteins localizing at tight junctions with no sequence similarity to occludin. *J Cell Biol.*1998;141(7):1539-50.

[17] Morita K; Sasaki H; Fujimoto K; Furuse M; Tsukita S. Caudin-11/OSP-based tight junctions of myelin sheaths in brain and Sertoli cells in testis. *J Cell Biol.* 1999;145(3):579-88.

[18] Furuse M; Hirase T; Itoh M; Nagafuchi A; Yonemura S; Tsukita S; et al. Occludin: a novel integral membrane protein localizing at tight junctions. *J Cell Biol.* 1993;123(6 pt2):1777-88.

[19] Hirase T; Staddon JM; Saitou M; Ando-Akatsuka Y; Itoh M; Fruse M; et al. Occludin as a possible determinant of tight junction permeability in endothelial cells. *J Cell Sci.* 1997;110(pt 14):1603-13.

[20] Martin-Pdaura I; Lostaglio S; Scheemann M; Williams L; Romano M; Frusecella P; et al. Junctional adhesion molecule, a novel member of the immunoglobulin superfamily that distributes at intercellular junctions and modulates monocyte transmigration. *J Cell Biol.* 1998;142(1):117-24.

[21] Haskins J; Gu L; Wittchen ES; Hibbard J; Stevenson BR. ZO-3, a novel member of the MAGUK protein family found at the tight junction, interacts with ZO-1 and occludin. *J Cell Biol.* 1998;141(1):199-208.

[22] Stevenson BR; Begg DA. Concentration-dependent effects of cytochalasin D on tight junctions and actin filaments in MDCK epithelial cells. *J Cell Sci.* 1994;107:367-75.

[23] Sakakibara A; Furuse M; Saitou M; Ando-Akatusuka Y; Tsukita S. Possible involvement of the phosphorylation of occluding in tight junction formation. *J Cell Biol.* 1997;137(6):1393-1404.

[24] Maher PA; Pasquale EB. Tyrosine phosphorylated proteins in different tissues during chick development. *J Cell Biol.* 1988;106(5):1747-55.

[25] Izumi Y; Hirose T; Tamai Y; Hirai S; Nagashima Y; Fujimoto T; et al. An atypical PKC directly associates and colocalizes at the epithelial tight junction with ASIP, a mammalian homologue of Caenorhabditis elegans polarity protein PAR-3. *J Cell Biol.* 1998;143(1):95-106.

[26] Rahman A; Anwar KN; Malik AB. Protein kinase C-zeta mediates TNF-alpha-induced ICAM-1 gene transcription in endothelial cells. *Am J Physiol Cell Physiol.* 2000;279(4):C906-C914.

[27] Jou TS; Nelson WJ. Effects of regulated expression of mutant RhoA and Rac1 small GTPases on the development of epithelial (MDCK) cell polarity. *J Cell Biol.* 1998;142(1):85-100.

[28] Pan W; Banks WA; Fasold MB; Bluth J; Kastin AJ. Transport of brain-derived neurotrophic factor across the blood-brain barrier. *Neuropharmcol.* 1998;37(12):1553-61.

[29] Pan W; Banks WA; Kastin AJ. Permeability of the blood-brain barrier to neurotrophins. *Brain Res.* 1998;778(1-2):87-94.

[30] Pan W; Kastin AJ. Entry of EGF into brain is rapid and saturable. *Peptides.* 1999;20(9):1091-8.

[31] Pan W; Vallance K; Kastin AJ. TGF alpha and the blood-brain barrier: accumulation in cerebral vasculature. *Exp Neurol.* 1999;160(2):454-9.

[32] Branks WA; Farr SA; La Scola ME; Morley JE. Intravenous human interleukin-1 alpha impairs memory processing in mice: dependence on blood-brain barrier transport into posterior division of the septum. *J Pharmacol Exp Ther.* 2001;299(2):536-41.

[33] Pan W; Banks WA; Kennedy MK; Gutierrez EG; Kastin AJ. Differential permeability of the BBB in acute EAE: enhanced transport of TNT-alpha. *Am J Physiol.* 1996;271:E636-E642.

[34] Ishida H; Takemori K; Dote K; Ito H. Expression of glucose transporter-1 and aquaporin-4 in the cerebral cortex of stroke-prone spontaneously hypertensive rats in relation to the blood-brain barrier function. *Am J Hypertens.* 2006;19(1):33-9.

[35] Calabria AR; Shusta EV. Blood-brain barrier genomics and proteomics: elucidating phenotype, identifying disease targets and enabling brain drug delivery. *Drug Discovery Today*. 2006;11(17/18):792-9.

[36] Zhu Z; Zhao B; Wang X; Zhu S; Zang Q; Xu Y; et al. Differentially expressed genes in hypertensive rats developing cerebral ischemia. *Life Sci.* 2004;74(15):1899-1909.

[37] Haqqani AS; Nesic M; Preston E; Baumann E; Kelly J; Stanimirovic D. Characterization of vascular protein expression patterns in cerebral ischemia/reperfusion using laser capture microdissection and ICAT-nanoLC-MS/MS. *FASEB J.* 2005;19(13):1809-21.

[38] Mark KS; Davis TP. Cerebral microvascular changes in permeability and tight junctions induced by hypoxia-reoxygenation. *Am J Physiol Heart Circ Physiol.* 2002;282(4): H1485-H1494.

[39] Brown RC; Mark KS; Egleton RD; Huber JD; Burroughs AR; Davis TP. Protection against hypoxia-induced increase in blood-brain barrier permeability: role of tight junction proteins and NFkappaB. *J Cell Sci.* 2003;116(Pt 4):693-700.

[40] Witt KA; Mark KS; Huber J; Davis TP. Hypoxia-inducible factor and nuclear factor kappa-B activation in blood-brain barrier endothelium under hypoxic/reoxygenation stress. *J Neurochem.* 2005;92(1):203-14.

[41] Mark KS; Burroughs AR; Brown RC; Huber JD; Davis TP. Nitric oxide mediates hypoxia-induced changes in paracellular permeability of cerebral microvasculature. *Am J Physiol Heart Circ Physiol.* 2004;286(1):H174-H180.

[42] Fischer S; Clauss M; Wiesnet M; Renz D; Schaper W; Karliczek GF. Hypoxia induces permeability in brain microvessel endothelial cells via VEGF and NO. *Am J Physiol.* 1999;276(4 Pt 1):C812-C820.

[43] Fischer S; Wiesnet M; Marti HH; Renz D; Schaper W. Simultaneous activation of several second messengers in hypoxia-induced hyperpermeability of brain derived endothelial cells. *J Cell Physiol.* 2004;198(3):359-69.

[44] Fischer S; Knoll R; Renz D; Karliczek GF; Schaper W. Role of adenosine in the hypoxic induction of vascular endothelial growth factor in porcine brain derived microvascular endothelial cells. *Endothelium.* 1997;5(3):155-65.

[45] Fischer S; Renz D; Wiesnet M; Schaper W; Karliczek GF. Hypothermia abolishes hypoxia-induced hyperpermeability in brain microvessel endothelial cells. *Brain Res Mol Brain Res.* 1999;74(1-2):135-44.

[46] Fischer S; Renz D; Schaper W; Karliczek GF. In vitro effects of dexamethasone on hypoxia-induced hyperpermeability and expression of vascular endothelial growth factor. *Eur J Pharmacol.* 2001;411(3):231-43.

[47] Fischer S; Renz D; Schaper W; Karliczek GF. Barbiturates decrease the expression of vascular endothelial growth factor in hypoxic cultures of porcine brain derived microvascular endothelial cells. *Brain Res Mol Brain Res.* 1998;60(1):89-97.

[48] Zhang W; Smith C; Howlett C; Stanimirovic D. Inflammatory activation of human brain endothelial cells by hypoxic astrocytes in vitro is mediated by IL-1beta. *J Cereb Blood Flow Metab.* 2000;20(6):967-78.

[49] Zhang W; Smith C; Shapiro A; Monette R; Hutchison J; Stanimirovic D. Increased expression of bioactive chemokines in human cerebromicrovascular endothelial cells and astrocytes subjected to simulated ischemia in vitro. *J Neuroimmunol.* 1999;101(2):148-60.

[50] Haorah J; Ramirez SH; Schall K; Smith D; Pandya R; Persidsky Y. Oxidative stress activates protein tyrosine kinase and matrix metalloproteinases leading to blood-brain barrier dysfunction. *J Neurochem.* 2007;101(2):566-76.

[51] Dimitrijevic OB; Stamatovic SM; Keep RF; Andjelkovic AV. Effects of the chemokine CCL2 on blood-brain barrier permeability during ischemia-reperfusion injury. *J Cereb Blood Flow Metab.* 2006;26(6):797-810.

[52] Brown RC; Mark KS; Egleton RD; Davis TP. Protection against hypoxia-induced blood-brain barrier disruption: changes in intracellular calcium. *Am J Physiol Cell Physiol.* 2004;286(5):C1045-C1052.

[53] Fischer S; Wiesnet M; Renz D; Schaper W. H2O2 induces paracellular permeability of porcine brain-derived microvascular endothelial cells by activation of the p44/42 MAP kinase pathway. *Eur J Cell Biol.* 2005;84(7):687-97.

[54] Witt KA; Mark KS; Sandoval KE; Davis TP. Reoxygenation stress on blood-brain barrier paracellular permeability and edema in the rat. *Microvasc Res.* 2008;75(1):91-6.

[55] Harris NG; Gauden V; Fraser PA; Williams SR; Parker GJ. MRI measurement of blood-brain barrier (BBB) permeability following spontaneous reperfusion the starch microsphere model of ischemia. *Magn Reson Imaging.* 2002;20(3):221-30.

[56] Knight RA; Nagesh V; Nagaraja TN; Ewing JR; Whitton PA; Bershad E; et al. Quantitation and localization of blood-to-brain influx by magnetic resonance imaging and quantitative autoradiography in a model of transient focal ischemia. *Magn Reson Med.* 2000;54(4):813-21.

[57] Petito CK. Early and late mechanisms of increased vascular permeability following experimental cerebral infarction. *J Neuropathol Exp Neurol.* 1979;38(3):222-34.

[58] Lopez-Otin C; Overall CM. Protease degradomics: a new challenge for proteomics. *Nat Rev Mol Cell Biol.* 2002;3(7):509-19.

[59] Nelson AR; Fingleton B; Rothenberg ML; Matrisian LM. Matrix metalloproteinases: biologic activity and clinical implications. *J Clin Oncol.* 2000;18(5):1135-49.

[60] Qi JH; Ebrahem Q; Moore N; Murphy G; Claesson-Welsh L; Bond M; et al. A novel function for tissue inhibitor of metalloproteinases-3 (TIMP3): inhibition for tissue inhibitor of angiogenesis by blockage of VEGF binding to VEGF receptor-2. *Nat Med.* 2003;9(4): 407-15.

[61] Brew K; Dinakarpandian D; Nagase H. Tissue inhibitors of metalloproteinases: evolution, structure and function. *Biochem Biophys Acta.* 2000;1477(1-2):267-83.

[62] Gottschall PE; Deb S. Regulation of matrix metalloproteinase expressions in astrocytes, microglia and neurons. *Neuroimmunomodulation.*1996;3(2-3):67-75.

[63] Gottschall PE; Yu X; Bing B. Increased production of gelatinase B (matrix metalloproteinase-9) and interleukin-6 by activated rat microglia in culture. *J Neurosci Res*. 1995;42(3):335-42.
[64] Ramos-DeSimone N; Hahn-Dantona E; Sipley J; Nagase H; French DL; Quigley JP. Activation of matrix metalloproteinase-9 (MMP-9) via a converging plasmin/stromelysin-1 cascade enhances tumor cell invasion. *J Biol Chem*. 1999;274(19):13066-76.
[65] Colton CA; Keri JE; Chen WT; Monsky WL. Protease production by cultured microglia: substrate gel analysis and immobilized matrix degradation. *J Neurosci*. 1993;35(3):297-304.
[66] Kuroiwa T; Ting P; Martinez H; Klatzo I. The biphasic opening of the blood-brain barrier to proteins following temporary middle cerebral artery occlusion. *Acta Neuropathol*. 1985;68(2):122-9. [Berlin].
[67] Rosenberg GA; Estrada EY; Dencoff JE. Matrix metalloproteinases and TIMPs are associated with blood-brain barrier opening after reperfusion in rat brain. *Stroke*. 1998;29(10):2189-95.
[68] Rosenberg GA; Cunningham LA; Wallace J; Alexander S; Estrada EY; Grossetete M; et al. Immunohistochemistry of matrix metalloproteinases in reperfusion injury to rat brain: activation of MMP-9 linked to stromelysin-1 and microglia in cell cultures. *Brain Res*. 2001;893(1-2):104-12.
[69] Wetzel M; Rosenberg GA; Cunningham LA. Tissue inhibitor of metalloproteinases-3 regulate neuronal sensitivity to doxorubicin-induced apoptosis. *Eur J Neurosci*. 2003;18(5):1050-60.
[70] Ahonen M; Poukkula M; Baker AH; Kashiwagi M; Nagase H; Eriksson JE; et al. Tissue inhibitor of metalloproteinases-3 induces apoptosis in melanoma cells by stabilization of death receptors. *Oncogene*. 2003;22(14):2121-34.
[71] Gu Z; Kaul M; Yan B; Kridel SJ; Cui Strongin A; Smith JW; et al. S-nitrosylation of matrix metalloproteinases: signaling pathway to neuronal cell death. *Science*. 2002;297(5584):1186-90.
[72] Huang CY; Fujimura M; Noshita N; Chang YY; Chan PH. SOD1 down-regulates NF-kappa B and e-Myc expression in mice after transient focal cerebral ischemia. *J Cereb Blood Flow Metab*. 2001;21(2):163-73.
[73] Huang CY; Fujimura M; Chang YY; Chan PH. Over-expression of copper-zinc superoxide dismutase attenuates acute activation of activator protein-1 after transient focal cerebral ischemia in mice. *Stroke*. 2001;32(3):741-7.
[74] Yang Y; Estrada EY; Thompson JF; Liu W; Rosenberg GA. Matrix metalloproteinase-mediated disruption of tight junction proteins in cerebral vessels is reversed by synthetic matrix metalloproteinase inhibitor in focal ischemia in rat. *J Cereb Blood Flow Metab*. 2007;27(4):697-709.
[75] Romanic AM; White RF; Arleth AJ; Ohlstein EH; Barone FC. Matrix metalloproteinase expression increases after cerebral focal ischemia in rats: inhibition of matrix metalloproteinase-9 reduces infarct size. *Stroke*. 1998;29(5):1020-30.
[76] Gasche Y; Fujimura M; Morita-Fujimura Y; Copin JC; Kawase M; Massengale J; et al. Early appearance of activated matrix metalloproteinase-9 after focal cerebral ischemia

in mice: a possible role in blood-brain barrier dysfunction. *J Cereb Blood Flow Metab.* 1999;19(9):1020-8.

[77] Acki T; Sumii T; Mori T; Wang X; Lo EH. Blood-brain barrier disruption and matrix metalloproteinase-9 expression during reperfusion injury: mechanical versus embolic focal ischemia in spontaneously hypertensive rats. *Stroke.* 2002;33(11):2711-17.

[78] Maier CM; Hsieh L; Yu F; Bracci P; Chan PH. Matrix metalloproteinase-9 and myeloperoxidase expression: quantitative analysis by antigen immunohistochemistry in a model of transient focal cerebral ischemia. *Stroke.* 2004;35(5):1169-74.

[79] Sood RR; Taheri S; Candelario-Jalil E; Estrada EY; Rosenberg GA. Early beneficial effect of matrix metalloproteinase inhibition on blood-brain barrier permeability as measured by magnetic resonance imaging countered by impaired long-term recovery after stroke in rat brain. *J Cereb Blood Flow Metab.* 2008;28(2):431-8.

[80] Planas AM; Sole S; Justicia C. Expression and activation of matrix metalloproteinase-2 and -9 in rat brain after transient focal cerebral ischemia. *Neurobiol Dis.* 2001;8(5):834-46.

[81] Asahi M; Wang X; Mori T; Sumii T; Jung JC; Moskowitz MA; et al. Effects of matrix metalloproteinase-9 gene knock-out on the proteolysis of blood-brain barrier and white matter components after cerebral ischemia. *J Neurosci.* 2001;21(19):7724-32.

[82] Amantea D; Russo R; Gliozzi M; Fratto V; Berliocchi L; Bagetta G; et al. Early upregulation of matrix metalloproteinase following reperfusion triggers neuroinflammatory mediators in brain ischemia in rat. *Int Rev Neurobiol.* 2007;82:149-69.

[83] Zhao BQ; Wang S; Kim HY; Storrie H; Rosen BR; Mooney DJ; et al. Role of matrix metalloproteinase in delayed cortical responses after stroke. *Nat Med.* 2006;12(4):441-5.

[84] Gursoy-Ozdemir Y; Can A; Dalkara T. Reperfusion-induced oxidative/ nitrative injury to neurovascular unit after focal cerebral ischemia. *Stroke.* 2004;35(6):1449-53.

[85] Liu R; Wen Y; Perez E; Wang X; Day AL; Simpkins JW; et al. 17beta-Estradiol attenuates blood-brain barrier disruption induced by cerebral ischemia-reperfusion in female rats. *Brain Res.* 2005;1060(1-2):55-61.

[86] Gidday JM; Gasche YG; Copin JC; Shah AR; Perez RS; Shapiro SD; et al. Leukocyte-derived matrix metalloproteinase-9 mediates blood-brain barrier breakdown and is proinflammatory after transient focal cerebral ischemia. *Am J Physiol Heart Circ Physiol.* 2005;289(2):H558-H568.

[87] Rosenberg GA; Estrada EY; Mobashery S. Effect of synthetic matrix metalloproteinase inhibitors on lipopolysaccharide-induced blood-brain barrier opening in rodents: differences in response based on strains and solvents. *Brain Res.* 2007;1133(1):186-92.

[88] Machado LS; Kozak A; Ergul A; Hess DC; Boriongan CV; Fagan SC. Delayed Minocycline inhibits ischemia-activated matrix metalloproteinase 2 and 9 after experimental stroke. *BMC Neurosci.* 2006;7:56.

[89] Reijerkerk A; Kooij G; van der Pol SM; Khazen S; Dijkstra CD; de Veries HE. Diapedesis of monocytes is associated with MMP-mediated occludin disappearance in brain endothelial cells. *FASEB J.* 2006;20(14):2550-2.

[90] Veltkamp R; Bieber K; Wagner S; Beynon C; Siebing DA; Veitkamp C; et al. Hyperbaric oxygen reduces basal lamina degradation after transient focal cerebral ischemia in rats. *Brain Res*. 2006;1076(1):231-7.

[91] Canelario-Jalil E; Taheri S; Yang Y; Sood R; Grossetete M; Estrada EY; et al. Cyclooxygenase inhibition limits blood-brain barrier disruption following intracerebral injection of tumor necrosis factor-alpha in the rat. *J Pharmacol Exp Ther*. 2007;323(2):488-98.

[92] Guo M; Cox B; Mahale S; Davis W; Carranza A; Hayes K; et al. Pre-ischemic exercise reduces matrix metalloproteinase-9 expression and ameliorates blood-brain barrier dysfunction in stroke. *Neuroscience*. 2008;151(2):340-51.

[93] Kamada H; Yu F; Nito C; Chan PH. Influence of hyperglycemia on oxidative stress and matrix metalloproteinase-9 activation after focal cerebral ischemia/reperfusion in rats: relation to blood-brain barrier dysfunction. *Stroke*. 2007;38(3):1044-9.

[94] Tsubokawa T; Solaroglu I; Yatsushige H; Cahill J; Yata K; Zhang JH. Cathepsin and calpain inhibitor E64d attenuates matrix metalloproteinase-9 activity after focal cerebral ischemia in rats. *Stroke*. 2006;37(7):1888-94.

[95] Zhang X; Winkles JA; Gongora MC; Polavarapu R; Michaelson JS; Hahm K; et al. TWEAK-Fm14 pathway inhibition protects the integrity of the neurovascular unit during cerebral ischemia. *J Cereb Blood Flow Metab*. 2007;27(3):534-44.

[96] Zhu W; Khachi S; Hao Q; Shen F; Young WL; Yang GY; et al. Upregulation of EMMPRIN after permanent focal cerebral ischemia. *Neurochem Int*. 2007. [Epub ahead of print].

[97] Wang Y; Deng XL; Xiao XH; Yuan BX. A non-steroidal anti-inflammatory agent provides significant protection during focal ischemic stroke with decreased expression of matrix metalloproteinase. *Curr Neurovasc Res*. 2007;4(3):176-83.

[98] Svedin P; Hagberg H; Savman K; Zhu C; Mallard C. Matrix metalloproteinase-9 gene knock-out protects the immature brain after cerebral hypoxia-ischemia. *J Neurosci*. 2007;27(7):1511-18.

[99] Sumii T; Lo EH. Involvement of matrix metalloproteinase in thrombolysis-associated hemorrhagic transformation after embolic focal ischemia in rats. *Stroke*. 2002;33(3): 831-6.

[100] Pfefferkorn T; Rosenberg GA. Closure of the blood-brain barrier by matrix metalloproteinase inhibition reduces rtPA-mediated mortality in cerebral ischemia with delayed reperfusion. *Stroke*. 2003;34(8): 2025-30.

[101] Tsuji K; Aoki T; Tejima E; Arai K; Lee SR; Atochin DN; et al. Tissue plasminogen activator promotes matrix metalloproteinase-9 upregulation after focal cerebral ischemia. *Stroke*. 2005;36(9):1954-59.

[102] Burggraf D; Martens HK; Dichgans M; Hamann GF. rt-PA causes a dose-dependent increase in the extravasation of cellular and non-cellular blood elements after focal cerebral ischemia. *Brain Res*. 2007;1164:55-62.

[103] Yang DY; Pan HC; Chen CJ; Cheng FC; Wang YC. Effects of tissue plasminogen activator on cerebral microvessel of rats during focal cerebral ischemia and reperfusion. *Neurol Res*. 2007;29(3):274-82.

[104] Kelly MA; Shuaib A; Todd KG. Matrix metalloproteinase activation and blood-brain barrier breakdown following thrombolysis. *Exp Neurol*. 2006;200(1):38-49.

[105] Gursoy-Ozdemir Y; Bolay H; Saribas O; Dalkara T. Role of endothelial nitric oxide generation and peroxynitrite formation in reperfusion injury after focal cerebral ischemia. *Stroke*. 2000;31(8): 1974-80.

[106] O'Neill MJ; Murray TK; McCarty DR; Hicks CA; Dell CP, Patrick KE; et al. ARL 17477, a selective nitric oxide synthase inhibitor, with neuroprotective effects in animal models of global and focal cerebral ischaemia. *Brain Res*. 2000;871(2):234-44.

[107] Jiang J; Wang W; Sun YJ; Hu M; Li F; Zhu DY. Neuroprotective effect of curcumin on focal cerebral ischemia rats by preventing blood-brain barrier damage. *Eur J Pharmacol*. 2007;561(1-3):54-62.

[108] Hu XM; Zhou MM; Hu XM; Zeng FD. Neuroprotective effects of scutellarin on rat neuronal damage induced by cerebral ischemia/reperfusion. *Acta Pharmacol Sin*. 2005;26(12):1454-9.

[109] Kahles T; Luedike P; Endres M; Galla HJ; Steinmetz H; Busse R; et al. NADPH oxidase plays a central role in blood-brain barrier damage in experimental stroke. *Stroke*. 2007;38(11):3000-6.

[110] Wang Y; Kilic E; Kilic U; Weber B; Bassetti CL; Marti HH; et al. VEGF overexpression induces post-ischaemic neuroprotection, but facilitates haemodynamic steal phenomena. *Brain*. 2005;128(Pt 1):52-63.

[111] Shimamura N; Matchett G; Solaroglu I; Tsubokawa T; Ohkuma H; Zhang J. Inhibition of integrin alphavbeta3 reduces blood-brain barrier breakdown in focal ischemia in rats. *J Neurosci Res*. 2006;84(8):1837-47.

[112] Shimamura N; Matchett G; Yatsushige H; Calvert JW; Ohkuma H; Zhang J. Inhibition of integrin alphavbeta3 ameliorates focal ischemic damage in the rat middle cerebral artery occlusion model. *Stroke*. 2006;37(7):1902-9.

[113] Zhang ZG; Zhang L; Tsang W; Soltanian-Zadeh H; Morris D; Zhang R; et al. Correlation of VEGF and angiopoietin expression with disruption of blood-brain barrier and angiogenesis after focal cerebral ischemia. *J Cereb Blood Flow Metab*. 2002;22(4):379-92.

[114] Li Y; Lu ZY; Ogle M; Wei L. Erythropoietin prevents blood-brain barrier damage induced by focal cerebral ischemia in mice. *Neurochem Res*. 2007;32(12):2132-41.

[115] Zhang AG; Zhang L; Croll SD; Chopp M. Angiopoietin-1 reduces cerebral blood vessel leakage and ischemic lesion volume after focal cerebral embolic ischemia in mice. *Neuroscience*. 2002;113(3):683-7.

[116] Zacharek A; Chen J; Cui X; Li A; Li Y; Roberts C; et al. Angiopoietina/Tie2 and VEGF/Flk1 induced by MSC treatment amplifies angiogenesis and vascular stabilization after stroke. *J Cereb Blood Flow Metab*. 2007;27(10):1684-91.

[117] Chi OZ; Liu X; Weiss HR. Effects of Endothelin-1 blood-brain barrier permeability during focal cerebral ischemia in rats. *Exp Brain Res*. 2001;141(1):1-5.

[118] Zhang Y; Pardridge WM. Neuroprotection in transient focal brain ischemia after delayed intravenous administration of brain-derived neurotrophic factor conjugated to a blood-brain barrier drug targeting system. *Stroke*. 2001;32(6):1378-84.

[119] Hornig CR; Busse O; Dorndorf W; Kaps M. Changes in CSF blood-brain barrier parameters in ischaemic cerebral infarction. *J Neurol.* 1983;229(1):11-16.

[120] Niebroj-Dobosz I; Mariam AG; Lukasiuk M; Ralatowska J. Blood-cerebrospinal fluid barrier integrity in cerebral infarction. *Neuropatol Pol.* 1992;30(1):29-33.

[121] Hornig CR; Busse O; Buettner T; Dorndorf W; Agnoli A; Akengin Z. CT contrast enhancement on brain scans and blood-CSF barrier disturbances in cerebral ischemic infarction. *Stroke.* 1985;16(2):268-73.

[122] Ito U; Tomita H; Kito K; Ueki Y; Inaba Y. CT enhancement after prolonged high-dose contrast infusion in the early stage of cerebral infarction. *Stroke.* 1986;17(3): 424-30.

[123] Kanner AA; Marchi N; Fazio V; Mayberg MR; Koltz MT; Siomin V; et al. Serum S100beta: a noninvasive marker of blood-brain barrier function and brain lesions. *Cancer.* 2003;97(11):2806-13.

[124] Bertsch T; Casarin W; Kretschmar M; Zimmer W; Walter S; Sommer C; et al. Protein S-100B: a serum marker for ischemic and infectious injury of cerebral tissue. *Clin Chem Lab Med.* 2001;39(4): 319-23.

[125] Aurell A; Rosengren LE; Karlsson B; Olsson JE; Zbornikova V; Haglid KG. Determination of S-100 and glial fibrillary acidic protein concentrations in cerebrospinal fluid after brain infarction. *Stroke.* 1991;22(10):1254-8.

[126] Foerch C; Wunderlich MT; Dvorak F; Humpich M; Kahles T; Goertler M; et al. Elevated serum S100B levels indicate a higher risk of hemorrhagic transformation after thrombolytic therapy in acute stroke. *Stroke.* 2007;38(9):2491-5.

[127] Tumani H; Nau R; Felgenhauer K. Beta-trace protein in cerebrospinal fluid: a blood-CSF barrier-related evaluation in neurological diseases. *Ann Neurol.*1998;44(6):882-9.

[128] Egelhoff T; Essig M; von Kummer R; Dorfier A; Winter R; Sartor K. Acute ischemic cerebral infarct: prospective serial observations by magnetic resonance imaging. *Rofo.* 1998;168(3):222-7. [Article in German].

[129] Maeda M; Maley JE; Crosby DL; Quets JP; Zhu MW; Lee GJ; et al. Application of contrast agents in the evaluation of stroke: conventional MR and echoplanar MR imaging. *J Magn Reson Imaging.* 1997;7(1):23-8.

[130] Henning EC; Latour LL; Warach S. Verification of enhancement of the CSF space, not parenchyma, in acute stroke patients with early blood-brain barrier disruption. *J Cereb Blood Flow Metab.* 2007 [Epub ahead of print].

[131] Merten CL; Knitelius HO; Assheuer J; Bergmann-Kurz B; Hedde JP; Bewermeyer H. MRI of acute cerebral infarcts, increased contrast enhancement with continuous infusion of gadolinium. *Neuroradiology.* 1999;41(4):242-8.

[132] Lorberboym M; Lampl Y; Sadeh M. Correlation of 99m Tc-DTPA SPECT of the blood-brain barrier with neurologic outcome after acute stroke. *J Nucl Med.* 2003;44(12):1898-1904.

[133] Lorberboym M; Blankenberg FG; Sadeh M; Lampl Y. In vivo imaging of apoptosis in patients with acute stroke: correlations with blood-brain barrier permeability. *Brain Res.* 2006;1103(1):13-19.

[134] Cordes M; Henkes H; Roll D; Eichstadt H; Christe W; Langer M; et al. Subacute and chronic cerebral infarction; SPECT and gandolinium-DTPA enhanced MR imaging. *J Comput Assist Tomogr.* 1989;13(4):567-71.

[135] Marks MP; de Crespigny A; Lentz D; Enzmann DR; Albers GW; Moseley ME. Acute and chronic stroke: navigated spin-echo diffusion-weighted MR imaging. *Radiology*. 1996;199(2):403-8.

[136] Mecocci P; Parnetti L; Reboldi GP; Santucci C; Gaiti A; Ferri C; et al. Blood-brain barrier in a geriatric population: barrier function in degenerative and vascular dementias. *Acta Neurol Scand*. 1991;84(3):210-13.

[137] Hassan A; Hunt BJ; O'Sullivan M; Parmar K; Bamford JM; Briley D; et al. Markers of endothelial dysfunction in lacunar infarction and ischaemic leukoaraiosis. *Brain*. 2003;126(Pt 2):424-32.

[138] Wallin A; Sjorgren M; Edman A; Blennow K; Regland B. Symptoms, vascular risk factors and blood-brain barrier function in relation to CT white-matter changes in dementia. *Eur Neurol*. 2000;44(4):229-35.

[139] Ergul A; Elgebaly MM; Middlemore ML; Li W; Elewa H; Switzer JA; et al. Increased hemorrhagic transformation and altered infarct size and localization after experimental stroke in a rat model type 2 diabetes. *BMC Neurol*. 2007;7:33.

[140] Kim EY; Na DG; Kim SS; Lee KH; Ryoo JW; Kim HK. Prediction of hemorrhagic transformation in acute ischemic stroke: role of diffusion-weighted imaging and early parenchymal enhancement. *AJNR Am J Neurolradiol*. 2005;26(5):1050-55.

[141] Latour LL; Kang DW; Ezzeddine MA; Chalela JA; Warach S. Early blood-brain barrier disruption in human focal brain ischemia. *Ann Neurol*. 2004;56(4):468-77.

[142] Bang OY; Buck BH; Saver JL; Alger JR; Yoon SR; Starkman S; et al. Prediction of hemorrhagic transformation after recanalization therapy using $T2^*$-permeability magnetic resonance imaging. *Ann Neurol*. 2007;62(2):170-6.

[143] Kassner A; Roberts T; Taylor K; Silver F; Mikulis D. Prediction of hemorrhage in acute ischemic stroke using permeability MR imaging. *AJNR Am J Neuroradiol*. 2005;26(9):2213-17.

[144] Bisdas S; Hartel M; Cheong LH; Koh TS. Detection of early vessel leakiness in acute ischemic stroke using computed tomography perfusion may indicate hemorrhagic transformation. *Acta Radiol*. 2007;48(3):341-4.

[145] Chen HY; Chen TY; Lee MY; Chen ST; Hsu YS; Kuo YL; et al. Melatonin decreases neurovascular oxidative/nitrosative damage and protects against early increases in the blood-brain barrier permeability after transient focal cerebral ischemia in mice. *J Pineal Res*. 2006;41(2):175-82.

[146] Dijkhuizen RM; Asahi M; Wu O; Rosen BR; Lo EH. Delayed rt-PA treatment in a rat embolic stroke model: diagnosis and prognosis of ischemic injury and hemorrhagic transformation with magnetic resonance imaging. *J Cereb Blood Flow Metab*. 2001;21(8):964-71.

[147] Neumann-Haefelin C; Brinker G; Uhlenkuken U; Pillekamp F; Hossmann KA; Hoehn M. Prediction of hemorrhagic transformation after thrombolytic therapy of clot embolism: an MRI investigation in rat brain. *Stroke*. 2002;33(5):1392-8.

[148] Dijkhuizen RM; Asahi M; Wu O; Rosen BR; Lo EH. Rapid breakdown of microvascular barriers and subsequent hemorrhagic transformation after delayed recombinant tissue plasminogen activator treatment in a rat embolic stroke model. *Stroke*. 2002;33(8):2100-4.

[149] Ding G; Jiang Q; Li L; Zhang L; Gang Zhang Z; Ledbetter KA; et al. Detection of BBB disruption and hemorrhage by Gd-DTPA enhanced MRI after embolic stroke in rat. *Brain Res*. 2006;1114(1):195-203.

[150] Kelly MA; Shuaib A; Todd KG. Matrix metalloproteinase activation and blood-brain barrier breakdown following thrombolysis. *Exp Neurol*. 2006;200(1):38-49.

[151] Warach S; Latour LL. Evidence of reperfusion injury, exacerbated by thrombolytic therapy, in human focal brain ischemia using a novel imaging marker of early blood-brain barrier disruption. *Stroke*. 2004;35(11 Supp 1):2659-61.

[152] Montaner J; Alvarez-Sabin J; Molina CA; Angles A; Abilleira S; Arenillas J; et al. Matrix metalloproteinase expression is related to hemorrhagic transformation after cardioembolic stroke. *Stroke*. 2001;32(12):2762-7.

[153] Hovsepyan MR; Haas MJ; Boyajyan AS; Guevorkyan AA; Mamikonyan AA; Myers SE; et al. Astrocytic and neuronal biochemical markers in the sera of subjects with diabetes mellitus. *Neurosci Lett*. 2004;369(3):224-7.

[154] Starr JM; Wardlaw J; Ferguson K; MacLullich A; Deary IJ; Marshall I. Increased blood-brain barrier permeability in type II diabetes demonstrated by gadolinium magnetic resonance imaging. *J Neurol Neurosurg Psych*. 2003;74(1):70-6.

[155] Hawkins BT; Lundeen TF; Norwood KM ; Brooks HL; Egleton RD. Increased blood-brain barrier permeability and altered tight junctions in experimental diabetes in the rat: contribution of hyperglycaemia and matrix metalloproteinase. *Diabetologia*. 2007;50(1):202-11.

[156] Chehade JM; Haas MJ; Mooradian AD. Diabetes-related changes in rat cerebral occludin and zonula occludens-I (ZO-1) expression. *Neurochem*. 2002;27(3):249-52.

[157] Huber JD; Vanglider RL; Houser KA. Streptozotocin-induced diabetes progressively increases blood-brain barrier permeability in specific brain regions in rats. *Am J Physiol Heart Circ Physiol*. 2006;291:H2660-H2668.

[158] Mooradian AD; Haas MJ; Batejko O; Hovsepyan M; Feman SS. Statins ameliorate endothelial barrier permeability changes in the cerebral tissue of streptozotocin-induced diabetic rats. *Diabetes*. 2005;54(10):2977-82.

[159] Mooradian AD. Blood-brain barrier choline transport is reduced in diabetic rats. *Diabetes*. 1987;36(10):1094-7.

[160] Hawkins BT; Ocheltree SM; Norwood KM; Egleton RD. Decreased blood-brain barrier permeability to fluorescein in streptozotocin-treated rats. *Neurosci Lett*. 2007;411(1):1-5.

[161] Kawai N; Keep RF; Betz AL; Nagao S. Hyperglycemia induces progressive changes in the cerebral microvasculature and blood-brain barrier transport during focal cerebral ischemia. *Acta Neurochir Suppl*. 1998;71:219-21.

[162] Ennis SR; Keep RF. Effects of sustained-mild and transient-severe hyperglycemia on ischemia-induced blood-brain barrier opening. *J Cereb Blood Flow Metab*. 2007;27(9):1573-82.

[163] Shima K; Ohashi K; Umezawa H; Chigasaki H; Okuyama S. Blood-brain barrier, cerebral blood flow, and brain edema in spontaneously hypertensive rats with chronic focal ischemia. *Acta Neurochi Suppl (Wien)*. 1994;60:271-3.

[164] Fredriksson K; Nordborg C; Kalimo H; Olsson Y; Johansson BB. Cerebral microangiopathy in stroke -prone spontaneously hypertensive rats. An Immunohistochemical and ultrastructural study. *Acta Neuropathol.* 1988;75(3):241-52.

[165] Sakaki T; Tsunoda S; Utsumi S. The influence of volume expansion with induced hypertension on vessel reactivities, the blood-brain barrier, and cerebral infarction in cats with one-hour occlusion of the middle cerebral artery. *Neurosurgery.* 1990;27(2):268-73.

[166] Del Bigio MR; Yan HJ; Kozlowski P; Sutherland GR; Peeling J. Serial magnetic resonance imaging of rt brain after induction of renal hypertension. *Stroke.* 1999;30(11):2440-7.

[167] Hazama F; Chue CH; Kataoka H; Sasahara M; Amano S. Pathogenesis of lacuna-like cyst formation and diffuse degeneration of the white matter in the brain of stroke-prone spontaneously hypertensive rats. *Clin Exp Pharmacol Physiol Suppl.* 1995;22(1):S260-S261.

[168] Lippoldt A; Kniesel U; Liebner S; Kalbacher H; Kirsch T; Wolburg H; et al. Structural alterations of tight junctions are associated with loss of polarity in stroke-prone spontaneously hypertensive rat blood-brain barrier endothelial cells. *Brain Res.* 2000;885(2):251-61.

[169] Hom S; Fleegal MA; Egleton RD; Campos CR; Hawkins BT; Davis TP. Comparative changes in the blood-brain barrier and cerebral infarction of SHR and WKY rats. *Am J Physiol Regul Integr Comp Physiol.* 2007;292(5):1881-92.

[170] Brown RC; Davis TP. Calcium modulation of adherens and tight junction function: a potential mechanism for blood-brain barrier disruption after stroke. *Stroke.* 2002;33(6):1706-11.

[171] Sakaki T; Tsunoda S; Morimoto T. The influence of the calcium antagonist nimodipine and induced hypertension on the behavior of the cerebral pial arteries, the blood-brain barrier, cerebral edema, and cerebral infarction in cats with one-hour occlusion of the middle cerebral artery. *Neurosurgery.* 1991;28(2):267-72.

[172] Banks WA; Coon AB; Robinson SM; Moinuddin A; Shultz JM; Nakaoke R; et al. Triglycerides induce leptin resistance at the blood-brain barrier. *Diabetes.* 2004;53(5):1253-60.

[173] Yepes M; Sandkvist M; Moore EG; Bugge TH; Strickland DK; Lawrence DA. Tissue-type plasminogen activator induces opening of the blood-brain barrier via the LDL receptor-related protein. *J Clin Invest.* 2003;112(10):1533-40.

[174] Liu XS; Zhang ZG; Zhang L; Morris DC; Kapke A; Lu M; et al. Atorvastatin downregulates tissue plasminogen activator-aggravated genes mediating coagulation and vascular permeability in single cerebral endothelial cells captured by laser microdissection. *J Cereb Blood Flow Metab.* 2006;26(6):787-96.

[175] Buttmann M; Lorenz A; Weishaupt A; Rieckmann P. Atorvastatin partially prevents an inflammatory barrier breakdown of cultured human brain endothelial cells at a pharmacologically relevant concentration. *J Neurochem.* 2007;102(4):1001-8.

In: The Blood-Brain Barrier
Editor: Tomas R. Helio

ISBN 978-1-60456-894-3

Chapter 5

CONSEQUENCES OF A DISRUPTED BLOOD-BRAIN BARRIER TO DRUG DELIVERY

Angela J. Monahan, Paul M. Carvey, Chaohui Zhao, Liaohai Chen and Zaodung Ling
Department of Pharmacology, Rush University
Medical Center, Chicago, IL 60521, USA.

ABSTRACT

There is emerging evidence that the blood brain barrier (BBB) is dysfunctional in neurodegenerative diseases such as Parkinson's disease (PD). Studies from our laboratory and others reveal that areas of BBB dysfunction occur in regions of the brain undergoing neuroinflammation including the substantia nigra and striatum. Thus, we have shown that several different tracers enter brain parenchyma in conjunction with microglia activation, cytokine release and up-regulation of integrins only expressed by angiogenic vessels [1] We have proposed that this BBB dysfunction contributes to disease progression by facilitating the entry of peripheral immune mediators producing a secondary immune response [2]. Such dysfunction would also facilitate the entry of dopamine (DA) neurotoxins into areas of active degeneration further contributing to disease progression. Such dysfunction similarly raises the possibility that our time-honored approach to delivering therapeutic treatments across an intact barrier by overcoming P-glycoprotein, utilizing existing transport mechanisms, or requiring high lipid solubility may be misguided. If our hypothesis is correct, we should be able to deliver neuroprotective agents that normally do not cross the BBB, directly to an area of active degeneration thereby providing targeted therapy. Since this treatment could be delivered at low circulating doses because of BBB dysfunction, it is likely that central side effects that might otherwise complicate treatment could be avoided.

Introduction

BBB Description

In 1904 Paul Ehrlich first demonstrated the existence of a blood-brain-barrier (BBB) by injecting water soluble dyes into the circulatory system. He found that all organs except the brain were stained by the dyes [3]. Following his study, others demonstrated that injections of dyes into the CSF resulted in staining of all cells within the CNS, but not the periphery [4]. Subsequent studies revealed overt differences between cerebral vasculature and peripheral vessels. Thus, although both capillary networks consist of a monolayer of endothelial cells, the cerebral vessels contain increased numbers of mitochondria [5] , lack fenestrations [6] , have minimal pinocytotic activity [7], and form tight junctions [8] . Despite these differences, the notion that the cerebral vasculature was a static structure became indoctrinated. Today our understanding of the BBB is beginning to broaden suggesting that the BBB is a more dynamic structure than we initially thought, yet, under tight control.

In humans, the BBB encompasses 100 billion capillaries totaling 400 miles in length with a combined surface area of brain capillary endothelium of approximately 20 m^2 [9]. This network requires tight regulation by elements of the peripheral blood (including vascular flow) and the CNS. The transport of nutrients between endothelial cells and nervous tissue is facilitated by interactions of the astrocytic end feet with the capillary walls. In addition, factors released from astrocytes are thought to signal endothelial cells to form tight junctions which thereby form a physical barrier [10-13]. Proteins making up the tight junctions include occludins, claudins, and junctional adhesion proteins [14-16]. The pericytes, which are mesenchymal-like cells and the endothelial cells, are embedded in a basement membrane composed of collagen type IV, heparin sulfate proteoglycans, laminin, fibronectin and other extracellular matrix proteins. Although the basement membrane provides mechanical support and anchorage, these embedded molecules also participate in communication between the endothelial cells and the nervous tissues [17]. The endothelial cells, astrocytes, pericytes, basement membrane and potentially products released from neurons therefore form the co-called "neurovascular unit" [18].

In addition to being a mechanical barrier, the endothelial cells that comprise the BBB also contain proteins that function as efflux pumps to exclude chemicals from the brain. For example, P-glycoprotein, a multi-drug resistant (MDR) protein, is present on the luminal surface of the endothelial cells and prevents access of chemotherapeutics, anti-epileptic as well as opiates. Expression of these proteins is found to be activated by tumor necrosis factor (TNF) and upregulated with long-term exposure to drugs [19,20]. There are also a number of biotransforming enzymes present that include members of the cytochrome P450 family which similarly contribute to barrier function by inactivating numerous chemicals and drugs before they reach brain parenchyma [21,22]. It is thus fair to characterize the BBB as both a physical and chemical barrier.

BBB Dysfunction in Parkinson's Disease

The integrity of barrier function is disrupted in certain conditions. For example, barrier function is compromised in bacterial meningitis, HIV infection and ischemia [23-25]. In diabetes, the midbrain, hippocampus, cortex and the basal ganglia endothelium exhibits enhanced leakage to sucrose whereas other regions show no change in permeability [26]. Physical trauma to the brain is also known to cause disruption of the barrier, but is usually re-established within ten days [27]. Stroke is also known to affect the integrity of the barrier. BBB disruption appears to be an early occurrence in the formation of white matter lesions found in multiple sclerosis [28]. Evidence for BBB disruption in AD has also emerged indicating increased permeability of serum protein into the brain parenchyma, irregular basement member and changes in protein expression on the endothelium [29]. Given that several conditions including neurodegenerative diseases lead to dysfunction of the BBB, it is not surprising that a growing literature has emerged to suggest disrupted function of the BBB in PD patients as well as models of PD.

PD is characterized by progressive loss of dopamine (DA) neurons in the substantia nigra (SN) associated with underlying neuroinflammation [30]. Recent studies in PD patients and its animal models point to microvascular changes in the SN and alterations in BBB markers [31-36] associated with areas of barrier disruption. We have demonstrated that exposure to the DA neurotoxin 6-hydroxydopamine (6-OHDA), leads to a compromised BBB in the SN and striatum such that albumin and horseradish peroxidase were able to enter brain parenchyma readily from the vasculature. These results were accompanied by loss of DA neurons, activation of microglia, up-regulation of p-glycoprotein and β3-integrin (an integrin expressed by angiogenic vessels) on the endothelial cells [1]. Another DA neurotoxin, 1-methyl-4-phenyl-1,2,3,6-tetrahydropyridine (MPTP), produced similar changes in mice in which compromise in the integrity of the BBB was thought to be caused by underlying neuroinflammation as a result of microglial activation [37,38]. We proposed that the neuroinflammatory consequences of toxin-induced DA neuron loss, leads to disruption of the BBB in areas of active inflammation. This barrier compromise does not affect the entire structure, but rather, is punctate and perhaps dynamic in that we cannot exclude the possibility that the areas of barrier compromise wax and wane in association with focal areas of active inflammation. If barrier function is compromised in this fashion, it is likely that drugs used to treat PD may not enter brain parenchyma homogeneously such that neurons adjacent to an area of punctate leakage may receive higher concentrations of drug than neurons adjacent to an intact BBB. Recent data from our laboratory suggests this may well be the case.

The most universally used and efficacious treatment for PD is levodopa. Systemically administered levodopa is transported by the large neutral amino acid (LNAA) transporter-1 (LAT1) across the BBB and into the brain [39,40]. Once in brain, levodopa is decarboxylated by aromatic amino acid decarboxylase (AAAD) in several locations where its active metabolite DA is taken up and recycled by DA terminals to replace the DA lost to the disease process [41,42]. The production of DA ameliorates the symptoms of PD, but can also create side effects such as dyskinesias or psychotic episodes [43,44]. However, systemically administered levodopa is also converted to DA in the periphery where it produces significant peripheral side effects (e.g., epigastric distress or nausea). To reduce these side effects, AAAD inhibitors that do not cross the BBB (carbidopa and benserazide) are given simultaneously with levodopa. These drugs significantly attenuate peripheral side effects, reduce first pass metabolism, and increase the amount of circulating levodopa available to the brain. The end result is increased potency and central anti-parkinsonian efficacy. Since the transport of LAT-1-mediated flux of levodopa and sequestration of peripheral AAAD inhibitors both depend upon proper function of the BBB, it is not surprising that growing evidence suggests abnormalities in levodopa delivery in animals exhibiting neuroinflammation.

Westin et al, (2006) demonstrated increased angiogenesis in levodopa treated animals that also developed dyskinesias following 6OHDA treatment [45]. They argued that toxicant exposure led to angiogenic changes and barrier compromise that resulted in dyskinesias. Since angiogenic vessels are leaky, this might suggest that inhomogeneous delivery of levodopa might lead to DA hot spots that could contribute to the abnormal movements [46,47]. Thus, too much levodopa may have entered some areas due to barrier dysfunction associated with increased conversion to DA. Alternatively, peripheral AAAD inhibitors might gain access to brain parenchyma, inhibit central AAAD, and reduce conversion of DA in that area. Since our laboratory had previously demonstrated that 6OHDA produced punctate areas of FITC-labeled albumin leakage into the SN and striatum where there was a concordant up-regulation of β3-integrin in the SN and striatum [1], we set out to test the entry of levodopa and benserazide in the striatum of animals with 6OHDA lesions.

Methods

We injected 6OHDA (8 μg/2μL) unilaterally into the medial forebrain bundle to produce a unilateral DA neuron loss. Ten days later and 30 minutes prior to sacrifice, the animals were treated systemically (i.p.) with the peripheral AAAD inhibitor, benserazide (50 mg/kg), followed by IV administration of levodopa methyl ester (200mg/kg). Just prior to sacrifice, we administered Evans Blue via the carotid artery and then perfused with ice-cold saline three minutes later to assess the patency of the BBB. We had hoped to dissect areas of striatum with parenchymal Evans Blue dye to determine if there were increases in DA, levodopa or benserazide. When we dissected the striata from the rat brains, we were able to visualize areas of Evans Blue dye in the ipsilateral striata suggesting disruption of barrier integrity. However, when we cut the striatum into 100 □m slabs, we were no longer able to discern areas of Evans Blue probably due to inadequate amounts in the thin sections. We then decided to cut the striatum into serial sections and passed them to HPLC analysis. The midbrain was post-fixed for subsequent DA neuron count assessment.

Results

Analysis of the midbrain revealed that the DA neuron loss on the ipsilateral side (verified using tyrosine hydroxylase immunoreactive cell counts) was associated with increased entry of levodopa and benserazide into the ipsilateral striatum (Figures 1 and 2) suggesting that DA degeneration-induced BBB dysfunction does in fact alter levodopa kinetics. Thus, the average levels of levodopa on the ipsilateral side across all sections were increased 51.10% (($t=3.52$, $p<0.05$) compared with the contralateral side, whereas the levels of benserazide were increased 75% ($t=4.65$, $p<0.05$). Examination of the ipsi-contralateral differences of each of tissue pieces revealed that virtually every section from the rostral regions of the striatum (low numbered sections) to the caudal regions (high numbered sections) had more levodopa and benserazide in them. Despite the increased levels of levodopa, DA levels on the ipsilateral were significantly reduced by 84.6% ($t=7.68$, $p<0.05$; Figure 3). Because the Evans Blue entry strategy did not work, the data is much more difficult to interpret. Thus, the reduced ipsilateral DA might suggest that the increased entry of benserazide led to reduced decarboxylation of levodopa, but could also reflect the fact that the DA neuron lesion led to a loss of striatal DA that could not be overcome by the levodopa administration. Similarly, the DA neuron lesion and its associated loss of DA terminals could have reduced the decarboxylation rate of levodopa producing the higher levels. Although the peripheral pharmacokinetics of levodopa are not altered by 6OHDA [48,49] it is also possible that the reduced food intake routinely observed in rats with 6OHDA lesions [50] may have depleted peripheral levels of other large neutral amino acids reducing competition at LAT1 and leading to increased levodopa entry [51]. However, the increased entry of benserazide into the ipsilateral striatum strongly suggests increased entry since its levels are likely independent of DA degeneration. We administered benserazide at 50 mg/kg because this dose is routinely used in animal studies, and at this dose, is detectable in brain [52]. This is consistent with the measurable levels on both the ipsi- and contralateral striata in our studies. However, the results in the lesioned animals were in stark contrast to sham operated animals where there were no ipsi-contra differences.

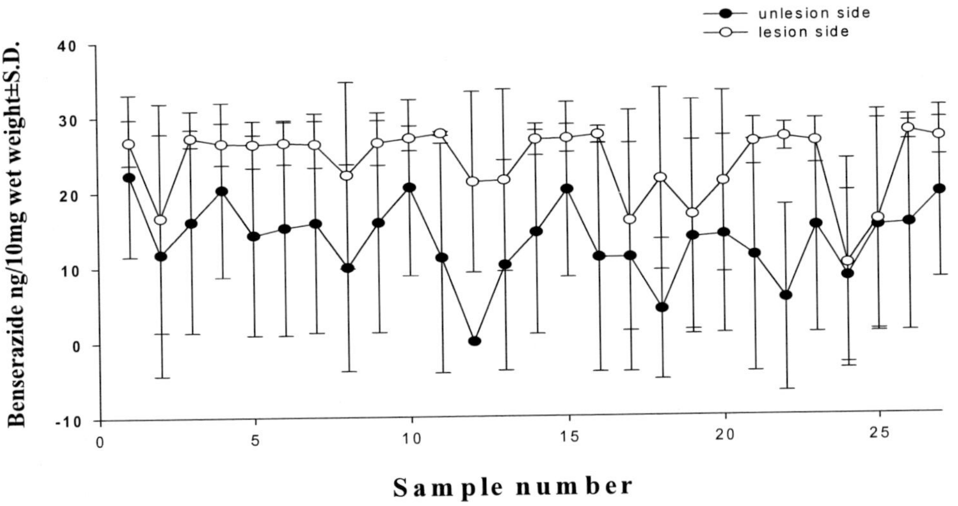

Figure 1. Levels of benserazide in the ipsi- (lesioned) and contralateral (unlesioned) straita after 6OHDA injection into the medial forebrain bundle. Depicted is the distribution of benserazide in striatum from the rostral regions (low numbered sections) to the caudal sections (higher numbered sections). The benserazide levels were elevated in every ipsilateral tissue section.

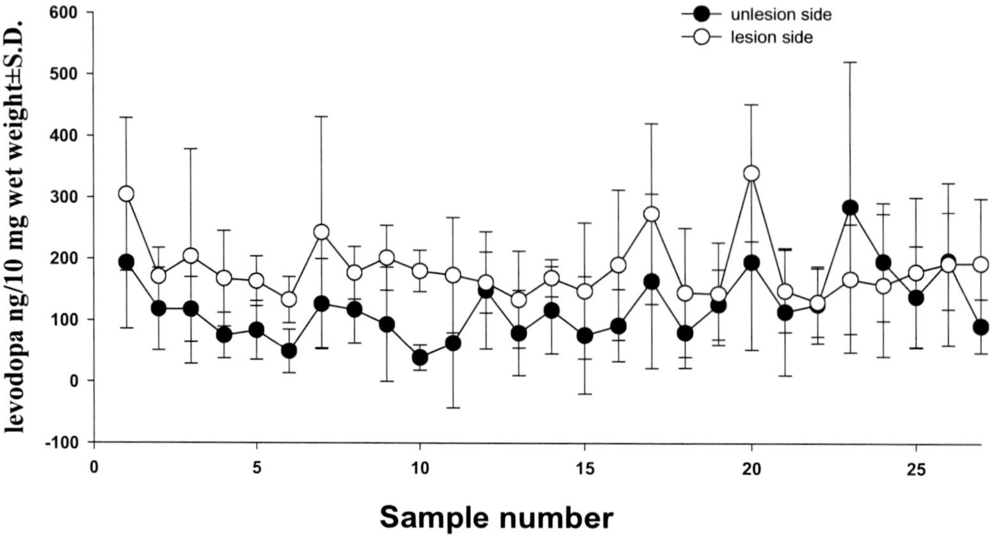

Figure 2. Levels of levodopa in the ipsi- (lesioned) and contralateral (unlesioned) straita after 6OHDA injection into the medial forebrain bundle. Depicted is the distribution of levodopa in striatum from the rostral regions (low numbered sections) to the caudal sections (higher numbered sections). The levodopa levels were elevated in almost every ipsilateral tissue section.

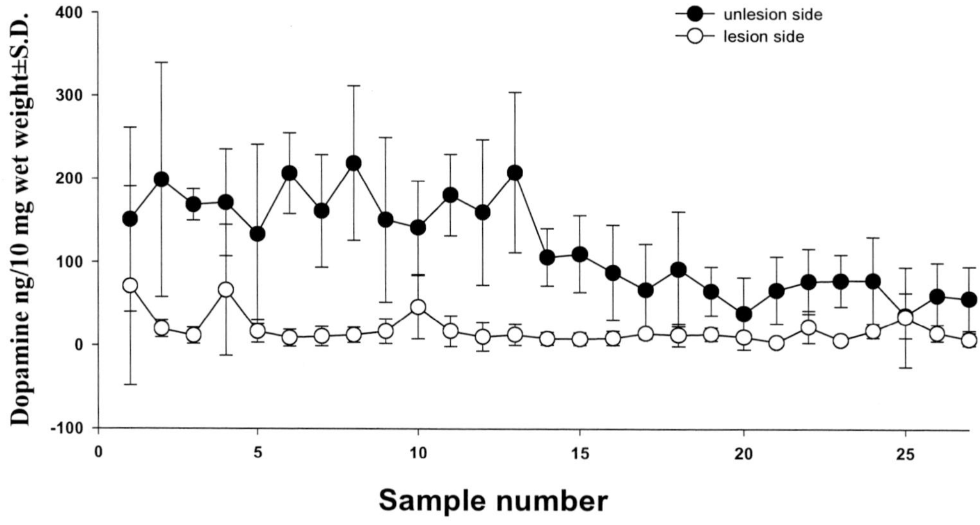

Figure 3. Levels of DA in the ipsi- (lesioned) and contralateral (unlesioned) straita after 6OHDA injection into the medial forebrain bundle. Depicted is the distribution of DA in striatum from the rostral regions (low numbered sections) to the caudal sections (higher numbered sections). The DA levels were reduced in every ipsilateral tissue section.

Although the increased levodopa observed on the ipsilateral side of the striatum could have been the result of increased entry into brain because of barrier compromise or increased benserazide entry or both, it was also possible that the barrier dysfunction led to alterations in the expression of the LAT1 transporter that normally carries levodopa into parenchyma. However, Western Blot analysis of LAT-1 protein revealed no ipsi-contra differences

($F_{3,16}$=0.655, p>0.05; Figure 4) suggesting that alterations in LAT-1 expression were not involved. Although LAT1 expression was unchanged, it is possible that its function could have been increased or that the newly discovered, highly active, Na+-dependent transporter (Na+-LNAA) present on the ablumenal side of the BBB and extrudes large neutral amino acids [53], could have been compromised. Regardless, taken together, these data suggest that the barrier dysfunction produced by 6OHDA did have functional consequences in terms of benserazide entry and further, that there may well be significant alterations in levodopa entry that could contribute to efficacy alterations and side effect production. Further studies are needed to clarify the interpretation of these data.

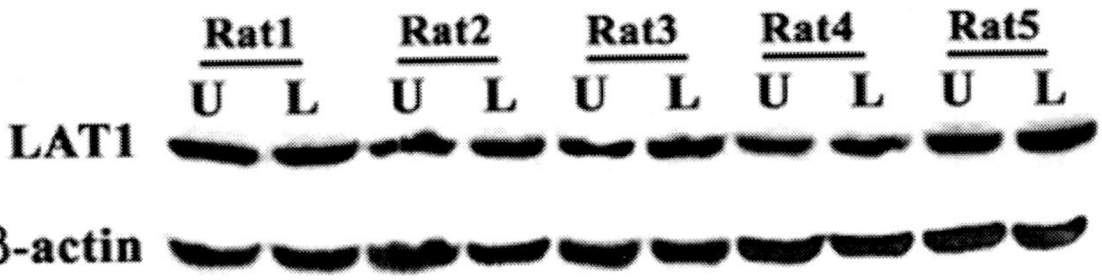

Figure 4. Western blot image of LAT1 and the loading controls of β-actin in the ipsilateral (L) and contralateral (U) striata of animals following 6OHDA injection into the medial forebrain bundle. The expression of the large neutral amino acid transporter-1 (LAT1) was not altered by 6OHDA .

It is important to appreciate that the BBB leakage seen in our prior 6OHDA and MPTP studies was not uniform across the striatum or SN, but rather punctuate [1,37]. Indeed, although there were numerous patchy areas of leakage, the majority of the BBB in the striatum was normal. Since the average ipsilateral levels of benserazide and levodopa were markedly higher than the contralateral side, it is likely that in areas of BBB leakage, these levels would have been considerably higher. This raises the interesting possibility that heterogeneous levels of benserazide and levodopa would likely occur at therapeutic dosages used in PD patients. These results are also consistent with our prior study where we observed increased entry of domperidone into the brains of animals with 6OHDA lesions. Thus, we performed intra-ventricular injections of 6OHDA into rats that produced unilateral DA neuron loss. After 14 days, we then injected the animals with apomorphine, a DA agonist that leads to intense stereotypic behaviors. We then injected domperidone systemically. This drug is a substrate for p-glycoprotein and is normally excluded from the brain and therefore useful in treating peripheral DA-mediated side effects in PD patients without compromising central DA replacement therapy efficacy. We demonstrated reductions in stereotypic behaviors in the 6OHDA animals compared with controls despite overt up-regulation of p-glycoprotein expression [1]. Apparently, disruption of barrier integrity led to what could be considered a compensatory response (i.e., increased p-glycoprotein), but this up-regulation was still not adequate to exclude domperidone from the brain since the apomorphine-induced stereotypic behavior was attenuated. This represents yet another example of BBB compromise leading to functional consequences.

Discussion

Overcoming the BBB to Deliver Therapeutics

Conventional thinking suggests that many drugs do not cross the BBB and are therefore not useful in treating CNS disease. Typically, only lipid soluble molecules with a low molecular mass of <500 Daltons are thought to enter brain parenchyma [54,55]. Although a molecule may meet one of these criteria, but not the other, usually means that the molecule will not penetrate the BBB. Histamine, for example, has a low molecular weight of 111 D but is limited in crossing the BBB by its hydrogen-bond-forming function groups [9]. Pharmacokinetic properties of a drug can also affect its BBB penetration. A drug with a large volume of distribution, rapid degradation or uptake by plasma proteins and a short half-life in circulation will not readily penetrate the BBB [56]. Enzymatic degradation in the endothelial cells of the BBB can also limit access of drug across the BBB [57]. It is also important to appreciate that the endothelial barrier is polarized. Some transporters are present on the abluminal side but not on the luminal side of the endothelial cells [58]. LAT-1, for instance, is located on the luminal surface and can carry levodopa into the endothelial cell but then needs to be transported into brain parenchyma by another transporter located on the ablumenal side of the endothelial cells. This points to the possibility that other unknown ablumenal transporters work in concert with other carrier-mediated transporters such as transferrin, GLUT1, LAT1, MCT1, CNT2, or active efflux transporters mechanisms such as P-glycoprotein, OATp2, or BSAT1 to mediate transport of molecules across the BBB.

Despite our current knowledge of the BBB, most strategies developed to overcome the BBB have centered around developing molecules that can take advantage of the numerous transport mechanisms present on the luminal side of the barrier. As clever as many of these strategies are, they are based on the notion that the BBB is intact in the diseased brain. Thus, water soluble drugs conjugated to lipid soluble carriers have been proposed. This pro-drug strategy presumes that the conjugate will be metabolized to the active drug once inside the CNS [9]. Drugs co-administered with a drug of interest can, for example, be used to inhibit the activity of efflux transporters such as P-glycoprotein which normally reduces the active drug's penetration. These traditional strategies have given way to more advanced techniques.

One current strategy involves the use of monoclonal antibodies acting as "Trojan horses" to deliver target specific drugs. Thus, peptidomimetic monoclonal antibodies (MAb) may cross the BBB via receptor mediated transport and can be used to deliver large molecule pharmaceuticals, including recombinant protein, RNA interference drugs or non-viral gene medicines [59]. Xia et al. recently demonstrated delivery of siRNA to rat brain tumors in vivo with the combined use of a receptor-specific monoclonal antibody and avidin-biotin technology [60]. In another study, glial cell line derived neurotrophic factor (GDNF; a large molecular weight neurotrophin with DA neurotrophic activity), that could potentially treat PD and stroke was similarly delivered. Human GDNF was re-engineered to fuse to a MAb to the human insulin receptor (HIRMAb). This fusion protein apparently bound to the human insulin receptor, triggered receptor-mediated transport across the BBB where GDNF was released to activate neuroprotection pathways [61].

The strategy of delivering genes across the BBB is also under development using gene targeting technology and molecular Trojan horses. In order to deliver a gene to the CNS, a non-viral super-coiled plasmid DNA is placed inside a 85 nm “pegylated” liposome. The liposome is then coated with a peptidomimetic MAb to form a pegylated immunoliposome (PIL). The MAb enables the PIL to become transcytosed across the BBB via receptor-mediated transcytosis, followed by receptor-mediated endocytosis across the neuronal cell membrane [62]. Thus, in the 6OHDA model of PD, a non-viral expression plasmid encoding rat TH was encapsulated in PILs and targeted to brain by murine MAb (OX26) producing a 100% normalization of striatal TH activity [63,64]. In another study, using a similar technology, a GDNF plasmid DNA non-viral gene was delivered IV in a PD model using Trojan horse liposomes fused with a MAb to the rat transferrin receptor. The results indicated a long lasting reduction in apormorphine-induced rotational behaviors which were correlated with a 19 fold increase in striatal TH enzyme activity [65]. These studies demonstrate the feasibility of these strategies in delivering large molecules across the BBB. But, what if the BBB was not intact in neurodegenerative diseases? Would these techniques be necessary? Moreover, did these studies work in disease based models because of the proposed mechanisms, or because the BBB was compromised by the disease process? Because conventional wisdom suggests that the BBB is intact in these diseases, one is forced to ask if systemic delivery of some of these molecules has ever been tried independent of these “penetration strategies?”

The advent of nanoparticles has also suggested another possible mechanism to deliver non-BBB penetrating drugs into the CNS. Nanoparticles conjugated to specific ligands that target receptors on the brain microvasculature have been proposed as a means of carrying drugs into the brain through receptor mediated transcytosis [66]. The major advantage here is that virtually any compound can be placed into the nanoparticles, although one has to determine how to open the particle once it is inside the brain. In our lab, we tested the feasibility of this technology.

We filled 50 nm nanoparticles with European which spontaneously fluoresces under UV light. Using MPTP lesioned mice, we infused these nanoparticles into the carotid artery along with FITC-labeled albumin as we have traditionally done in our previous BBB studies. Three minutes later we sacrificed the animals. The results revealed that the vasculature was intact in the sham controls as evidenced by vessels filled with FITC (Figure 5). As we have seen in every animal study that examined the integrity of the BBB following DA neurotoxin exposure, animals treated with MPTP exhibited FITC-labeled albumin leakage into brain parenchyma suggesting barrier compromise. Interestingly, the nanoparticles did not enter brain parenchyma in the saline controls. This is consistent with the notion that there is little pinocytosis in the brain vasculature and the tight junctions present are much smaller than 50 nM. In the MPTP mice however, there was significant immunofluorescence in brain parenchyma that was highly concordant with areas of FITC-labeled albumin leakage in the adjacent tissue section. This again suggests that the BBB is physically compromised in association with DA neuron degeneration although the notion that MPTP exposure up-regulated pinocytotic function in brain capillaries cannot be ruled out. This study serves to further illustrate the assumption that delivery strategies that do not use a targeting strategy (e.g., MAb) may enter a diseased brain because of barrier compromise.

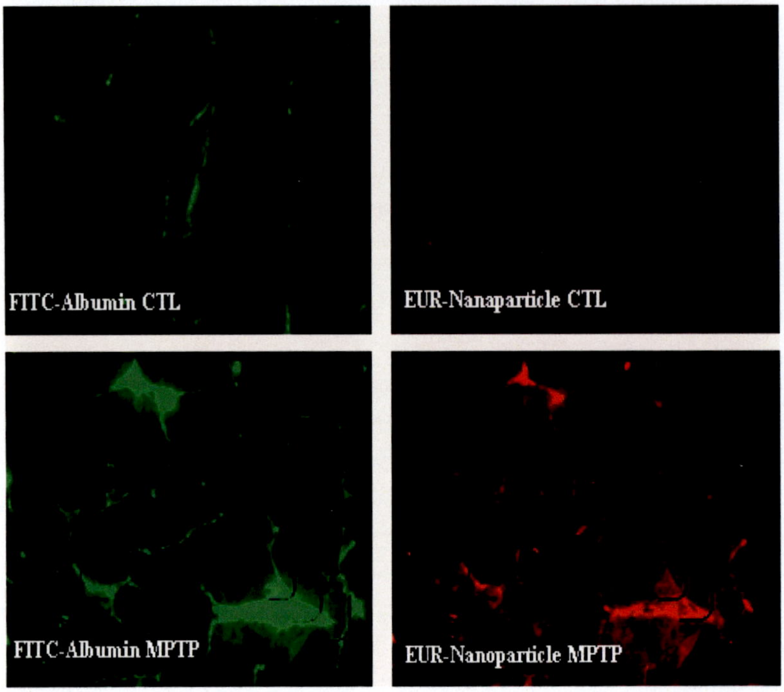

Figure 5. Delivery of EUR-nanoparticle in an MPTP treated animal. As indicated in the figure, FITC-Albumin leakage is seen in the MPTP treated animal compared to the saline treated control animal. The EUR-nanoparticle leakage is also present in the MPTP treated animal but not the Saline control animal.

Implications of Barrier Compromise in PD for Targeted Delivery

Emerging evidence from several laboratories appears to suggest BBB dysfunction in animal models of PD that produce functional consequence (i.e., increased drug entry or dyskinesias). Although these observations raise the specter that drugs not normally considered capable of entering brain because of the BBB may do so in PD, it also raises the issue of targeted delivery. If our observations in animals are correct and the barrier compromise is punctate due to regional areas of neuroinflammation, then the barrier is likely to be compromised only in those areas. Thus, only active areas of active neurodegeneration would be capable of opening the BBB. This has a number of implications for targeted delivery in PD.

First, neuroprotective strategies are presumed to rescue remaining DA neurons to stop disease progression. If punctate barrier compromise occurs, systemic delivery of non- or poor BBB penetrating drugs could be delivered systemically and only or primarily enter, respectively, areas of active degeneration. (Figure 6) Given that the physical barrier is likely compromised, this would lead to targeted delivery of high concentrations of active neuroprotective agent. In contrast, punctate leakage would also lead to high concentrations of neurotoxic substances that could exacerbate DA neuron loss. As we have discussed elsewhere, this would also allow for entry or peripheral immune mediators that might contribute to disease progression [2]. Alternatively, breakdown of the BBB might facilitate the exit of tropic chemokines that direct peripheral immune mediators to areas of active degeneration. Second, since high concentrations of drugs may be achieved in areas of barrier compromise, systemically delivered drugs dosages could be reduced as a result of this targeted delivery. Third, the focal barrier compromise may lead to expression of certain antigens that could serve as homing targets for systemically administered antibodies designed to target these punctate sites. Finally, systemic nanoparticle delivery to the punctate region of barrier compromise could utilize neuroinflammatory mediators to open them and deliver their contents.

The available data to date strongly suggests the need to explore the role of neuroinflammation mediated barrier compromise further. Clearly, more work needs to be done to establish the validity, magnitude and mechanism of this phenomenon. However, it does appear to be time to question the conventional wisdom behind the notion that chemicals delivered to the brains of patients with PD, or other neurodegenerative diseases associated with neuroinflammation for that matter, need to be manipulated in some fashion to enter the diseased brain.

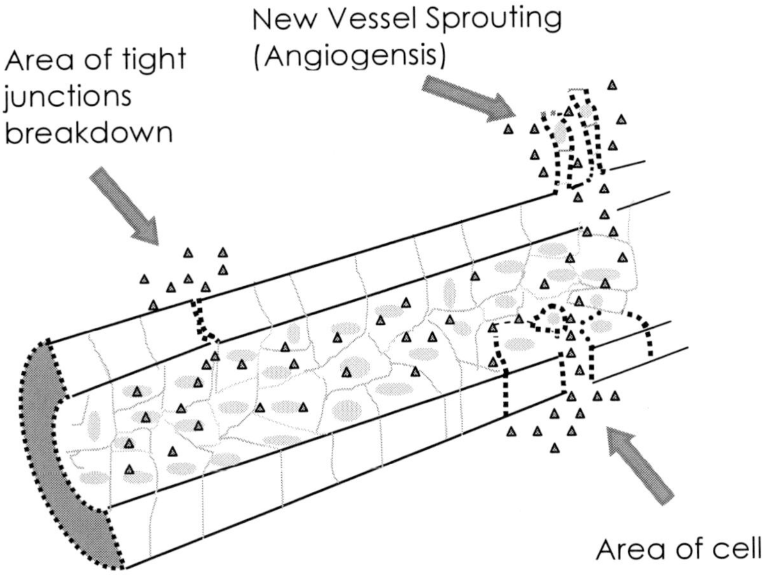

Figure 6. Mechanisms by which drug delivery could be compromised during disease states with a known altered blood-brain-barrier. During the process of angiogenesis, new vessel sprouting occurs which can lead to leaky vessels and region specific delivery of drug. Also, areas of endothelial cell necrosis result in loss of tight junctions, cell shrinkage and leakage of drug. Areas of tight junction breakdown also lead to leaky vessels and an increase in drug delivery to the parenchyma. Thus, given a disrupted BBB during diseases such as PD, therapeutics used to treat the disease may in fact be acting in localized areas, creating unwanted side effects.

References

[1] Carvey PM, Zhao CH, Hendey B, Lum H, Trachtenberg J, Desai BS et al. 6-Hydroxydopamine-induced alterations in blood-brain barrier permeability. *Eur J Neurosci* 2005; 22(5):1158-1168.

[2] Monahan AJ, Carvey PM. Neuroinflammation and Peripheral Immune Infiltration in Parkinson's disease: An autoimmune hypothesis. *Cell Transplantation* 2008; 17:1-10.

[3] Ehrlich P. Ueber die beziehungen von chemischer constitution, verteilung und pharmakologischer wirkung. *Gesammelte Arbeiten zur Immunitaetsforschung* 1904; 574.

[4] Goldmann E. Vitalfarbung am zentralnervensystem. *Abhandl Konigl preuss Akad Wiss* 1913; 1:1-60.

[5] Oldendorf W.H., Cornford ME, Brown W.J. The large appent work capability of the blood-brain barrier: A study of the mitochondrial content of capillary endothelial cells in brain and other tissues of the rat. *Ann Neurol* 1977; 1 :409-417.

[6] Fenstermacher J, Kaye T. Drug "diffusion" within the brain. *Ann N Y Acad Sci* 1988; 531:29-39.

[7] Sedlakova R, Shivers RR, Del Maestro RF. Ultrastructure of the blood-brain barrier in the rabbit. *J Submicrosc Cytol Pathol* 1999; 31(1):149-161.

[8] Kniesel U, Wolburg H. Tight junctions of the blood-brain barrier. *Cell Mol Neurobiol* 2000; 20(1):57-76.

[9] Pardridge WM. *Brain Drug Targeting: The Future of Brain Drug Development.* Cambridge, U.K.: Cambridge University Press, 2001.

[10] Abbott NJ. Astrocyte-endothelial interactions and blood-brain barrier permeability. *J Anat* 2002; 200(6):629-638.

[11] Bauer HC, Bauer H. Neural induction of the blood-brain barrier: still an enigma. *Cell Mol Neurobiol* 2000; 20(1):13-28.

[12] Gaillard PJ, van dS, I, Voorwinden LH, Vu D, Nielsen JL, de Boer AG et al. Astrocytes increase the functional expression of P-glycoprotein in an in vitro model of the blood-brain barrier. *Pharm Res* 2000; 17(10):1198-1205.

[13] Haseloff RF, Blasig IE, Bauer HC, Bauer H. In search of the astrocytic factor(s) modulating blood-brain barrier functions in brain capillary endothelial cells in vitro. *Cell Mol Neurobiol* 2005; 25(1):25-39.

[14] Kniesel U, Wolburg H. Tight junctions of the blood-brain barrier. *Cell Mol Neurobiol* 2000; 20(1):57-76.

[15] Rubin LL, Staddon JM. The cell biology of the blood-brain barrier. *Annu Rev Neurosci* 1999; 22:11-28.

[16] Stevenson BR, Keon BH. The tight junction: morphology to molecules. *Annu Rev Cell* Dev Biol 1998; 14:89-109.

[17] Farkas E, Luiten PG. Cerebral microvascular pathology in aging and Alzheimer's disease. *Prog Neurobiol* 2001; 64(6):575-611.

[18] Hawkins BT, Davis TP. The blood-brain barrier/neurovascular unit in health and disease. *Pharmacol Rev* 2005; 57(2):173-185.

[19] Yu C, Kastin AJ, Tu H, Waters S, Pan W. TNF activates P-glycoprotein in cerebral microvascular endothelial cells. *Cell Physiol Biochem* 2007; 20(6):853-858.

[20] Yang HW, Liu HY, Liu X, Zhang DM, Liu YC, Liu XD et al. Increased P-glycoprotein function and level after long-term exposure of four antiepileptic drugs to rat brain microvascular endothelial cells in vitro. *Neurosci Lett* 2008; 434(3):299-303.

[21] Al Anizy M, Horley NJ, Kuo CW, Gillett LC, Laughton CA, Kendall D et al. Cytochrome P450 Cyp4x1 is a major P450 protein in mouse brain. *FEBS J* 2006; 273(5):936-947.

[22] Granberg L, Ostergren A, Brandt I, Brittebo EB. CYP1A1 and CYP1B1 in blood-brain interfaces: CYP1A1-dependent bioactivation of 7,12-dimethylbenz(a)anthracene in endothelial cells. *Drug Metab Dispos* 2003; 31(3):259-265.

[23] Kago T, Takagi N, Date I, Takenaga Y, Takagi K, Takeo S. Cerebral ischemia enhances tyrosine phosphorylation of occludin in brain capillaries. *Biochem Biophys Res Commun* 2006; 339(4):1197-1203.

[24] Toborek M, Lee YW, Flora G, Pu H, Andras IE, Wylegala E et al. Mechanisms of the blood-brain barrier disruption in HIV-1 infection. *Cell Mol Neurobiol* 2005; 25(1):181-199.

[25] Van der FM, Hoppenreijs S, van Rensburg AJ, Ruyken M, Kolk AH, Springer P et al. Vascular endothelial growth factor and blood-brain barrier disruption in tuberculous meningitis. *Pediatr Infect Dis J* 2004; 23(7):608-613.

[26] Huber JD, Campos CR, Mark KS, Davis TP. Alterations in blood-brain barrier ICAM-1 expression and brain microglial activation after lambda-carrageenan-induced inflammatory pain. *Am J Physiol Heart Circ Physiol* 2006; 290(2):H732-H740.

[27] Reynolds DS, Morton AJ. Changes in blood-brain barrier permeability following neurotoxic lesions of rat brain can be visualised with trypan blue. *J Neurosci Methods* 1998; 79(1):115-121.

[28] van Horssen J, Brink BP, de Vries HE, van d, V, Bo L. The blood-brain barrier in cortical multiple sclerosis lesions. *J Neuropathol Exp Neurol* 2007; 66(4):321-328.

[29] Kalaria RN. The blood-brain barrier and cerebral microcirculation in Alzheimer disease. *Cerebrovasc Brain Metab Rev* 1992; 4(3):226-260.

[30] McGeer PL, McGeer EG. Glial reactions in Parkinson's disease. *Mov Disord* 2007.

[31] Barcia C, Emborg ME, Hirsch EC, Herrero MT. Blood vessels and parkinsonism. *Front Biosci* 2004; 9:277-282.

[32] Faucheux BA, Bonnet AM, Agid Y, Hirsch EC. Blood vessels change in the mesencephalon of patients with Parkinson's disease. *Lancet* 1999; 353(9157):981-982.

[33] Barcia C, Emborg ME, Hirsch EC, Herrero MT. Blood vessels and parkinsonism. *Front Biosci* 2004; 9:277-282.

[34] Faucheux BA, Bonnet AM, Agid Y, Hirsch EC. Blood vessels change in the mesencephalon of patients with Parkinson's disease. *Lancet* 1999; 353(9157):981-982.

[35] Kortekaas R, Leenders KL, van Oostrom JC, Vaalburg W, Bart J, Willemsen AT et al. Blood-brain barrier dysfunction in parkinsonian midbrain in vivo. *Ann Neurol* 2005; 57(2):176-179.

[36] Kortekaas R, Leenders KL, van Oostrom JC, Vaalburg W, Bart J, Willemsen AT et al. Blood-brain barrier dysfunction in parkinsonian midbrain in vivo. *Ann Neurol* 2005; 57(2):176-179.

[37] Zhao CH, Ling ZD, Newman MB, Bhatia A, Carvey PM. TNF-Alpha Knockout and Minocycline Treatment Attenuates Blood Brain Barrier Leakage in MPTP-Treated Mice. *Neubiology of Disease*. In press.

[38] Zhao C, Ling Z, Newman MB, Bhatia A, Carvey PM. TNF-alpha knockout and minocycline treatment attenuates blood-brain barrier leakage in MPTP-treated mice. *Neurobiol Dis* 2007; 26(1):36-46.

[39] Killian DM, Chikhale PJ. Predominant functional activity of the large, neutral amino acid transporter (LAT1) isoform at the cerebrovasculature. *Neurosci Lett* 2001; 306(1-2):1-4.

[40] Killian DM, Chikhale PJ. Predominant functional activity of the large, neutral amino acid transporter (LAT1) isoform at the cerebrovasculature. *Neurosci Lett* 2001; 306(1-2):1-4.

[41] Kageyama T, Nakamura M, Matsuo A, Yamasaki Y, Takakura Y, Hashida M et al. The 4F2hc/LAT1 complex transports L-DOPA across the blood-brain barrier. *Brain Res* 2000; 879(1-2):115-121.

[42] Kageyama T, Nakamura M, Matsuo A, Yamasaki Y, Takakura Y, Hashida M et al. The 4F2hc/LAT1 complex transports L-DOPA across the blood-brain barrier. *Brain Res* 2000; 879(1-2):115-121.

[43] Graybiel AM, Canales JJ, Capper-Loup C. Levodopa-induced dyskinesias and dopamine-dependent stereotypies: a new hypothesis. *Trends Neurosci* 2000; 23(10 Suppl):S71-S77.

[44] Braak H, Ghebremedhin E, Rub U, Bratzke H, Del Tredici K. Stages in the development of Parkinson's disease-related pathology. *Cell Tissue Res* 2004; 318(1):121-134.

[45] Westin J, Nyholm D, Groth T, Dougherty MS, Yerramsetty PK, Palhagen SE. Outcome prediction of enteral levodopa/carbidopa infusion in advanced Parkinson's disease. *Parkinsonism Relat Disord* 2006; 12(8):509-513.

[46] Bankiewicz KS, Daadi M, Pivirotto P, Bringas J, Sanftner L, Cunningham J et al. Focal striatal dopamine may potentiate dyskinesias in parkinsonian monkeys. *Exp Neurol* 2006; 197(2):363-372.

[47] Bankiewicz KS, Daadi M, Pivirotto P, Bringas J, Sanftner L, Cunningham J et al. Focal striatal dopamine may potentiate dyskinesias in parkinsonian monkeys. *Exp Neurol* 2006; 197(2):363-372.

[48] Carta M, Lindgren HS, Lundblad M, Stancampiano R, Fadda F, Cenci MA. Role of striatal L-DOPA in the production of dyskinesia in 6-hydroxydopamine lesioned rats. *J Neurochem* 2006; 96(6):1718-1727.

[49] Carta M, Lindgren HS, Lundblad M, Stancampiano R, Fadda F, Cenci MA. Role of striatal L-DOPA in the production of dyskinesia in 6-hydroxydopamine lesioned rats. *J Neurochem* 2006; 96(6):1718-1727.

[50] Salamone JD, Mahan K, Rogers S. Ventrolateral striatal dopamine depletions impair feeding and food handling in rats. *Pharmacol Biochem Behav* 1993; 44(3):605-610.

[51] Hellenbrand W, Boeing H, Robra BP, Seidler A, Vieregge P, Nischan P et al. Diet and Parkinson's disease. II: A possible role for the past intake of specific nutrients. Results from a self-administered food-frequency questionnaire in a case-control study. *Neurology* 1996; 47(3):644-650.

[52] Jonkers N, Sarre S, Ebinger G, Michotte Y. Benserazide decreases central AADC activity, extracellular dopamine levels and levodopa decarboxylation in striatum of the rat. *J Neural Transm* 2001; 108(5):559-570.

[53] Hawkins RA, Mokashi A, Simpson IA. An active transport system in the blood-brain barrier may reduce levodopa availability. *Exp Neurol* 2005; 195(1):267-271.

[54] Levin VA. Relationship of octanol/water partition coefficient and molecular weight to rat brain capillary permeability. *J Med Chem* 1980; 23(6):682-684.

[55] Banks WA, Kastin AJ. Peptides and the blood-brain barrier: lipophilicity as a predictor of permeability. *Brain Res Bull* 1985; 15(3):287-292.

[56] Banks WA. Delivery of peptides to the brain: Emphasis on therapeutic development. *Biopolymers* 2008.

[57] Pardridge WM. BBB-Genomics: creating new openings for brain-drug targeting. *Drug Discov Today* 2001; 6(8):381-383.

[58] Hawkins RA, O'Kane RL, Simpson IA, Vina JR. Structure of the blood-brain barrier and its role in the transport of amino acids. *J Nutr* 2006; 136(1 Suppl):218S-226S.

[59] Pardridge WM. Drug targeting to the brain. Pharm Res 2007; 24(9):1733-1744.

[60] Xia CF, Zhang Y, Zhang Y, Boado RJ, Pardridge WM. Intravenous siRNA of brain cancer with receptor targeting and avidin-biotin technology. *Pharm Res* 2007; 24(12):2309-2316.

[61] Boado RJ, Zhang Y, Zhang Y, Wang Y, Pardridge WM. GDNF fusion protein for targeted-drug delivery across the human blood-brain barrier. *Biotechnol Bioeng* 2007.

[62] Zhang YF, Boado RJ, Pardridge WM. Absence of toxicity of chronic weekly intravenous gene therapy with pegylated immunoliposomes. *Pharm Res* 2003; 20(11):1779-1785.

[63] Shi N, Pardridge WM. Noninvasive gene targeting to the brain. *Proc Natl Acad Sci U S A* 2000; 97(13):7567-7572.

[64] Zhang Y, Calon F, Zhu C, Boado RJ, Pardridge WM. Intravenous nonviral gene therapy causes normalization of striatal tyrosine hydroxylase and reversal of motor impairment in experimental parkinsonism. *Hum Gene Ther* 2003; 14(1):1-12.

[65] Xia CF, Boado RJ, Zhang Y, Chu C, Pardridge WM. Intravenous glial-derived neurotrophic factor gene therapy of experimental Parkinson's disease with Trojan horse liposomes and a tyrosine hydroxylase promoter. *J Gene Med* 2008; 10(3):306-315.

[66] Kabanov AV, Batrakova EV. New technologies for drug delivery across the blood brain barrier. *Curr Pharm Des* 2004; 10(12):1355-1363.

In: The Blood-Brain Barrier
Editor: Tomas R. Helio
ISBN 978-1-60456-894-3

Chapter 6

IMAGING OF THE BLOOD-BRAIN BARRIER IN ACUTE NEUROLOGICAL EVENTS: DIAGNOSTIC AND PROGNOSTIC IMPLICATIONS

Mordechai Lorberboym[1,*] and Yair Lampl[2]
[1]Department of Nuclear Medicine and the [2]department of Neurology of the Edith Wolfson Medical Center, Sackler Faculty of Medicine, Tel Aviv University, Tel Aviv, Israel.

INTRODUCTION

The blood brain barrier (BBB) is a highly selective barrier of brain microvascular endothelial cells that shields the brain from toxic substances in the blood, supplies brain tissues with nutrients, and filters harmful compounds from the brain back to the bloodstream [1]. Transport across the BBB is strictly limited through both physical (tight junctions) and metabolic barriers (enzymes, diverse transport systems). BBB breakdown or alterations in transport systems play an important role in the pathogenesis of many CNS diseases (HIV-1 encephalitis, Alzheimer's disease, ischemia, tumors, multiple sclerosis, and Parkinson's disease).

The BBB in Ischemia

Cerebral ischemia leads to disruption of blood flow, increased BBB permeability, and is associated with rapid depletion of essential nutrients and oxygen [2,3]. Using in vitro models of BBB, Mark and Davis [4] demonstrated that hypoxia and reoxygenation increased BBB

* Correspondence concerning this article should be addressed to: Mordechai Lorberboym, M.D., Department of Nuclear Medicine, Edith Wolfson Medical Center, Holon, 58100 Israel. Phone: 011-972-544-630930; Fax: 011-972-3-5358494; Email: mvlorber@zahav.net.il.

permeability and were associated with tight junctions impairment. Vascular endothelial growth factor VEGF and nitric oxide (NO) mediate in part tight junctions alterations caused by hypoxia [4]. VEGF blocking diminished postischemic edema and tissue damage in vivo [5], indicating that tight junctions disruption is likely involved in the progression of ischemic brain injury.

THE BBB IN ACUTE ISCHEMIC STROKE

Experimental studies on animal models were performed in order to define the effect of BBB disruption in acute stroke [6-8]. Studies in rats demonstrated preservation of the BBB for the first 2-3 hours post middle cerebral artery (MCA) occlusion and progressive disruption following the first 6 hours [6]. Siegel et al [9] used a multiple tracer assessment of ischemic brain injury in rats including Tc-99m-pertechnetate. He proposed that abnormal molecular permeability of the BBB most likely results from damage to the endothelial cells or the intercellular junctions of the capillaries.

Only a few studies were designed in humans in order to compare the degree of BBB changes and the neurological outcome after a stroke. The most significant stage of BBB breakdown occurs in humans within 48-72 hours post infarction and is accompanied by increased brain edema volume. One study which examined cerebral spinal fluid (CSF) and serum albumin ratios as a parameter for the degree of BBB opening, found no difference between patients with a large or with a small infarct [10].

CT is used to detect hemorrhage and mass effect after a stroke, however, it is not sensitive at detecting brain ischemia in the acute stage of an infarct [11]. MRI is more sensitive than CT, but it may fail to detect hyperacute ischemia [12,13]. Perfusion-weighted and diffusion-weighted magnetic resonance imaging have been widely used to detect and quantify ischemia in experimental models [14]. Diffusion weighted MRI is sensitive to the translational motion of water protons and provides an image of apparent diffusion coefficients (ADCs). A mismatch between diffusion- and perfusion-weighted MRI is thought to define tissue at risk of infarction. This concept is based on the assumption that diffusion slowing of and decreases in the ADC serve as indicator of tissue proceeding to infarction. However, ADC decreases do not reliably indicate tissue infarction [15] and diffusion abnormalities probably correspond to early changes of both reversible and irreversible ischemia [16]. Moreover, MRI is expensive and has practical limitations in many patients with surgical implants and pacemakers.

Most positron emission tomography (PET) studies in stroke aimed to visualize changes in blood flow and energy metabolism. Marchal et al [17] used positron emission tomography (PET) with combined imaging of cerebral blood flow and oxygen consumption to distinguish three different uptake patterns after first MCA stroke, each associated with a different outcome.

Tc-99m-DTPA (Diethylenetriamine- pentacetic acid) brain scintigraphy is a useful technique for the assessment of BBB disruption. Is has been used in the past to localize areas within the cranium which had been disrupted by infection, neoplasms, trauma or stroke [18,19]. For the SPECT study each patient receives 740 MBq Tc-99m-DTPA and a SPECT study is performed 60-9- minutes later (Figure 1). A dual head or a triple head gamma camera is usually used, equipped with high resolution collimators.

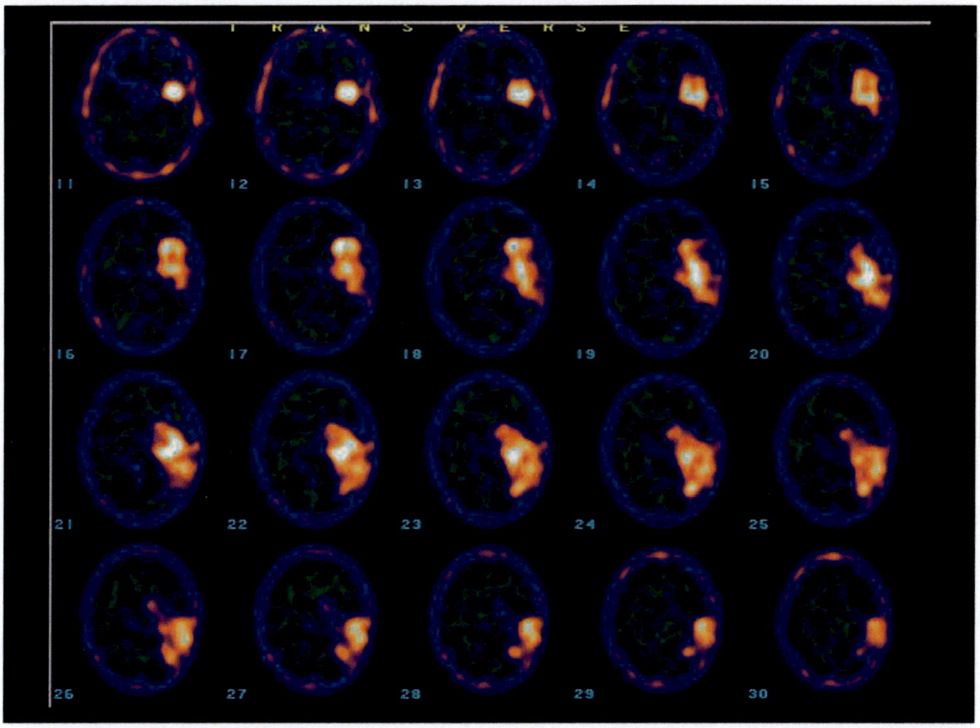

Figure 1. Transaxial DTPA SPECT slices from a 59 year-old female with a stroke in the territory of the left middle cerebral artery.

For quantitative analysis the transaxial slice with the most extensive DTPA uptake is selected, and a region of interest (ROI) is traced around the DTPA activity. A ROI of similar size and shape is drawn on the opposite side in a corresponding location. A quantitative index of BBB breakdown (disruption index, DI) is defined as the ratio of mean count/pixel in the infarcted region compared to the mean count/pixel in the contralateral non-affected hemisphere.

In a recent human study thirty consecutive patients with acute stroke of the middle cerebral artery occurring more than 24 hours and less than 48 hours before admission were investigated [20]. A CT scan was performed on all patients to determine the volume of stroke and the integrity of the BBB was evaluated using technetium-99m-DTPA brain SPECT. SPECT perfusion imaging was also performed with Tc-99m-HMPAO. The study showed that the magnitude of disruption of the BBB was negatively correlated with the change in neurological status with a sensitivity of 95% and a specificity of 89%. Perfusion abnormalities on the HMPAO SPECT studies which ranged between 12-90% (mean 37.6±17.8 %) compared to the contralateral non-affected side had no correlation to the neurological status, infarct volume by CT, or magnitude of BBB disruption. Interestingly, a significant proportion of patients with stroke (23%) had no gross evidence of BBB disruption, all of them with very good prognosis.

THE BBB IN HEMORRHAGIC STROKE

Among the victims of intracerebral hemorrhagic (ICH) stroke, 15%-20% have primary brain bleeding which varies in frequency from country to country [21-23]. The outcomes of hemorrhagic and ischemic strokes differ from one another. Hemorrhagic stroke, as opposed to ischemic stroke, has no formation of an ischemic penumbra surrounding the bleeding [24,25]. The perihematomal edema formation and the duration of its persistence are dependent upon the concentration of various blood degradation factors of the blood clot and its effect on the BBB [26-30]. Three main phases can be observed in the animal model during formation of the perihematomal edema: (1) the very early phase taking place during the first few hours involving the hydrostatic pressure and clot retraction; (2) second phase continuing on day 1 and 2 due to activation of the coagulation cascade and thrombin production; and (3) the third phase occurring on day 3 or later when the edema is induced by blood lysis and the hemoglobin toxic effect on neuron tissue [31,32]. Lee et al. showed that BBB permeability post bleeding increases significantly prior to occurrence of surrounding edema [33]. Xi et al. [34] and Bhasin et al. [35] showed a disruption of BBB during the first day after the infusion of lysed red blood cells and a multi-intense degree of disruption three days after packed red blood cells. Since the significance of the influence of BBB alone in human primary brain bleeding is not yet clear, we examined its clinical outcome in ICH in correlation both to the DTPA radioisotope examination and the bleeding itself as measured using neuroradiologic methods.

We conducted a study on twenty seven consecutive patients (17 men and 10 women, mean age 62.1 ± 10.1) with spontaneous intracerebral hemorrhage diagnosed by CT scan. Each patient underwent a complete neurological examination, including scoring of neurological deficit according to the NIH score [36] performed on days 1, 7 and 30 after the bleeding. Modified Rankin score [37,38] was used performed on days 90 and 180. The integrity of the BBB was evaluated using ^{99m}Tc-DTPA SPECT brain scintigraphy, as described (Figure 2). The volume of hemorrhage was calculated according to the method of Kothari et al [39]. The results of this preliminary study showed that the BBB disruption was in significant correlation with the late functional outcome, but not with the early neurological deficits. The volume of blood, as measured on CT scan, had no correlation to the BBB disruption degree and late functional outcome, but a significant correlation to the early neurological scores. The non correlation between the CT findings and the SPECT imaging data reflects the non correlation between the blood volume hemorrhage blood volume and the BBB disruption. This also reinforces preliminary animal study data, which show there are additional important factors dealing with the content of the hemorrhage, besides the volume itself [26-28]. It seems that the degree of BBB disruption of the ICH surrounding area varies from patient to patient and is only indirectly related to the mass of the blood damage of the perihematomal edema occurring independently of the early stage neurological deficits.

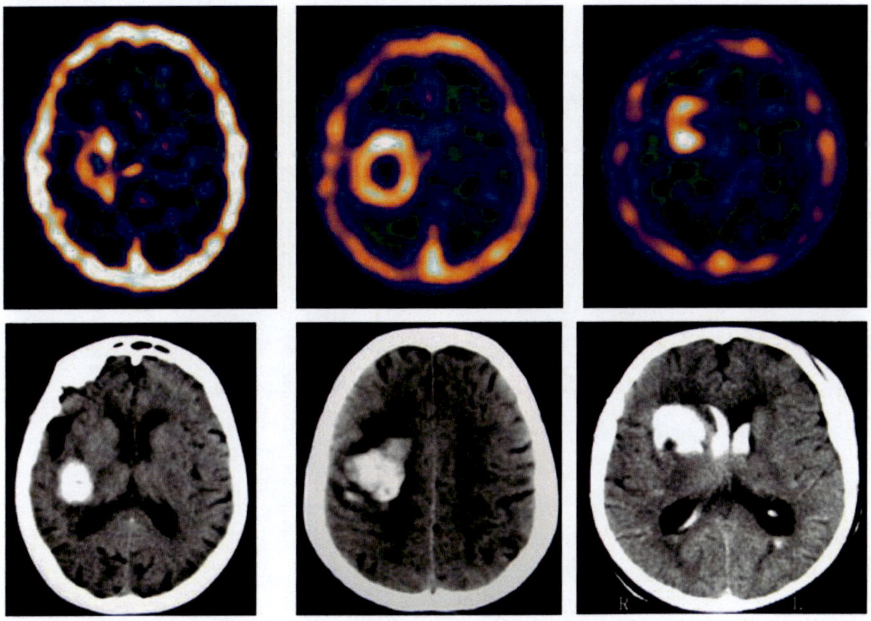

Figure 2. Three different patients with acute hemorrhagic stroke in the right MCA distribution. Note the rim of DTPA activity representing BBB disruption surrounding the core of bleeding.

The BBB in Malignant MCA Infarction

Malignant middle cerebral artery (MMCA) infarction is defined as a development of severe brain edema in the surrounding area of a large middle cerebral artery (MCA) infarction. The edema may lead to a rapid deterioration of consciousness, increase of intracranial pressure, brain midline shift and finally, herniation. The time peak of MMCA is on day 2-4 post stroke, with mortality rate up to 80% [40]. Treatment methods of decompressive craniotomy are very promising and lower the mortality rate significantly [41]. However, the reduction of this rate is dependent upon early intervention [41]. Studies on various methods have been published searching after an early prognostic marker to predict the development of MMCA using clinical techniques [42,43], CT scan findings [43,44], perfusion parameters [45] and different criteria of diffusion perfusion weighted MRI [46,47]. However, these methods have their limitations, either low sensitivity rate or management difficulties.

In order to find an efficient and easy to perform method which may predict the evolution of a large MCA infarct into a MMCA early in the course of a stroke, we examined the correlation between the degree of the blood brain barrier (BBB) permeability and MMCA. The results were compared to the clinical findings and to concurrent CT volume measurements.

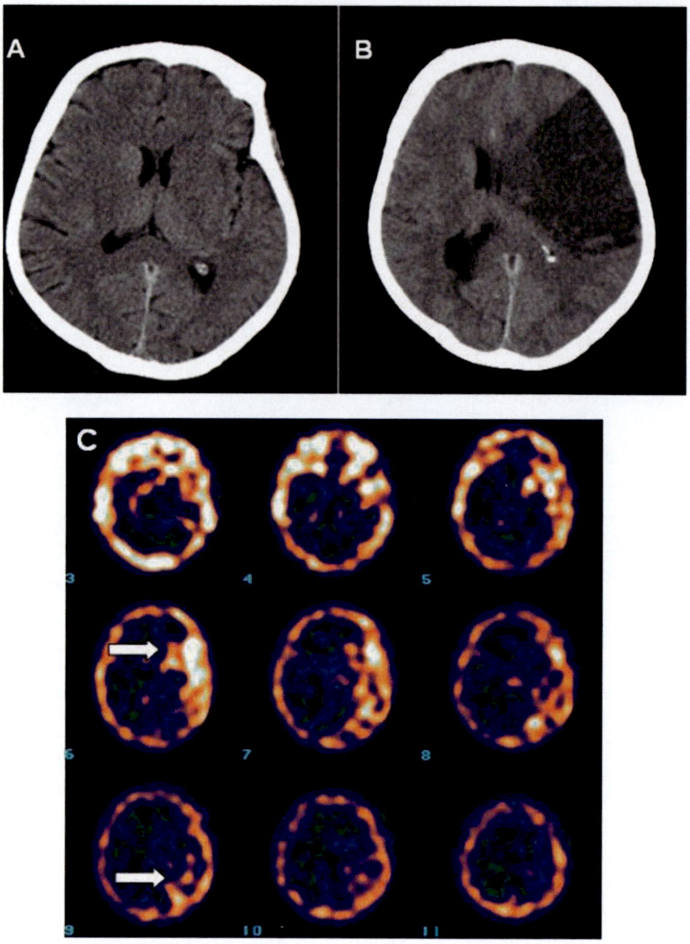

Figure 3. A patient with a left MCA stroke shows the CT on admission (A) resulting in brain herniation and death (B). There is characteristic widespread disruption of the BBB (C), invading the ACA and PCA territories (arrows).

The integrity of the BBB was evaluated using brain scintigraphy with technetium-99m DTPA at 36 hours after the stroke. Twenty five consecutive patients (17 men and 8 women, mean age 62.1 ± 10.1) were included in the study. The mean volume of stroke was 138 ± 87 cm^3. The mean DTPA disruption index was 6.6 ± 4.6 (range 1.0-21.0). The mean NIHSS score was 14 ± 4, with no significant difference between MMCA and non MMCA patients ($p=0.2$). Among the 25 patients 15 had a left hemispheric infarction, and 10 had a right hemispheric infarction. Five of 25 patients had brain herniation as evidenced on brain CT (Figure 3). In all five patients the clinical deterioration was characterized by decrease of consciousness, anisocoria and respiratory distress. The Glasgow Coma Score declined to a maximum score of 6. All patients were treated with intravenous Manitol. Four of the five patients died whereas one patient was rescued and remained with severe neurological deficits. Statistical analysis by T-Test continuous variables showed that the volume of stroke was only marginally elevated in patients with herniation ($p=0.062$).

All patients showed significant, inverse correlation between NIHSS score and DTPA uptake ($r=-0.43$, $p=0.033$). There was a significant correlation between the extent of DTPA distribution (more than one vascular territory) and the occurrence of herniation ($p<0.001$). In this study the DTPA-SPECT technique was an excellent predictor for the emergence of MMCA. The SPECT data showed a characteristic pattern not found in non MMCA patients: (1) the degree of BBB breakdown was significantly larger in the MMCA patients and (2) the area of distribution of BBB breakdown which occurred in the MMCA patients extended beyond the MCA region and clearly invaded the territories of other arteries.

It is noteworthy that none of our patients had clinical or imaging criteria compatible with MMCA infarct at the time of DTPA-SPECT imaging. Since no correlation was found between the area of BBB disruption and neurological deficit in any of the MMCA patients, it seems that the “malignant” extension of BBB disruption in MMCA is not only caused by the intensity of the stroke, but is also related to cascadic nuclear events leading to clinical deterioration and development of MMCA. Knowing that BBB breakdown has a role in the progress of MMCA may promote developing of medication to decrease this BBB disruption.

The BBB and Apoptosis in Acute Stroke

Apoptosis is an essential component of normal human growth and development, frequently described as "programmed cell death" (PCD). Apoptosis causes susceptible cells to undergo a series of enzymatic and morphologic changes encoded by the human genome. Apoptosis plays a significant role in the pathogenesis of many disorders including malignancy, organ and bone marrow transplant rejection, and tumor response to chemotherapy and radiation [48]. Evidence for apoptosis, including DNA fragmantation and TUNEL staining and protaction by p53 was found in epilepsy and traumtic brain injury [49,50], as well as in neurodegenerative diseases such as Alzheimer disease, Parkinson disease and amyotrophic lateral sclerosis [51,52]. The role of apoptosis in the cascade of brain ischemia was highlighted by findings of DNA fragmantation in vitro and in vivo [53,54], findings charecteristics of apoptosis in ultrastructural morphology [55], protection by Bcl-2 overexpression [56] and protection by p53 attenuation [57]. In vivo studies in animals show apoptotic cells 30 minutes after onset of the ischemic cascade, reaching a peak after 24-48 hours and remaining for 4 weeks [53].

Annexin V is an endogenous human protein which binds to membrane-bound phosphatidylserine (PS), a constitutive anionic membrane phospholipid [58]. PS is normally restricted to the inner leaflet of the plasma membrane lipid bilayer, but is exposed on the surfaces of cells as they undergo apoptosis Annexin V can be used in vitro to detect apoptosis before other well described morphologic or nuclear changes associated with apoptosis [48]. Labeled with fluorescein dye, annexin has been used to detect PS expression in hematopoietic cell lines, neurons, fibroblasts, endothelial cells, smooth muscle cells, carcinomas, lymphomas, and all embryonic cell types, [59]. Quantitative annexin-V tumor uptake values correlate well with the mean number of apoptotic cells.

Blankenberg and colleagues utilized radiolabeled annexin to detect apoptosis in vivo in animal models of transplant rejection, hypoxic cerebral injury, tumor therapy and Fas induced apoptosis [48,60]. In a rat model of cerebral ischemia moderate to severe injury was associated with remarkable focal radiolabeled annexin uptake, without evidence of BBB breakdown. Other studies on animal models have shown that reduced blood flow to the brain can alter the BBB permeability and regulatory transport functions [61,62].

Understanding the pattern and distribution of apoptosis in stroke may elucidate the mechanisms of neuronal injury and repair and promote new therapies that may prevent neuronal loss.

We conducted a study on humans in order to determine the ability of exogenously administered radiolabeled annexin V to concentrate at sites of apoptotic cell death in patients with acute cerebral strokes. The results were compared to the findings of BBB imaging using Tc-99m-DTPA SPECT and to concurrent CT volume measurements. Twelve consecutive patients (7 male and 5 female; mean age 66, range 36-83 years) with acute nonhemorrhagic stroke had a complete neurological examination, including the NIH stroke scale and the Glasgow coma scale (GCS). A CT scan was performed on all patients to determine the volume of stroke. A brain SPECT was obtained in all patients 2 hours after injection of annexin V. The integrity of the BBB was evaluated in seven patients using Tc-99m-DTPA brain SPECT at 24 hours after the annexin study. A quantitative index of apoptosis (AI) and of blood-brain barrier breakdown (DI) was calculated. Image fusion of the annexin V and DTPA studies was also performed.

Eight of 12 patients had abnormal increased uptake of annexin V corresponding to the pathological infarct regions identified by CT. The mean AI was 3.6 (range 1-15.6). The uptake was either focal or multifocal in all cases. In five of eight patients with abnormal studies foci of apoptosis were noted contralateral to the affected hemisphere as well.

All seven patients with DTPA SPECT showed breakdown of the BBB. The mean DI was 10.9 (range 3.2-26.3). DTPA ratio was significantly and positively associated with the NIH score ($r=0.80$, $p=0.01$) and inversely associated with GCS ($r=-0.89$, $p=-0.03$). In all cases image fusion showed only partial overlap between annexin and DTPA activity (Figure 4) with more widespread distribution of DTPA except for one case.

Annexin uptake showed a lack of correlation with the volume of stroke and it demonstrated multifocal distribution as opposed to the more diffuse and widespread DTPA distribution. These findings suggest a more specific role to annexin in imaging only the apoptotic regions and excluding areas with edema, and perhaps with necrosis.

Blankenberg have shown that moderate to severe injury, without evidence of blood-brain barrier breakdown, is associated with remarkable focal radiolabeled annexin uptake in an adult rat model of ischemic/reperfusion hemispheric injury [63,64]. Abnormal, bilateral, multifocal uptake of 99mTc-annexin V in each cerebral hemisphere was seen by both SPECT and autoradiography. Cell death, however, was not observed in the contralateral (normal) hemisphere in any of the brains studied. Blankenberg suggested that neuronal stress may play a role in the response of the brain to focal injury and be responsible for annexin V uptake outside the region of ischemic insult. Since the BBB was noted to be intact on the side of ischemic injury, disruption of the BBB was an unlikely mechanism for the significant increase in annexin V uptake within the brain.

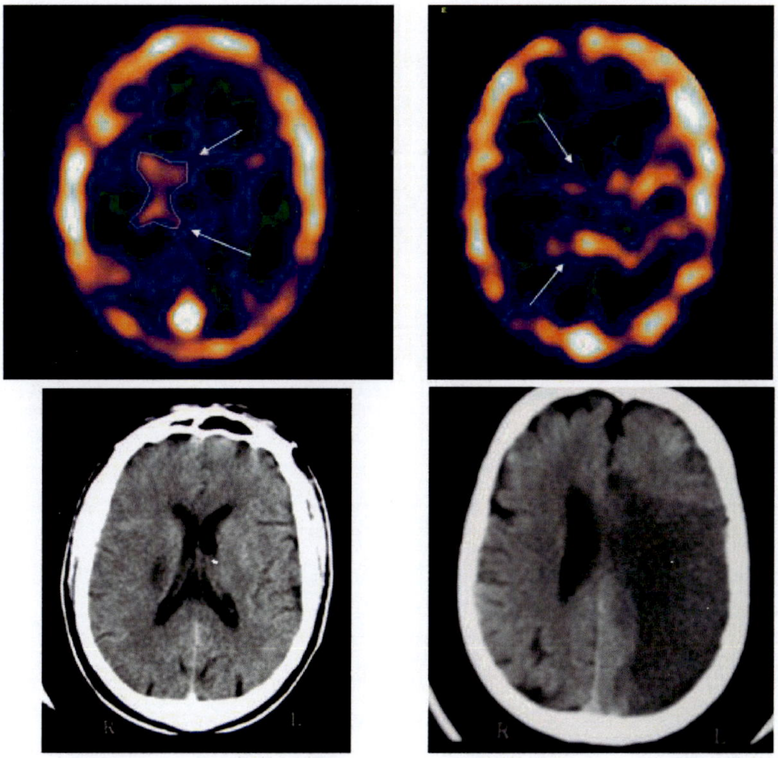

Figure 4. Annexin V brain SPECT in a patient with a right peri-ventricular stroke (left), showing a wider distribution of annexin (top, arrows) compared to the CT findings (bottom). Another patient with a cortical stroke localized to the left MCA region (right), shows extensive stroke on CT (bottom) with selective uptake of annexin in the same region (top, arrows), crossing the midline.

References

[1] Persidsky Y, Ramirez SH, Haorah J, Kanmogne GD. Blood-brain barrier: structural components and function under physiologic and pathologic conditions. *J Neuroimmune Pharmacol* 2006;1:223-236.

[2] del Zoppo GJ, Hallenbeck JM (2000) Advances in the vascular pathophysiology of ischemic stroke. *Thromb Res 98*:73–81

[3] Petty MA, Wettstein JG (2001) Elements of cerebral microvascular ischaemia. *Brain Res Rev 36*:23–34

[4] Mark KS, Davis TP (2002) Cerebral microvascular changes in permeability and tight junctions induced by hypoxia-reoxygenation. *Am J Physiol Heart Circ Physiol 282*:H1485–H1494

[5] van Bruggen N, Thibodeaux H, Palmer JT, Lee WP, Fu L, Cairns B, Tumas D, Gerlai R, Williams SP, van Lookeren Campagne M, Ferrara N (1999) VEGF antagonism reduces edema formation and tissue damage after ischemia/reperfusion injury in the mouse brain. *J Clin Invest 104*:1613–1620

[6] Belayev L, Busto R, Zhao W, Ginsberg MD. Quantitative evaluation of blood brain barrier permeability following middle cerebral artery occlusion in rats. *Brain Res.* 1996;739:88-96.

[7] Kuroiwa T, Shibutani M, Okeda R. Blood-brain barrier disruption and exacerbation of ischemic brain edema after restoration of blood flow in experimental focal cerebral ischemia. *Acta Neuropathol.* 1988;76:62-70.

[8] Yang BY, Betz AL. Reperfusion-induced injury to the blood-brain barrier after middle cerebral artery occlusion in rats. *Stroke*. 1994;25:1658-1664, discussion 1664-1665.

[9] Siegel BA, Meidinger R, Elliott AJ, et al. Experimental cerebral microembolism. Multiple tracer assessment of brain edema. *Arch Neurol.* 1972;26:73-77.

[10] Al-Kassab S, Skyhoj-Olsen T, Skriver EB. Blood-brain barrier integrity in patients with cerebral infarction investigated by computed tomography and serum-CSF-albumin. *Acta Neurol Scand.* 1981;64: 438-445.

[11] Lansberg MG, Albers GW, Beaulieu C, Marks MP. Comparison of diffusion-weighted MRI and CT in acute stroke. *Neurology*. 2000;54:1557-1561.

[12] Bryan RN, Levy LM, Whitlow WD, Killian JM, Preziosi TJ, Rosario JA. Diagnosis of acute cerebral infarction: comparison of CT and MR imaging. *Am J Neuroradiol.* 1991;12:611-620.

[13] Perkins CJ, Kahya E, Roque CT, Roche PE, Newman GC. Fluid-attenuated inversion recovery and diffusion- and perfusion-weighted MRI abnormalities in 117 consecutive patients with stroke symptoms. *Stroke*. 2001;32:2774-2781.

[14] Hossmann KA, Hoehn-Berlage M. Diffusion and perfusion MR imaging of cerebral ischemia. *Cerebrovasc Brain Metab Rev*. 1995;7:187-217.

[15] Fiehler J, Foth M, Kucinski T, et al. Severe ADC decreases do not predict irreversible tissue damage in humans. *Stroke*. 2002;33:79-86.

[16] Ringer TM, Neumann-Haefelin T, Sobel RA, Moseley ME, Yenari M. Reversal of early diffusion-weighted magnetic resonance imaging abnormalities does not necessarily reflect tissue salvage in experimental cerebral ischemia. *Stroke*. 2001;32:2362-2369.

[17] Marchal G, Serrati C, Rioux P, et al. PET imaging of cerebral perfusion and oxygen consumption in acute ischaemic stroke: relation to outcome [see comments]. *Lancet*. 1993;341:925-927.

[18] Barth A, Haldemann AR, Reubi JC, et al. Noninvasive differentiation of meningiomas from other brain tumours using combined 111Indium-octreotide/99mtechnetium-DTPA brain scintigraphy. *Acta Neurochir Wien*. 1996;138:1179-1185.

[19] Inoue Y, Momose T, Machida K, et al. Delayed imaging of Tc-99m-DTPA-HSA SPECT in subacute cerebral infarction. *Radiat Med.* 1993;11:214-216.

[20] 20. Peters KD, Kochanek KD, Murphy SL. Deaths: final data for 1996. *Natl Vital Stat Rep.* 1998;47:1-100.

[21] Kunitz SC, Gross CR, Heyman A, et al. The pilot stroke data bank: definition, design and data. *Stroke* 1984;15:740-746.

[22] Ingall T. Stroke – incidence, mortality, morbidity and risk. *J Insur Med* 2004;36:143-152.

[23] Ovary C, Suzuki K, Nagy Z. Regional differences in incidence rates, outcome predictors and survival of stroke. *Neuroepidemiology* 2004;23:240-246.
[24] Qureshi AI, Wilson DA, Hanley DF, Traystman RJ. No evidence for an eschemic penumbra in a massive experimental intracerebral hemorrhage. *Neurology* 1999;52:266-272.
[25] Schellinger PD, Fiebach JB, Hoffman K, Becker K, Orakcioglu B, Kollmar R, Juttler E, Schramm P, Schwab S, Sartor K, Hacke W. Stroke MRI intracerebral hemorrhage: is this perihemorrhagic penumbra? *Stroke* 2003;34:1674-1679.
[26] Lee KR, Betz AL, Kim S, Keep RF, Hoff JT. The role of the coagulation cascade in brain edema formation after intracerebral hemorrhage. *Acta Neurochir (Wein)* 1996;138:396-400.
[27] Lee KR, Kawai N, Kim S, Sagher O, Hoff JT. Mechanisms of edema formation after intracerebral hemorrhage: effects of thrombin on cerebral brain flow, blood-brain barrier permeability and cerebral survival in a rat model. *J Neurosurg* 1997;86:272-278.
[28] Koeppen AH, Dickson AC, Smith J. Heme oxygenase in experimental intracerebral hemorrhage: the benefit of tin-mesoporphyrine. *J Neuropathol Exp Neurol* 2004;63:587-597.
[29] Xi G, Reiser G, Keep RF. The role of thrombin and thrombin receptors in ischemic, hemorrhagic and traumatic brain injury deleterious or protective? *J Neurochem* 2003;84:3-9.
[30] Hoff JT, Xi G. Brain edema from intracerebral hemorrhage. *Acta Neurochir Suppl* 2003;86:11-15.
[31] Xi G, Keep RF, Hoff JT. Pathophysiology of brain edema formation. *Neurosurg Clin N Am* 2002;13:371-383.
[32] Tomita H, Ito U, Ohno K, Hirakawa K. Chronological changes in brain edema induced by experimental intracerebral hematoma in cats. *Acta Neurochir Suppl (Wein)* 1994;60:558-560.
[33] Lee EJ, Hung YC, Lee MY. Early alterations in cerebral hemodynamics brain metabolism and blood-brain barrier permealbility in experimental intracerebral hemorrhage. *J Neurosurg* 1999;91:1013-1019.
[34] Xi G, Hua Y, Bhasin RR, Ennis SR, Keep RF, Hoff JT. Mechanisms of edema formatin after intracerebral hemorrhage: effects of extravasated red blood cells on blood flow and blood-brain barrier integrity. *Stroke* 2001;32:2932-2938.
[35] Bhasin RR, Xi G, Hua Y, Keep RF, Hoff JT. Experimental intracerebral hemorrhage: effect of lysed erythrocytes on brain edema and blood-barrier permeability. *Acta Neurochir Suppl* 2002;81:249-251.
[36] Goldstein LB, Bertels C, Davis JN. Interrater reliability of the NIH stroke scale. *Arch Neurol* 1989;46:660-662.
[37] Burn JP. Reliability of the modified Rankin Scale. *Stroke* 1991;22(10):1242-1244.
[38] Wolfe CD, Taub NA, Woodrow ED, Burney PG. Assessment of scales of disability and handicapped stroke patients. *Stroke* 1991;22:1242-1244.
[39] Kothari RU, Brott T, Broderick JP, Barsan WG, Sauerbeck LR, Zuccarello M, Khoury J. The ABCs of measuring intracerebral hemorrhage. *Stroke* 1996;27:1304-1305.

[40] Hacke W, Schwab S, Horn M, Spranger M, De Georgia M, von Kummer R. 'Malignant' middle cerebral artery territory infarction: clinical course and prognostic signs. *Arch Neurol* 1996;53:309-315.

[41] Schwab S, Steiner T, Aschoff A, et al. Early hemicraniectomy in patients with complete middle cerebral artery infarction. *Stroke* 1998;29:1888-1893.

[42] Krieger DW, Demchuk AM, Kasner SE, Jauss M, Hantson L. Early clinical and radiological predictors of fatal brain swelling in ischemic stroke. *Stroke* 1999 ;30:287-292.

[43] Haring HP, Dilitz E, Pallua A, et al. Attenuated corticomedullary contrast: An early cerebral computed tomography sign indicating malignant middle cerebral artery infarction. A case-control study. *Stroke* 1999;30:1076-1082.

[44] von Kummer R, Meyding-Lamade U, Forsting M, et al. Sensitivity and prognostic value of early CT in occlusion of the middle cerebral artery trunk. *AJNR* 1994;15:9-15.

[45] Berrouschot J, Barthel H, von Kummer R, Knapp WH, Hesse S, Schneider D. 99m technetium-ethyl-cysteinate-dimer single-photon emission CT can predict fatal ischemic brain edema. *Stroke* 1998;29:2556-2562.

[46] Oppenheim C, Samson Y, Manai R, et al. Prediction of malignant middle cerebral artery infarction by diffusion-weighted imaging. *Stroke* 2000;31:2175-2181.

[47] Thomalla GJ, Kucinski T, Schoder V, et al. Prediction of malignant middle cerebral artery infarction by early perfusion- and diffusion-weighted magnetic resonance imaging. *Stroke* 2003 ;34:1892-1899.

[48] Blankenberg FG, Katsikis PD, Tait JF, Davis RE, Naumovski L, Ohtsuki K, Kopiwoda S, Abrams MJ, Darkes M, Robbins RC, Maecker HT, Strauss HW. In vivo detection and imaging of phosphatidylserine expression during programmed cell death. *Proc Natl Acad Sci U S A.* 1998;95:6349-6354.

[49] Rink A, Fung KM, Trojanowski JQ, Lee VM, Neugebauer E, McIntosh TK. Evidence of apoptotic cell death after experimental traumatic brain injury in the rat. *Am J Pathol* 1995;147:1575-1583.

[50] Pollard H, Cantagrel S, Charriaut-Marlangue C, Moreau J, Ben Ari Y. Apoptosis associated DNA fragmentation in epileptic brain damage. *Neuroreport* 1994;5:1053-1055.

[51] Rabizadeh S, Gralla E, Borchelt D, Gwinn R, Valentine J, Sisodia S, Wong P, Lee M, Hahn H, Bredesen D. Mutations associated with ALS convert superoxide dismutase from an anti-apoptotic gene to a pro-apoptotic gene: studies in yeast and neural cells. *Proc Natl Acad Sci USA* 1995;92:3024-3028.

[52] Loo D, Copani A, Pike C, Whittemore E, Walencewicz A, Cotman C. Apoptosis is induced by β-amyloid in cultured central nervous system neurons. *Proc Natl Acad Sci USA* 1993;90:7951-7955.

[53] Li Y, Chopp M, Jiang N, Yao F, Zaloga C. Temporal profile of in situ DNA fragmentation after transient middle cerebral artery occlusion in the rat. *J Cereb Blood Flow Metab* 1995;15:389-397.

[54] Kihara S, Shiraishi Y, Nakagawa S, Toda K, Tabuchi K. Visualization of DNA double strand breaks in the gerbil hippocampal CA1 following transient ischemia. *Neurosci Lett* 1994;175:133-136.

[55] Li Y, Sharov VG, Jiang N, Zalong C, Sabbah HN, Chopp M. Ultrastructural and light microscopic evidence of apoptosis after middle cerebral artery occlusion in the rat. *Am J Pathol* 1995;146:1045-1051.

[56] Linnik MD, Zahos P, Geschwing MD, Federoff HJ. Expression of *bcl*-2 from a defective herpes simplex virus-1 vector limits neuronal death in focal cerebral ischemia. *Stroke* 1995;26:1670-1675.

[57] Crumrine RC, Thomas AL, Morgan PF. Attenuation of p53 expression protects against focal ischemic damage in transgenic mice. *J Cereb Blood Flow Metab* 1994;14:887-891.

[58] van Heerde WL, de Groot PG, Reutelingsperger CPM. The complexity of the phospholipid binding protein annexin V. *Thromb Haemost* 1995;73:172–179.

[59] O'Brien IEW, Reutingsperger CPM, Holdaway KM. Annexin-V and TUNEL use in monitoring the progression of apoptosis in plants. *Cytometry* 1997;29:28–33.

[60] Blankenberg FG, Katsikis PD, Tait JF, Davis RE, Naumovski L, Ohtsuki K, Kopiwoda S, Abrams MJ, Strauss HW. Imaging of apoptosis (programmed cell death) with 99mTc annexin V. *J Nucl Med* 1999;40:184–191.

[61] Belayev L, Busto R, Zhao W, Ginsberg MD. Quantitative evaluation of blood brain barrier permeability following middle cerebral artery occlusion in rats. *Brain Res.* 1996;739:88-96.

[62] Kuroiwa T, Shibutani M, Okeda R. Blood-brain barrier disruption and exacerbation of ischemic brain edema after restoration of blood flow in experimental focal cerebral ischemia. *Acta Neuropathol.* 1988;76:62-70.

[63] Mari C, Karabiyikoglu M, Goris ML, Tait JF, Yenari MA, Blankenberg FG. Detection of focal hypoxic-ischemic injury and neuronal stress in a rodent model of unilateral MCA occlusion/reperfusion using radiolabeled annexin V. *Eur J Nucl Med Mol Imaging* 2004;31:733-739.

[64] Blankenberg FG, Tait JF, Strauss HW. Apoptotic cell death: its implications for imaging in the next millennium. *Eur J Nucl Med.* 2000;27:359-367.

In: The Blood-Brain Barrier
Editor: Tomas R. Helio

ISBN 978-1-60456-894-3

Chapter 7

Astrocytes and Astrocyte-Derived Factors in the Blood-Brain Barrier in Health and Diseases

Shucui Jiang*[*], *Caixin Su and David Ballok
Departments of Surgery (Neurosurgery, Neurobiology),
Hamilton Neurorestorative Group,
McMaster University, Health Sciences Centre, West Hamilton,
ON L8N 3Z5, Canada.

Abstract

Since the meninges, cerebrospinal fluid (CSF), and the blood-brain barrier (BBB) effectively shield the central nervous system from other tissues, it was once believed that the brain was an "immunologically privileged" organ. Over the last two decades, however, various resident cells have been shown to mount a full immune response during CNS trauma, infection and disease, and thus the long-standing view that the brain was exempt from processes observed in the periphery has been re-examined and revised. How astroglial cells affect the induction and maintenance of the BBB under physiological and pathological conditions remains an area that requires much attention. More specifically, the potential involvement of astrocytes in neurodegenerative conditions and in neurorestorative attempts appears to be important, but more intense experimentation is required to elucidate the precise role of these cells. For example, astrocytes are clearly implicated in the initiation, maintenance, and suppression of immune responses, and appear to propagate both CNS damage and repair, depending on the milieu of the micro-environment. Various factors produced and released by astroglia can also influence the properties of the BBB (e.g., sustaining tight junctions), however, these same factors may contribute to a compromised BBB when dysregulated. Therefore,

[*] Correspondence concerning this article should be addressed to: Shucui Jiang, Telephone: (905) 521 2100 x76628; Fax: (905) 521 9992; E-mail: jiangs@mcmaster.ca.

the objective of this chapter is to review recent evidence of connections between, and bi-directional signaling among, astrocytes and other resident brain cells, as well as examining the part played by astrocyte-derived factors in modulating the integrity of the BBB in health and during CNS disease.

INTRODUCTION

An intact blood-brain barrier (BBB) and normal production, circulation, and absorption of cerebrospinal fluid are critical for normal brain function. Brain capillary endothelial cells form the BBB. Various cell types, particularly astrocytes, but also pericytes and neurons, are located in close proximity to the capillary endothelial cells and these cells may influence the formation and function of the BBB (Zlokovic 2008). This paper discusses aspects of these cells surrounding brain capillary endothelial cells with focus on the role of astrocytes in the formation and maintenance of the BBB.

Howastroglial cells affect the induction and maintenance of the BBB under physiological as well as pathological conditions is discussed. Astrocyte end-feet processes come into close contact with cerebral capillaries, and a number of astroglial-derived mediators and factors contribute to inducing and maintaining BBB functions (Kacem et al., 1998; Wolburg and Lippoldt, 2002). Although how these molecular mediators work is not fully understood, similar interactions likely exist between astroglia and epithelial cells in the choroid plexus and arachnoid forming a glial limitans (Choi, 1994). Various factors produced and released by astroglia can induce barrier properties in both endothelial and epithelial layers. For example, increased expression of barrier-relevant proteins (e.g., tight junction proteins) in the presence of astrocyte-derived factors exists, and many studies demonstrate the improvement of physiological parameters, such as increased transendothelial resistance and decreased paracellular permeability, in different models of the BBB (Gaillard et al., 2001; Dehouck et al., 1990; Iwasaki et al., 1999).

Although the literature presents manifold evidence for a variety of astroglial effects, controversies exist. The different cellular models and experimental conditions used may account for some of these apparent discrepancies (Hasseloff et al., 2005). Moreover, the interaction of brain endothelial cells and astrocytes is bi-directional, and other cell types surrounding the brain microvasculature also contribute to both the function and dysfunction of the BBB (Zlokovic 2008). Therefore, it is expected that current and future research focused on molecular mechanisms and bi-directional signaling pathways will produce new and exciting insights into BBB regulation.

NEUROVASCULAR UNITS

In the fully differentiated neurovascular system, the BBB is a highly specialized brain endothelial structure that separates components of circulating blood from neurons (Huber et al., 2001). The endothelial barrier consists of an extensive network of endothelial cells, pericytes, microglia, and astrocytes, which collectively forms functional "neurovascular units" (Iadecola, 2004; Hawkins and Davis, 2005; Zlokovic, 2005). These organizations of cells are important in maintaining a precisely regulated micro-environment (i.e. chemical composition) in the central nervous system (CNS) for reliable neuronal activity. More specifically, the BBB is a selective diffusion barrier characterized by tight junctions between endothelial cells, having specific active transporters and lacking fenestrations (Kniesel and Wolburg, 2000; Oldendorf et al., 1977; Fenstermacher et al., 1988). These characteristics are important in maintaining the proper neuronal "milieu" necessary for the continuous energetic functioning of neuronal circuits, synaptic transmission, synaptic remodeling, angiogenesis, and neurogenesis seen in healthy adult brains (Deane and Zlokovic, 2007; Lok et al., 2007) . Overall, the close proximity of different non-neuronal cell types (e.g., pericytes, astrocytes, and microglia) to each other and to neurons allows for effective paracrine regulations that are critical for normal CNS functioning.

The breakdown of the BBB due to disruption of the tight junctions, altered bi-directional transport of molecules between blood and brain, vessel regression, aberrant angiogenesis, brain hypo-perfusion, and/or inflammatory responses may initiate a disease process. It can also contribute to a vicious cycle of progressive synaptic and neuronal dysfunction and brain cell death. Substantial evidence now supports the hypothesis that in many patients, dysregulation of neurovascular components leading to a compromised BBB is the primary pathogenic event underlying such conditions as Parkinson's disease, Alzheimer's disease, neuropsychiatric lupus erythematosus, amyotrophic lateral sclerosis, multiple sclerosis, and others.

While the role of astrocytes was minimized in the past , studies have shown that these cells are critical in BBBformation and maintenance over the last two decades. Although various cell types are located closely to CNS capillary endothelial cells, astrocytic end-foot processes surround these: a membrane composed of collagen type IV, laminin, fibronectin, and heparin sulfate proteoglycan surround endothelial cells and pericytes (Farkas and Luiten, 2001), which is ensheathed by astrocyte end-foot processes. Therefore, given their anatomical associations with endothelial cells, it appears that astrocytes play a role the development, maintenance in the breakdown of the BBB (Zlokovic 2008). The integrity of the BBB may be largely astrocyte dependent. Mutual interactions between astrocytes, endothelial cells, and neurons are also required. While undifferentiated neurons can be in contact with endothelial cells during development, neurons do not make contact with these cells in the adult CNS. Instead, astrocytes mediate the neurovascular connection (Pardridge, 1999).

Although the specialized communication between astrocytes and endothelial cells is increasingly recognized, a comprehensive understanding of the structural and functional relationships is not yet known. Through better understanding, the mutual interactions between astrocytes and endothelial cells in both physiological and pathological conditions, new therapeutic approaches may be created for treating chronic neurodegenerative disorders associated with disruption of the BBB.

Cells Comprising the BBB

Endothelial Cells

The prominent characteristic of CNS endothelial cells is the tight junction, which results from the triangular relationship among endothelial cells, glial cells, and neurons (Dermietzel and Krause, 1991). Tight junctions are the most critical structure in the barrier function and prevent all molecules larger than 400 daltons (as well as most smaller molecules) from crossing the BBB (Pardridge, 2002). The tight junction complex includes two classes of transmembrane molecules: occludin and claudins. These molecules interact with transmembrane proteins on adjacent endothelial cells to form a physical barrier to paracellular diffusion (Hirase et al., 1997; Furuse et al., 1998). Accessory proteins, such as members of the zonula occludens family (ZO-1 and ZO-2), are the most widely studied (Haskins et al., 1998; Reichert et al., 2000) and interact with occludin and claudins, as well as actin cytoskeleton (Fanning et al., 1998; Itoh et al., 1999). The cytoplasmic tails of the occludin-claudin complex are linked to the actin cytoskeleton via the accessory proteins and anchor the transmembrane adhesion proteins to the endothelial cell cytoskeletal scaffold. Therefore, the tight junction functions not only as a physical blockade, but also as a segregator of the apical and basal domains in the endothelium (Engelhardt and Wolburg, 2004). The endothelial cells also provide protection from ongoing changes in the vascular system and serve CNS nutritional demands. The endothelial cells of the BBB have three types of transporters including receptor-mediated transporters, carrier-mediated and active efflux; the firstis for large molecules, and the last two are for the delivery of small molecules. These CNS cells also have transporters to supply neurons with nutrients, which includes GLUT1 glucose carriers, LAT1 amino acid carriers, and transporters for nucleosides, nucleobases, as well as other substances (Begley and Brightman, 2003). Interestingly, endothelial cells in the CNS are resistant to inflammation and thus limit the inflammatory response (Hickey, 2001).

Neuron, Pericyte and Microglia

Blood vessels are closely linked to neuronal activity. Consequently, blood flow increases in response to local neuron activation (Iadecola, 1993). However, the cellular mechanisms are not completely understood (Leybaert, 2005). The breakdown of BBB is often followed by pathological changes in blood flow and perfusion pressure, which would be a compensatory mechanism rather than the simple anatomic disruption (Lee et al., 1999). Pericytes are in close proximity to endothelial cells and are separated only by a shared basement membrane. Interactions between pericytes and endothelial cells are mediated by endothelin-1 (Dehouck et al., 1997). Pericytes have contractile proteins that contract capillaries to regulate blood flow (Bandopadhyay et al., 2001), and they induce or maintain the BBB of endothelial cells in a manner similar to astrocytes (Hori et al., 2004). While not much is known about the function of pericytes in the BBB, hypoxia and trauma (associated with the BBB breakdown), disrupt pericyte-endothelial interactions (Dore-Duffy et al., 2000; Gonul et al., 2002).

Microglia cells (regarded as endogenous immune cells in the brain) originate from blood-borne cells and conglomerate with endothelial cells in the CNS. Although it has been suggested that these cells trap foreign materials (Xu and Ling, 1994) or guide monocytes across endothelial cells (Persidsky et al., 1999), their role in the maintenance and breakdown of the BBB also requires further study.

Astrocyte

Astrocytes were once considered to be scaffolds in neuronal development and interactions and were coined the "glue of CNS". Recently, however, astrocytes have been found to have other important functions. These include control of CNS vascular tone, neurogenesis, and synaptogenesis (Zlokovic, 2008), but more knowledge into astrocyte function is needed into their precise role in BBB formation, maintenance, and breakdown (Janzer and Raff, 1987). Currently known, astrocytes ensheath endothelial cells and the attached pericytes (almost entirely) by end-foot processes (Kacem et al., 1998), and these processes are also closely surrounded by CNS capillaries. Astrocytic end-feet have a high density of the water channel aquaporin 4 and the potassium channel Kir4.1 (Neely et al., 1999; Connors et al., 2004). The precise localization of these channels in the end-feet appears to contribute to the inductive influences between astrocytes and endothelial cells (Wolburg and Lippoldt, 2002). In addition, astrocytes interconnect endothelial cells with surrounding neurons. Studies have confirmed that mutual interactions between astrocytes, endothelial cells and neurons are required to maintain BBB integrity (Davson and Oldendorf, 1967). Interestingly, astrocytes can induce junctional tightening and up-regulation of tight junction proteins (i.e. induce barrier properties) in non-CNS endothelial cells (Dehouck et al., 1990; Hurst and Fritz, 1996; Hayashi et al., 1997; Kuchler-Bopp et al., 1999) as well as the up regulation of transporters such as GLUT1 (McAllister et al., 2001). These studies highlight the importance of astrocytes anatomical association with neural endothelial cells and suggest that astrocytes have an intrinsic potential to play a role as a barrier-supportive cell.

More comprehensive studies on the structural and functional relationships between astrocytes, endothelia, and neurons are required to better understand the specialized communication among them. Mi et al (2001) recently suggested endothelial cells induce growth and differentiation of astrocytes. Considering the interaction between neighboring cells, such as endothelial cells and neurons, astrocytes secrete several astrocyte-derived factors associated with cell to cell interaction for BBB formation. More specifically, angiopoietin-1 (ang-1) seems to be responsible for this recruiting and sustaining of peri-endothelial support cells and for contributing to the impermeability of blood vessels (Risau et al., 1998; Thurston et al., 1999). The secretion of ang-1 from perivascular astrocytes has also been found to bind to the receptor, found on endothelial cells, Tie-2 (Hori et al., 2004; Zacharek et al., 2007). Recently, it has been shown that src-suppressed C-kinase substrate (SSeCKS) stimulates astrocytic expression and secretion of ang-1, which leads to the increased expression of tight junction proteins and decreases in the permeability of endothelial cells (Lee et al., 2003). Future studies should lead to a clearer understanding of signaling factors and their relevance between astrocytes and endothelial cells.

ASTROGLIA FACTORS IN THE BBB

In traumatic injury or stroke, the BBB breakdown and astrocyte activation (i.e. "reactive gliosis") is a consequence of the disease (Pekny and Nilsson, 2005), whereas, in neuropsychiatric lupus or multiple sclerosis, it appears to be the precipitating factor (Abbott et al., 2003; Floris et al., 2004). In other conditions, such as in Alzheimer's, the relationship between dysfunction of the BBB and disease are not definite (Wardlaw et al., 2003). As astrocytes are positioned at the interface between the blood and the CNS, they are poised to influence not only hematogenous cell entry into the CNS, but also the activity of invading cells (Mucke and Eddleston, 1993). Astrocytes respond to CNS infection and inflammatory demyelinating disease in a rapid fashion, which is generally detectable within 24 hours (Molina-Holgado et al., 1999). Activated astrocytes produce a number of cytokines, hence the implication that they may participate in mediation of immune responses within the CNS.

Interleukin (IL)-1, a 17-kDa polypeptide, is synthesized and secreted by both microglia and astrocytes (Benveniste, 1994). Astrocytes stimulated with IL-1 secrete both granulocyte colony-stimulating factor (G-CSF) and granulocyte-macrophage colony-stimulating factor (GM-CSF) (Malipiero et al., 1990; Benveniste, 1994). G-CSF and GM-CSF enhance a number of functional activities of mature macrophages (e.g. phagocytic, cytotoxic, and microbicidal activities). Locally produced G-CSF and GM-CSF (by astrocytes) may therefore provide an essential element for the recruitment and activation of blood-borne immune cells., IL-1 also stimulates astrocytic growth, as well as astrocytic differentiation and maturation (Giulian and Lachman, 1985)., IL-1 promotes glial scaring or astrogliosis when injected into the CNS (Giulian et al., 1988) and may thus mediate astrocytic hypertrophy following neuronal damage (Giulian et al., 1988)., activation of astrocytes by IL-1 leads to synthesis of the nerve growth factor (NGF) (Yoshida and Toya, 1997). IL-1 increases intracellular adhesion molecule (ICAM)-1 expression. which is antagonized by cyclic AMP-dependent protein kinase-mediated signaling pathways, indicating that it may have a role in antigen presentation (Frohman et al., 1989; Ballestas and Benveniste, 1997).

IL-1 also plays a key role in inducing astrocytic nitric oxide (NO) production. NO is a reactive nitrogen intermediate that plays an important role in host -defense and injury (Hu et al., 1995). Anti-inflammatory cytokines such as IL-4 and IL-10 suppresse the IL-1 plus interferon (IFN) gamma potentiated NO production, while transforming growth factor beta (TGF-b) preferentially inhibits IL-1b plus TNF-alpha potentiated production of NO (Ballestas and Benveniste, 1997; Hellendall and Ting, 1997). In addition, IL-1 enhances both release of ciliary neurotrophic factor from and expression of high-molecular weight basic fibroblast growth factor (FGF) in astrocytes (Yoshida and Toya, 1997) suggesting that in the early phase following brain injury, IL-1-activated astrocytes may rescue the damaged neurons via neurotrophic factors and other biologically active molecules. IL-1 has also been shown to stimulate secretion of tumor necrosis factor (TNF)-alpha and IL-6 from astrocytes (Norris and Benveniste, 1993). While IL-6 functions prominently in induction of terminal differentiation of activated B cells into immunoglobulin-secreting plasma cells, it also has a mitogenic effect on astrocytes, and therefore may contribute to reactive gliosis (Selmaj et al., 1990). Interestingly, astrocytes respond to IL-6 by secreting nerve growth factor (NGF), which induces neuronal differentiation.

TNF-alpha (a 17-kDa polypeptide) is synthesized and secreted both by astrocytes and microglia (Benveniste, 1994). This cytokine increases endothelial cell permeability, facilitating the adhesion of neutrophils, monocytes and lymphocytes to the capillary surface (Pober et al., 1986; Pohlman et al., 1986; Brett et al., 1989). Similar to the effects of IL-1, TNF-alpha also stimulates astrocytes to release IL-6, G-CSF, and GM-CSF (Malpiero et al., 1990) and produces endothelial endothelin-1, which leads to the release of IL-1beta from astrocytes (Deli et al., 1995). Astrocytes producing G-CSF and GM-CSF (in response to TNF-alpha stimulation) can increase inflammatory responses by facilitating the migration of both macrophages and granulocytes to sites of injury, by promoting their survival, and by increasing their effector functions in the CNS. Astrocytes stimulated with TNF-alpha also express TNF-alpha mRNA, which suggests a positive feedback loop for TNF-alpha expression (Benveniste, 1994). This autocrine mechanism exists for IL-1 as well and similarly acts to maintain these brain cytokines at an optimum level (Benveniste, 1994). TNF-alpha stimulates astrocyte platelet-derived growth factor (PDGF) production (Silberstein et al., 1996). This cytokine has been shown to regulate immune responses by modulating the expression of Class I major histocompatibility complex (MHC) molecules in astrocytes (Lavi et al., 1988; Mauerhoff et al., 1988). Also similar to IL-1, TNF-alpha enhances the expression of various adhesion molecules (i.e. ICAM-1 expression) on astrocytic cells, which together with MHC, are important in antigen presentation (Frohman et al., 1989).

CNS Diseases: The Role of Astrocytes

In the development and progression of CNS diseases, dysfunction of the BBB is a critical event and astroglia have the potential to release mediators that compromise the BBB during pathological conditions (Haseloff et al., 2005). In the experimentally induced absence of astrocytes around injury sites, however, the traumatically damaged blood–brain barrier can still repair (Willis et al., 2004). Also, following a period of hypoxia, astrocytes exposed to oxygenation are found to release thrombospondin-1, or TSP-1 (Song et al., 2002). TSP-1 is known to activate tumor growth factor (TGF)-beta, which is thought to upregulate tight junctions and glycoproteins of endothelial cells, both important in maintaining the integrity of the BBB (Abbott, 2002). Thus, factors released by astroglia have a varied potential to influence CNS barrier functions in health and disease.

In CNS tumors, the BBB is usually impaired. When the permeability of BBB increases, and following the decrease of tight junction proteins and associated proteins (i.e. opening of paracellular pathways), edema is formed around the tumor. In the developing stage of tumor, the BBB appears to be preserved due to relatively adequate vascular endothelial growth factor (VEGF) secretion for tumor parenchyma (Lund et al., 2006). With the progression of the tumor, however, the BBB appears to become more permeable not only due to an over-expression of VEGF, but also as a result of the loss of astrocytic end-foot effacement and abnormalities of the tumor vessels (Machein et al., 1999; Rascher et al., 2002).

Due to a loss of blood flow, oxygen, nutrients, and other molecules, ischemia is considered to be a combined insult (Mark and Davis, 2002). Endothelial cells are vulnerable to ischemia, which results in genotoxic damage, disruption of tight junction proteins, and apoptosis. Interestingly, astrocytes are less responsive to ischemia because they have the capacity for anaerobic glycolysisy, as well as high antioxidant activity (Schroeter et al., 1999). Nevertheless, in ischemic conditions, astrocytes become more reactive, similar to neonatal astrocytes (Stanimirovic et al., 1997). While the function of astrocytes in the ischemia is still unclear, it has been found that endothelial cells are less responsive to hypoxic stress when co-cultured with astrocytes (Plateel et al., 1995). However, transcellular permeability of endothelial cells increases in a co-culture with glial cells under ischemia (Brillault et al., 2002). While more studies are needed in this area, astrocytes may be important in maintaining BBB integrity following hypoxic insults.

In the etiology of autoimmune disorders of the CNS, the local production of the cytokine IFN-gamma by astrocytes (as well as microglia) has been implicated. While IFN-gamma is predominantly produced by activated T cells, it is normally absent from the brain. This pleiotropic cytokine has antiviral activity, anti-proliferative effects, and immunomodulatory abilities. Its immune functions include activation of macrophages, enhancement of oxygen radical formation by macrophages, and differentiation of both T cells and B cells. It also modulates Class I and Class II MHC expression (Wong et al., 1984; Suzumura et al., 1986; Hellendall and Ting, 1997). It is possible that enhanced MHC Class I antigen expression on astrocytes (ollowing IFN-gamma stimulation renders them susceptible to lysis by Class-I-restricted cytotoxic T lymphocytes (CTL) (Skias et al., 1987) once the integrity of the BBB is compromised. Thus, the local production of IFN-gamma by astrocytes has been implicated in the pathogenesis of astrocyte-involved autoimmune diseases of the CNS.

Unless accompanied by CNS pathology, peripheral inflammation alone does not compromise the BBB (Abbott et al., 1999). Tight junction disruption leading to a failure of the BBB, however, is characteristic of general inflammatory CNS diseases (Petty and Lo, 2002). Once compromised, many inflammatory mediators can then influence the permeability of BBB, and these inflammatory mediators can differentially act on the various BBB cell complex. For example, although bradykinin directly acts on endothelial cells, it can also activate nuclear factor-kappa B (NF-kB) in astrocytes to release IL-6 (Schwaninger et al., 1999). Importantly, neuronal-glial interactions appear to determine the activation threshold of astrocytes to inflammatory cytokines. More specifically, the response of human astrocytes to cytokines, i.e., inducing the synthesis of additional astrocytic-derived cytokines, varies greatlydependent upon the presence or absence of neurons in a culture system (Aloisi et al., 1995). While most cytokines may play an important role in the initiation and maintenance of immune responses within the CNS, recent evidence suggests that specific cytokines are involved in different CNS diseases at different stages (Otten et al., 2000). Future studies in this field will undoubtedly provide novel information on the molecular basis of these events, and the role of astrocytes and astrocyte-derived cytokines in breakdown of the BBB during immune responses of the CNS.

Conclusions and Future Directions

Recent progress of neuroscience research for molecular and cellular mechanisms of the BBB has given us insights into understanding physiology and pathology of CNS. However, the ability to treat CNS diseases is incongruous with the progression in the neuroscience. Many CNS drugs have been discovered, but none have been successful in correcting BBB dysfunctions. It is now known that astrocyte-endothelial cell interactions influence the BBB in both physiological and pathological conditions. However, further studies are needed to clarify the exact nature of BBB formation, maintenance, and disruption. Gaps also need to be bridged between molecular biology, cellular biology and clinical practice if mutual interactions between astrocytes and endothelial cells are to be better understood. Deciphering the crosstalk between non-neuronal cell types, i.e. microglia and glia, cells of the vessel wall, i.e. pericytes and endothelium, neurons with other neurons, and neurons with peripheral hematopoetic cells remains an imperative challenge before effective treatments can be developed to correct BBB irregularities. More specifically, identifying how these cells respond to, process, or synthesize different receptors and identifying the ligands that mediate their interactions is critical to understanding how these cells regulate the "neuronal milieu" (Zlokovic 2008).

References

Abbott, N.J., Chugani, D.C., Zaharchuk, G., Rosen, B.R., Lo, E.H. (1999). Delivery of imaging agents into brain. *Adv. Drug Deliv. Rev. 37*, 253-277.

Abbott, N.J. (2002). Astrocyte-endothelial interactions and blood-brain barrier permeability. *J. Anat. 200*, 629-38.

Abbott, N.J., Mendonca, L.L., Dolman, D.E. (2003). The blood-brain barrier in systemic lupus erythematosus. *Lupus. 12*, 908-915.

Aloisi, F., Borscllino, G., Care, A., Testa, U., Gallo, P., Russo, G., Peschle, C., Levi, G. (1995). Cytokine regulation of astrocyte function: in-vitro studies using cells from the human brain. *Int. J. Dev. Neurosci. 13*, 265-274.

Ballestas, M.E. & Benveniste, E.N. (1997). Elevation of cyclic AMP levels in astrocytes antagonizes cytokine-induced adhesion molecule expression. *J. Neurochem. 69*, 1438-1448.

Bandopadhyay, R., Orte, C., Lawrenson, J.G., Reid, A.R., De Silva, S., Allt, G. (2001). Contractile proteins in pericytes at the blood-brain and blood-retinal barriers. *J. Neurocytol. 30*, 35-44.

Begley, D.J. & Brightman, M.W. (2003). Structural and functional aspects of the blood-brain barrier. *Prog. Drug Res. 61*, 39-78.

Benveniste, E.N. (1994). Cytokine circuits in brain. Implications for AIDS dementia complex. *Res. Publ. Assoc. Res. Nerv. Ment. Dis. 72*, 71-88.

Brett, J., Gerlach, H., Nawroth, P., Steinberg, S., Godman, G., Stern, D. (1989). Tumor necrosis factor/cachectin increases permeability of endothelial cell monolayers by a mechanism involving regulatory G proteins. *J. Exp. Med. 169*, 1977-1991.

Brillault, J., Berezowski, V., Cecchelli, R., Dehouck, M.P. (2002). Intercommunications between brain capillary endothelial cells and glial cells increase the transcellular permeability of the blood-brain barrier during ischaemia. *J. Neurochem. 83*, 807-817.

Choi, B.H. (1994). Role of the basement membrane in neurogenesis and repair of injury in the central nervous system. *Microsc. Res. Tech. 28*, 193-203.

Connors, N.C., Adams, M.E., Froehner, S.C., Kofuji, P. (2004). The potassium channel Kir4.1 associates with the dystrophin-glycoprotein complex via alpha-syntrophin in glia. *J. Biol. Chem. 279*, 28387-28392.

Davson, H. & Oldendorf, W.H. (1967). Symposium on membrane transport. Transport in the central nervous system. *Proc. R. Soc. Med. 60*, 326-329.

Deane, R. & Zlokovic, B.V. (2007). Role of the blood-brain barrier in the pathogenesis of Alzheimer's disease. *Curr. Alzheimer Res. 4*, 191-197.

Dehouck, M.P., Méresse, S., Delorme, P., Fruchart, J.C., Cecchelli, R. (1990). An easier, reproducible, and mass-production method to study the blood-brain barrier in vitro. *J. Neurochem. 54*, 1798-1801.

Dehouck, M.P., Vigne, P., Torpier, G., Breittmayer, J.P., Cecchelli, R., Frelin, C. (1997). Endothelin-1 as a mediator of endothelial cell-pericyte interactions in bovine brain capillaries. *J. Cereb. Blood Flow Metab. 17*, 464-469.

Deli, M.A., Descamps, L., Dehouck, M.P., Cecchelli, R., Joo, F., Abraham, C.S., Torpier, G. (1995). Exposure of tumor necrosis factor-alpha to luminal membrane of bovine brain capillary endothelial cells cocultured with astrocytes induces a delayed increase of permeability and cytoplasmic stress fiber formation of actin. *J. Neurosci. Res. 41*, 717-726.

Dermietzel, R. & Krause, D. (1991). Molecular anatomy of the blood-brain barrier as defined by immunocytochemistry. *Int. Rev. Cytol. 127*, 57-109.

Dore-Duffy, P., Owen, C., Balabanov, R., Murphy, S., Beaumont, T., Rafols, J.A. (2000). Pericyte migration from the vascular wall in response to traumatic brain injury. *Microvasc. Res. 60*, 55-69.

Eddleston M. & Mucke, L. (1993). Molecular profile of reactive astrocytes--implications for their role in neurologic disease. *Neuroscience. 54*, 15-36.

Engelhardt, B. & Wolburg, H. (2004). Mini-review: Transendothelial migration of leukocytes: through the front door or around the side of the house? *Eur. J. Immunol. 34*, 2955-2963.

Fanning, A.S., Jameson, B.J., Jesaitis, L.A., Anderson, J.M. (1998). The tight junction protein ZO-1 establishes a link between the transmembrane protein occludin and the actin cytoskeleton. *J. Biol. Chem. 273*, 29745-2953.

Farkas, E. & Luiten, P.G. (2001). Cerebral microvascular pathology in aging and Alzheimer's disease. *Prog. Neurobiol. 64*, 575-611.

Fenstermacher, J., Gross, P., Sposito, N., Acuff, V., Pettersen, S., Gruber, K. (1988). Structural and functional variations in capillary systems within the brain. *Ann. N. Y. Acad. Sci. 529*, 21-30.

Floris, S., Blezer, E.L., Schreibelt, G., Dopp, E., van der Pol, S.M., Schadee-Eestermans, I.L., Nicolay, K., Dijkstra, C.D., de Vries, H.E. (2004). Blood-brain barrier permeability and monocyte infiltration in experimental allergic encephalomyelitis: a quantitative MRI study. *Brain 127*, 616-627.

Frohman, E.M., Frohman, T.C., Dustin, M.L., Vayuvegula, B., Choi, B., Gupta, A., van den Noort S., Gupta S. (1989). The induction of intercellular adhesion molecule 1 (ICAM-1) expression on human fetal astrocytes by interferon-gamma, tumor necrosis factor alpha, lymphotoxin, and interleukin-1: relevance to intracerebral antigen presentation. *J. Neuroimmunol. 23*, 117-124.

Furuse, M., Fujita, K., Hiiragi, T., Fujimoto, K., Tsukita, S. (1998). Claudin-1 and -2: novel integral membrane proteins localizing at tight junctions with no sequence similarity to occludin. *J. Cell Biol. 29*, 1539-1550.

Gaillard, P.J., Voorwinden, LH., Nielsen, J.L., Ivanov, A., Atsumi, R., Engman, H., Ringbom, C., de Boer, A.G., Breimer, D.D. (2001). Establishment and functional characterization of an in vitro model of the blood-brain barrier, comprising a co-culture of brain capillary endothelial cells and astrocytes. *Eur. J. Pharm. Sci. 12*, 215-22.

Giulian, D. & Lachman, L.B. (1985). Interleukin-1 stimulation of astroglial proliferation after brain injury. *Science. 228*, 497-499.

Giulian, D., Young, D.G., Woodward, J., Brown, D.C., Lachman, L.B. (1988b). Interleukin-1 is an astroglial growth factor in the developing brain. *J. Neurosci. 8*, 709-714.

Giulian, D., Woodward, J., Young, D.G., Krebs, J.F., Lachman, L.B. (1988a). Interleukin-1 injected into mammalian brain stimulates astrogliosis and neovascularization. *J. Neurosci. 8*, 2485-2490.

Gonul, E., Duz, B., Kahraman, S., Kayali, H., Kubar, A., Timurkaynak, E. (2002). Early pericyte response to brain hypoxia in cats: an ultrastructural study. *Microvasc. Res. 64*, 116-119.

Haseloff, R.F., Blasig, I.E., Bauer, H.C., Bauer, H. (2005). In search of the astrocytic factor(s) modulating blood-brain barrier functions in brain capillary endothelial cells in vitro. *Cell Mol. Neurobiol. 25*, 25-39.

Haskins, J., Gu, L., Wittchen, E.S., Hibbard, J., Stevenson, B.R. (1998). ZO-3, a novel member of the MAGUK protein family found at the tight junction, interacts with ZO-1 and occludin. *J. Cell Biol. 141*, 199-208.

Hawkins, B.T. & Davis, T.P. (2005). The blood-brain barrier/neurovascular unit in health and disease. *Pharmacol. Rev. 57*, 173-185.

Hayashi, Y., Nomura, M., Yamagishi, S., Harada, S., Yamashita, J., Yamamoto, H. (1997). Induction of various blood-brain barrier properties in non-neural endothelial cells by close apposition to co-cultured astrocytes. *Glia. 19*, 13-26.

Hellendall, R.P. & Ting, J.P. (1997). Differential regulation of cytokine-induced major histocompatibility complex class II expression and nitric oxide release in rat microglia and astrocytes by effectors of tyrosine kinase, protein kinase C, and cAMP. *J. Neuroimmunol. 74*, 19-29.

Hickey, M.J. (2001). Role of inducible nitric oxide synthase in the regulation of leucocyte recruitment. *Clin. Sci. (Lond). 100*, 1-12.

Hirase, T., Staddon, J.M., Saitou, M., Ando-Akatsuka, Y., Itoh, M., Furuse, M., Fujimoto, K., Tsukita, S., Rubin, L.L. (1997). Occludin as a possible determinant of tight junction permeability in endothelial cells. *J. Cell Sci. 110*, 1603-13.

Hori, S., Ohtsuki, S., Hosoya, K., Nakashima, E., Terasaki, T. (2004). A pericyte-derived angiopoietin-1 multimeric complex induces occludin gene expression in brain capillary endothelial cells through Tie-2 activation in vitro. *J. Neurochem. 89*, 503-513.

Hu, S., Sheng, W.S., Peterson, P.K., Chao, C.C. (1995). Differential regulation by cytokines of human astrocyte nitric oxide production. *Glia. 15*, 491-494.

Huber, J.D., Egleton, R.D., Davis, T.P. (2001). Molecular physiology and pathophysiology of tight junctions in the blood-brain barrier. *Trends Neurosci., 24*, 719-725.

Hurst, R.D. & Fritz, I.B. (1996). Properties of an immortalised vascular endothelial/glioma cell co-culture model of the blood-brain barrier. *J. Cell Physiol. 167*, 81-8.

Iadecola, C. (1993). Regulation of the cerebral microcirculation during neural activity: is nitric oxide the missing link? *Trends Neurosci. 16*, 206-214.

Iadecola, C. (2004). Neurovascular regulation in the normal brain and in Alzheimer's disease. *Nat. Rev. Neurosci. 5*, 347-360.

Itoh, M., Morita, K., Tsukita, S. (1999). Characterization of ZO-2 as a MAGUK family member associated with tight as well as adherens junctions with a binding affinity to occludin and alpha catenin. *J. Biol. Chem. 274*, 5981-5986.

Iwasaki, T., Kanda, T., Mizusawa, H. (1999). Effects of pericytes and various cytokines on integrity of endothelial monolayer originated from blood-nerve barrier: an in vitro study. *J. Med. Dent. Sci. 46*, 31-40.

Janzer, R.C. & Raff, M.C. (1987). Astrocytes induce blood-brain barrier properties inendothelial cells. *Nature. 325*, 253-257.

Kacem, K., Lacombe, P., Seylaz, J., Bonvento, G. (1998). Structural organization of the perivascular astrocyte endfeet and their relationship with the endothelial glucose transporter: a confocal microscopy study. *Glia. 23*, 1-10.

Kniesel, U. & Wolburg, H. (2000). Tight junctions of the blood-brain barrier. *Cell Mol. Neurobiol. 20*, 57-76.

Kuchler-Bopp, S., Delaunoy, J.P., Artault, J.C., Zaepfel, M., Dietrich, J.B. (1999). Astrocytes induce several blood-brain barrier properties in non-neural endothelial cells. *Neuroreport. 10*, 1347-1353.

Lavi, E., Suzumura, A., Murasko, D.M., Murray, E.M., Silberberg, D.H., Weiss, S.R. (1988). Tumor necrosis factor induces expression of MHC class I antigens on mouse astrocytes. *J. Neuroimmunol. 18*, 245-253.

Lee, E.J., Hung, Y.C., Lee, M.Y. (1999). Early alterations in cerebral hemodynamics, brain metabolism, and blood-brain barrier permeability in experimental intracerebral hemorrhage. *J. Neurosurg. 91*, 1013-1019.

Lee, S.W., Kim, W.J., Choi, Y.K., Song, H.S., Son, M.J., Gelman, I.H., Kim, Y.J., Kim, K.W. (2003). SSeCKS regulates angiogenesis and tight junction formation in blood-brain barrier. *Nat. Med. 9*, 900-906.

Leybaert, L. (2005). Neurobarrier coupling in the brain: a partner of neurovascular and neurometabolic coupling? *J. Cereb. Blood Flow Metab. 25*, 2-16.

Lok, J., Gupta, P., Guo, S., Kim, W.J., Whalen, M.J., van Leyen, K., Lo, E.H. (2007). Cell-cell signaling in the neurovascular unit. *Neurochem. Res. 32*, 2032-2045.

Lund, C.V., Nguyen, M.T., Owens, G.C., Pakchoian, A.J., Shaterian, A., Kruse, C.A., Eliceiri, B.P. (2006). Reduced glioma infiltration in Src-deficient mice. *J. Neurooncol. 78*, 19-29.

Mark, K.S. & Davis, T.P. (2002). Cerebral microvascular changes in permeability and tight junctions induced by hypoxia-reoxygenation. *Am. J. Physiol. Heart Circ. Physiol. 282*, H1485-H1494.

Machein, M.R., Kullmer, J., Fiebich, B.L., Plate, K.H., Warnke, P.C. (1999). Vascular endothelial growth factor expression, vascular volume, and, capillary permeability in human brain tumors. *Neurosurgery. 44*, 732-740.

Mauerhoff, T., Pujol-Borrell, R., Mirakian, R., Bottazzo, G.F. (1988). Differential expression and regulation of major histocompatibility complex (MHC) products in neural and glial cells of the human fetal brain. *J. Neuroimmunol. 18*, 271-289.

Molina-Holgado, F., Hernanz, A., De la Fuente, M., Guaza, C. (1999). N-Acetyl-cysteine inhibition of encephalomyelitis Theiler's virus-induced nitric oxide and tumour necrosis factor-alpha production by murine astrocyte cultures. *Biofactors. 10*, 187-193.

Malipiero, U.V., Frei, K., Fontana, A. (1990). Production of hemopoietic colony-stimulating factors by astrocytes. *J. Immunol. 144*, 3816-3821.

McAllister, M.S., Krizanac-Bengez, L., Macchia, F., Naftalin, R.J., Pedley, K.C., Mayberg, M.R., Marroni, M., Leaman, S., Stanness, K.A., Janigro, D. (2001). Mechanisms of glucose transport at the blood-brain barrier: an in vitro study. *Brain Res. 904*, 20-30.

Mi, H., Haeberle, H., Barres, B.A. (2001). Induction of astrocyte differentiation by endothelial cells. *J. Neurosci. 21*, 1538-1547.

Neely, J.D., Christensen, B.M., Nielsen, S., Agre, P. (1999). Heterotetrameric composition of aquaporin-4 water channels. *Biochemistry. 38*, 11156-11163.

Norris, J.G. & Benveniste, E.N. (1993). Interleukin-6 production by astrocytes: induction by the neurotransmitter norepinephrine. *J. Neuroimmunol. 45*, 137-145.

Oldendorf, W.H., Cornford, M.E., Brown, W.J. (1977). The large apparent work capability of the blood-brain barrier: a study of the mitochondrial content of capillary endothelial cells in brain and other tissues of the rat. *Ann. Neurol. 5*, 409-417.

Otten, U., März, P., Heese, K., Hock, C., Kunz, D., Rose-John, S. (2000). Cytokines and neurotrophins interact in normal and diseased states. *Ann. N. Y. Acad. Sci. 917*, 322-30.

Plateel, M., Dehouck, M.P., Torpier, G., Cecchelli, R., Teissier, E. (1995). Hypoxia increases the susceptibility to oxidant stress and the permeability of the blood-brain barrier endothelial cell monolayer. *J. Neurochem. 65*, 2138-2145.

Pober, J.S., Bevilacqua, M.P., Mendrick, D.L., Lapierre, L.A., Fiers, W., Gimbrone, M.A. (1986). Two distinct monokines, interleukin 1 and tumor necrosis factor, each independently induce biosynthesis and transient expression of the same antigen on the surface of cultured human vascular endothelial cells. *J. Immunol. 136*, 1680-1687.

Pohlman, T.H., Stanness, K.A., Beatty, P.G., Ochs, H.D., Harlan, J.M. (1986). An endothelial cell surface factor(s) induced in vitro by lipopolysaccharide, interleukin 1, and tumor necrosis factor-alpha increases neutrophil adherence by a CDw18-dependent mechanism. *J. Immunol. 136*, 4548-4553.

Pekny, M. & Nilsson, M. (2005). Astrocyte activation and reactive gliosis. *Glia 50*, 427-434.

Persidsky, Y., Ghorpade, A., Rasmussen, J., Limoges, J., Liu, X.J., Stins, M., Fiala, M., Way, D., Kim, K.S., Witte, M.H., Weinand, M., Carhart, L., Gendelman, H.E. (1999). Microglial and astrocyte chemokines regulate monocyte migration through the blood-brain barrier in human immunodeficiency virus-1 encephalitis. *Am. J. Pathol. 155*, 1599-1611.

Petty, M.A. & Lo, E.H. (2002). Junctional complexes of the blood-brain barrier: permeability changes in neuroinflammation. *Prog. Neurobiol. 68*, 311-23.

Pardridge, W.M. (1999). Blood-brain barrier biology and methodology. *J. Neurovirol. 5*, 556-569.

Pardridge, W.M. (2002). Drug and gene delivery to the brain: the vascular route. *Neuron 36*, 555-558.

Rascher, G., Fischmann, A., Kroger, S., Duffner, F., Grote, E.H., Wolburg. H. (2002). Extracellular matrix and the blood-brain barrier in glioblastoma multiforme: spatial segregation of tenascin and agrin. *Acta. Neuropathol. 104*, 85-91.

Reichert, M., Müller T, Hunziker W. (2000). The PDZ domains of zonula occludens-1 induce an epithelial to mesenchymal transition of Madin-Darby canine kidney I cells. Evidence for a role of beta-catenin/Tcf/Lef signaling. *J. Biol. Chem. 275*, 9492-9500.

Risau, W., Esser, S., Engelhardt, B. (1998). Differentiation of blood-brain barrier endothelial cells. *Pathol. Biol. (Paris). 46*, 171-175.

Silberstein, F.C., De Simone, R., Levi, G., Aloisi, F. (1996). Cytokine-regulated expression of platelet-derived growth factor gene and protein in cultured human astrocytes. *J. Neurochem. 66*, 1409-1417.

Schwaninger, M., Sallmann, S., Petersen, N., Schneider, A., Prinz, S., Libermann, T.A., Spranger, M. (1999). Bradykinin induces interleukin-6 expression in astrocytes through activation of nuclear factor-kappaB. *J. Neurochem. 73*, 1461-1466.

Skias, D.D., Kim, D.K., Reder, A.T., Antel, J.P., Lancki, D.W., Fitch, F.W. (1987). Susceptibility of astrocytes to class I MHC antigen-specific cytotoxicity. *J. Immunol. 138*, 3254-3258.

Schroeter, M.L., Mertsch, K., Giese, H., Muller, S., Sporbert, A., Hickel, B., Blasig, I.E. (1999). Astrocytes enhance radical defence in capillary endothelial cells constituting the blood-brain barrier. *FEBS Lett. 449*, 241-244.

Stanimirovic, D.B., Ball, R., Durkin, J.P. (1997). Stimulation of glutamate uptake and Na,K-ATPase activity in rat astrocytes exposed to ischemia-like insults. *Glia. 19*, 123-134.

Suzumura, A., Silberberg, D.H., Lisak, R.P. (1986). The expression of MHC antigens on oligodendrocytes: induction of polymorphic H-2 expression by lymphokines. *J. Neuroimmunol. 11*, 179-190.

Song, H.S., Son, M.J., Lee, Y.M., Kim, W.J., Lee, S.W., Kim, C.W., Kim, K.W. (2002). Oxygen tension regulates the maturation of the blood-brain barrier. *Biochem. Biophys. Res. Commun. 290*, 325-331

Selmaj, K.W., Farooq, M., Norton, W.T., Raine, C.S., Brosnan, C.F. (1993). Proliferation of astrocytes in vitro in response to cytokines. A primary role for tumor necrosis factor. *J. Immunol. 144*, 129-135.

Thurston, G., Suri, C., Smith, K., McClain, J., Sato, T.N., Yancopoulos, G.D., McDonald, D.M. (1999). Leakage-resistant blood vessels in mice transgenically overexpressing angiopoietin-1. *Science. 286*, 2511-2514.

Wolburg, H. & Lippoldt, A. (2002). Tight junctions of the blood-brain barrier: development, composition and regulation. *Vascul. Pharmacol. 38*, 323-337.

Willis, C.L., Nolan, C.C., Reith, S.N., Lister, T., Prior, M.J., Guerin, C.J., Mavroudis, G., Ray, D.E. (2004). Focal astrocyte loss is followed by microvascular damage, with subsequent repair of the blood-brain barrier in the apparent absence of direct astrocytic contact. *Glia. 45*, 325-337.

Wardlaw, J.M., Sandercock, P.A., Dennis, M.S., Starr, J. (2003). Is breakdown of the blood-brain barrier responsible for lacunar stroke, leukoaraiosis, and dementia? *Stroke 34*, 806-812.

Wong, G.H., Bartlett, P.F., Clark-Lewis, I., Battye, F., Schrader, J.W. (1984). Inducible expression of H-2 and Ia antigens on brain cells. *Nature. 310*, 688-691.

Xu, J. & Ling, E.A. (1994). Studies of the ultrastructure and permeability of the blood-brain barrier in the developing corpus callosum in postnatal rat brain using electron dense tracers. *J. Anat. 184*, 227-237.

Yoshida, K. & Toya, S. (1997). Neurotrophic activity in cytokine-activated astrocytes. *Keio. J. Med. 46*, 55-60.

Zacharek, A., Chen, J., Cui, X., Li, A., Li, Y., Roberts, C., Feng, Y., Gao, Q., Chopp, M. (2007). Angiopoietin1/Tie2 and VEGF/Flk1 induced by MSC treatment amplifies angiogenesis and vascular stabilization after stroke. *J. Cereb. Blood Flow Metab. 27*, 1684-1691.

Zlokovic, B.V. (2005). Neurovascular mechanisms of Alzheimer's neurodegeneration. *Trends Neurosci. 28*, 202-208.

Zlokovic, B.V. (2008). The blood-brain barrier in health and chronic neurodegenerative disorders. *Neuron 57*, 178-201.

In: The Blood-Brain Barrier
Editor: Tomas R. Helio

ISBN 978-1-60456-894-3

Chapter 8

LIPOPROTEINS AND APOLIPOPROTEINS IN HUMAN CEREBROSPINAL FLUID: A NEW ROLE OF LIPOPROTEIN(A) AND APOLIPOPROTEIN(A) IN THE NEUROLOGICAL DISEASES CHARACTERIZED BY BLOOD-CEREBROSPINAL FLUID BARRIER DYSFUNCTION

Gabriella Pepe[1,2,*] and Guglielmina Chimienti[1]
[1]Department of Biochemistry and Molecular Biology, University of Bari, Italy;
[2]Institute of Bioenergetics and Biomembranes of Bari, CNR, Italy.

ABSTRACT

The barrier between blood and CSF contributes to homeostasis of the CNS and protects it from potentially harmful substances present in the blood.

Lipoproteins present in the CSF are clearly distinct from their plasma counterparts. Human CSF lipoproteins contain mainly Apo AI and Apo E, the former deriving mostly from plasma after crossing the blood–cerebrospinal fluid barrier, the latter being also produced by CNS. Apo AI and E containing lipoproteins in the brain are key players in transport and delivery of lipids, cholesterol homeostasis, and are also involved in CNS remodeling mechanisms. On the other hand, the isoform apo E4 represents the most important genetic risk factor for sporadic and familial late-onset Alzheimer's disease and is involved in brain injury and neurodegenerative diseases.

Apo B containing lipoproteins are not produced by CNS and the characterization of normal human CSF lipoproteins did not allowed the isolation of low density lipoproteins.

* Correspondence concerning this article should be addressed to: Gabriella Pepe, g.pepe@biologia.uniba.it.

Lipoprotein(a) is a low density lipoprotein-like particle with the unique protein apo(a), which is characterized by a dimensional polymorphism. Lipoprotein(a) is a well known risk factor for athero-thrombosis. The pathological role of Lipoprotein(a) is strictly associated with its plasma concentrations and the size of apo(a) isoforms, with inverse relation. The pathophysiology of Lipoprotein(a) in cardio and cerebrovascular system is widely studied. Recently, we demonstrated that, in neuroinflammatory and neurodegenerative disorders, Lipoprotein(a) can cross a dysfunctional blood-CSF barrier and be found in the CSF.

This chapter focuses on the physiological presence of the lipoproteins in CNS, on the pathological aspects deriving from their isoforms, and in particular on the anomalous presence in CSF of Lipoprotein(a).

INTRODUCTION

Lipoprotein particles, Lps, are macromolecular complexes composed by a lipid core and a apolipoprotein moiety, apo. Lps circulate in blood maintaining the lipid homeostasis and providing the cells of source of energy, precursors for the synthesis of biomembrane, and molecules such as steroid hormones and vitamins for many physiological processes.

The barrier between blood and cerebrospinal fluid, called blood-CSF barrier, contributes to the homeostasis of the central nervous system, CNS, and protects it from potentially harmful substances present in the blood.

Lps present in the CSF are clearly distinct from their plasma counterparts.

The first report of the presence of Lps in human CSF was published 40 years ago [1] and the characterization of human CSF apos in terms of dimension and concentration with respect to their plasma counterparts dates from 1979 [2].

To date only some Lps have been isolated in human CSF and only few apos have been found synthesized in the brain, as apo E [3-7], while others derive from blood after crossing the blood-CSF barrier, as apo AI [8]. Neither apo B mRNA nor the protein nor the low density lipoproteins, LDLs, were found in human CSF, indicating that apo B-containing Lps are not produced in CNS [2,3,9,10]. Just recently we described for the first time the presence of the Lipoprotein(a), Lp(a), in CSF of patients affected by neurological diseases characterized by blood-CSF barrier dysfunction [11].

While the synthesis and metabolism of plasma Lps are well characterized, the presence of Lps in CSF and their role in the brain metabolism have not yet been fully elucidated.

However, increased interest on the topic has been stimulated by the finding of the association of some Lps with pathological processes in CNS.

This chapter intends to highlights the physiological presence of the Lps in CNS, but especially the pathological roles deriving from their isoforms. In particular we want to focus on the anomalous presence in CSF of Lp(a), due to the crossing of the blood-CSF barrier, possibly affecting the normal activity of CNS.

Presence and Physiological Activity of Lipoproteins in CNS

Among the apos known in human plasma, apo AI and E are the most abundant found in human CSF. However, also apo AII, AIV, CI, CII, CIII, D, and J have been isolated and characterized in CSF by ultracentrifugation and gel chromatography analyses [7]. Table 1 summarizes the approximate content in lipids and the major apos of the Lps in human CSF and their percentage with respect to plasma level.

Table 1. Components of human CSF lipoproteins and percentage with respect to plasma concentration

	Concentration (μg/ml)	%	References
Phospholipids	6.0	0.3	[10,17]
Total cholesterol	4.0	0.2	[10,17]]
Triglycerides	0.2	0.02	[17]
apo E	3.0	4.0	[2,10]
apo AI	4.0	0.3	[2,10]

On the basis of cholesterol, phospholipids, and triglycerides content as well as apos presence, Lps can be distinct in two main classes relatively enriched for apo AI or apo E and other two classes characterized by the presence of the other Lps [2,3,9,10]. The Lps present in human CSF are mostly spherical and discoidal, in form of a $\rho < 1.210$ g/l fraction, similar in size to plasma high density lipoproteins, HDLs [2,3,9,12]. Three possibilities have been considered on the origin of Lps in CSF: free apos deriving from plasma can combine with lipids in the CSF; whole Lps are transferred to CSF with a mechanism different from that responsible for the transfer of other plasma proteins; finally apos can be synthesized in the CNS [2].

The fact that apo E is present in CSF at concentrations exceeding what would be expected for a filtered plasma protein (4-5% of that present in plasma) [2], indicates that apo E is a secretory product of the brain. Apo E is synthesized and secreted primarily by the liver, but, unlike other apos, it is also synthesized and secreted, to a lesser extent, by many other tissues. The brain is among those tissues with the highest concentrations of apo E mRNA in all animals tested, including humans [3-6]. Direct evidence for apo E synthesis within the brain was obtained by immunocytochemistry: Boyles et al. [6] demonstrated that in rat all types of astrocytes contain high concentrations of apo E mRNA and protein and are able to secrete it. The expression of apo E mRNA in rat microglia was also demonstrated [4]. Apo D and apo J also are synthesized in rat and human astrocytes [13-15]. Other CSF apos apparently are incorporated into the brain. For example, there is no significantly detectable mRNA for apo AI, apo AII, or apo AIV in neurons or glia, although these proteins have been localized in brain endothelial and epithelial cells [8,16-18]. In contrast to the periphery, there is not detectable apo B mRNA or protein in the normal CNS and investigation of apo B-containing Lps in normal human CSF failed to confirm the presence of LDLs [2,3,9,10]. Similarly, neither apo(a) nor Lp(a) were found in normal human CSF.

The presence of apos and Lps in normal brain and CSF suggests that they are involved in lipid transport and play a role in the cholesterol homeostasis in the CNS. The expression of apo B, E(LDL) receptors by brain cells, as the mediator of Lps internalization, implies for CNS mechanisms similar to that of other tissues [3].

The brain derives cholesterol both from plasma and from *de novo* synthesis: thus, cholesterol homeostasis in brain cells is maintained by the perfect balance between cholesterol influx through the apo E receptor family and cholesterol synthesis, in a way that the adult brain does not accumulate cholesterol. The Lps in CSF, in particular those containing apo E, could provide the mechanism to redistribute cholesterol to the cells and remove its excess with the flow of the CSF. The apo AI-containing Lps in CSF might also remove cholesterol from the brain [3,19].

Furthermore, apo E produced by the astrocytes contributes to regulate neurotransmission, growth factor release and immune response, thus acting as a critical and multifunctional signaling molecule in the brain [20-26].

Apo E secretion and accumulation in the regenerating peripheral nerve has been also demonstrated. This observation suggests that apo E plays a central role in transport of lipids necessary in axon regeneration, *de novo* axon growth, and nerve maturation [27-29]. In fact, from *in vitro* and animal studies apo E-containing Lps have been associated with the process of the CNS cholesterol recycling, in response to acute brain injury [30-31].

APO E IN NEUROLOGICAL DISEASES

Human apo E is unique among apos in having a special relevance to the central and peripheral nervous systems.

An important biochemical characteristic of human apo E stems from the polymorphism of its gene having three different common alleles: *APO E*-ε2, *APO E*-ε3, and *APO E*-ε4 that account for three major isoforms, apo E2, apo E3, and apo E4. The isoforms are distinguishable by having different combinations of the amino acids arginine and cysteine at positions 112 and 158. The amino acid changes result in distinctive physical and biochemical properties, such as the domain interaction and protein stability [32-33].

APO E-ε3 allele is predominant in all populations, while *APO E*-ε4 allele is the less common allele [34] and is associated with poor clinical outcome in patients with a variety of acute brain injuries, such as traumatic injury, intracerebral haemorrhage, aneurismal subarachnoid haemorrhage [35-39], and with chronic and age-related neurodegenerative diseases, such as Alzheimer's disease, AD. Whereas *APO E*-ε2 allele is considered protective [40,41], *APO E*-ε4 is a major susceptibility allele for sporadic and familial late-onset AD [42-46]. *APO E*-ε4 allele affects with a clear gene-dose effect the rate of the disease progression, the extent of the neuronal cell loss, the beta amyloid production and deposition of amyloid plaques in the brain of AD subjects [42]. AD apo E4 carriers exhibit poor synaptic remodelling and defective compensatory plasticity in brain areas [47,48]. There is an inverse relationship between *APO E*-ε4 allele copy number and brain cholinergic activity in the brains of subjects with AD [49].

Protein instability and misfolding are important component of neurodegenerative diseases: apo E4 is the least stable of the apo E isoforms, and exists as a partially folded intermediate, called molten globule, and in apo E4, but not to the same extent in the other two isoforms, the N-domain and C-domain interact. These structural properties of apo E4 confer characteristics to this isoform that associate it to neuropathology. Domain interaction increases beta amyloid production and deposition, leading to plaque formation [50,51]. Apo E4 can undergo neuron-specific proteolytic cleavage that produces C-terminal fragments that disrupt the cytoskeleton of neuron, interfere with the mitochondrial functions, and cause cell death, thus promoting neurodegeneration [33,50].

Moreover, the therapeutic response to drugs in AD resulted genotypic-specific, since the apo E 4/4 carriers are the worst responders to conventional treatments [49,52]. Based on these data, another aspect to be considered is the possible role of apo E as a therapeutic target for AD. Since *APO E*-ε4 allele affects cholinergic activity in the brain of subjects with AD, as well as the drug response to cholinomimetic agents, the utility of the pharmacogenomics has been highlighted for drug therapies in central nervous system [49,52].

Regarding the mechanisms underlying the link between *APO E*-ε4 allele and AD, it is still not completely clear. It has been postulated that it is related to disturbance in brain Lps metabolism [53], or even in one of the other neurobiological roles attributed to apo E isoforms, including stabilizers of microtubules, molecular chaperones of amyloidogenic peptides, immunomodulatory molecules, antioxidants and neurotrophins [20,24-26,54-57].

Lps in CSF from AD patients have different concentrations, lipid content and apos composition with respect to plasma Lps [18]. Apo E and apo AI can also exist in a subclass of very high density Lps, poor in lipid, not represented in the ρ <1.210 g/ml fraction, and rarely seen in the normal plasma [58]. Although the reports are conflicting, the association between lower levels of apo E-containing Lps and apo E4 isoform has been proven in AD brain tissues [18,44]. It was proposed that together with the qualitative modification of the apo E structure due to the *APO E*-ε4 allele, quantitative variations of *APO E* mRNA expression played a major role in risk determination. A polymorphism in the *APO E* regulatory region was found to modify significantly *APO E* allelic mRNA expression levels in human AD brain tissue and was associated with the risk of developing AD [59]. The association between ε4 allele and apo E levels may be the results of a linkage disequilibrium between the E4 allele and promoter variants controlling the apo E production [60]. The quantitative alteration of apo E levels seems to be crucial to the correct lipid homeostasis in brain, thus contributing to the pathology. As a confirm, experiments with animal models demonstrated, in apo E knockout mice, that the complete absence of apo E in the brain compromises synaptic density and reinnervation in the adult mice, strongly suggesting the potential role of apo E in the maintenance of synaptic integrity and plasticity in the CNS [61]. Further, results on apo E-/- transgenic mice showed that apo E deficiency contributes to the formation of a leaky blood-brain barrier consequent to brain injuries, neurodegenerative diseases, such as AD, and age-related changes, and indicated that apo E is crucial for maintaining the integrity of the blood-brain barrier and for its effective recovery [62].

It is also important to note that in CSF of AD patients polyunsatured fatty acids have significantly decreased levels: since they are the lipids most labile to free radical-mediated damage, it has been hypothesized that in this situation Lps are exposed to greater oxidative stress than in normal individuals, and are more susceptible to lipid peroxidation [18]. It has been demonstrated that oxidized plasma Lps can be toxic to a variety of cells in culture, including neurons. In particular, LDL and its major protein, apo B, is prone to oxidation in circulation and the resultant oxidized LDL is internalized by several types of cells, to which it is cytotoxic [63]. Although neither apo B mRNA nor the protein is present in normal human CNS, in the cases of injury to brain, increased oxidative stress, in association with disruption of the blood-brain barrier, raises the possibility of exposing the CNS to oxidized LDL that may activate innate immunity and thereby influence indirectly neuronal survival [64]. Indeed, Apo B and oxidized LDLs have been found in the CNS of patients with ischemic injury, with a positive correlation between their concentration and CSF/serum albumin ratio, the main index of damaged blood-brain barrier. It has been demonstrated with *in vitro* experiments that oxidized LDLs can be internalized by cultured astrocytes, thereby stimulating IL-6 secretion and influencing the neuronal survival [62]. In similar way, Lps in CSF of AD patients, subjected to increased lipid peroxidation, can become deleterious to neuronal cells [65].

APO E-ε4 allele has also been supposed to be associated with the risk of Parkinson disease, PD, and with the presence of some clinical features in PD patients. However, the role of *APO E*-ε4 allele in risk of PD remains unclear. In most of the studies, no significant association between *APO E*-ε4 allele and PD was found. Probably because of the multifactorial aetiology of PD, a susceptibility gene would be expected to have only a modest association with the disease, that requires the analysis of very large study groups [66,67]. By using meta-analysis criteria, *APO E*-ε4 allele appears to be associated with a higher prevalence of dementia in PD [68].

The possible association between apo E and multiple sclerosis, MS, has been also considered. As repair of nerve tissue and immunomodulation are essential for the restoration of CNS function after MS relapses, *APO-E* genotype could influence the risk for development or clinical progression of MS. The available results indicate that *APO*-ε4 does not immediately bias the development of MS, but it can be considered a predisposing factor to a faster disease progression. Overall, these findings do not definitively support a role for *APO E* in MS, and underscore the importance of using large sample sizes to detect modest genetic effects, particularly in studies of genotype-phenotype relationships [69-71].

Table 2 summarizes the principal roles of apo E isoforms in normal and diseased CNS.

Table 2. Roles of apo E isoforms in CNS

		References
Protective effects of apo E3	Lipid transport and cholesterol homeostasis	[19]
	Immune response	[24-26]
	Neuron growth and axon regeneration	[27-29]
	Antioxidant effect	[55,56]
Pathological effects of apo E4	Altered lipid metabolism	[53]
	Amyloid β production and deposition	[50,51]
	Mitochondrial function interference	[50]
	Lysosomal leakage and apoptosis	[50]
	Cytoskeleton disruption	[54]

Finally, because of its influence on the outcome in acute and chronic neurological diseases, by down-regulating glial activation and neuroinflammatory response, it has been proposed that apo E can be used for therapeutic purposes. Based on the knowledge of the unique conformational and biophysical properties of apo E4, domain interaction and molten globule formation, a new therapeutic strategy could be to identify small molecules to modulate the neuropathological structure of apo E4 and convert it to an apo E3-like molecule. Other possibility would be to inhibit the apo E-cleaving enzyme to prevent the generation of toxic apo E4 fragments [33,50].

Another potential therapeutic strategy is based on the administration of intact apo E3 to patients with CNS diseases or injury. This seems to be successful in animal models. However, such method is too invasive; furthermore, the entire protein has difficulty to cross the blood-brain barrier and it is unlikely that it would readily enter the CNS compartment. Thus, a novel approach would be synthesizing smaller peptides derived from the receptor binding region of apo E that mimic the functional anti-inflammatory and neuroprotective effects of the intact apo E protein. These apo E-derived therapeutic peptides are able to cross the blood-brain barrier and have been demonstrated to improve functional and histological outcomes in murine models of brain injury [25].

Lp(a), Structure and Pathophysiology

Lp(a) is an LDL-like lipoprotein having the distinctive apo(a) linked to apo B-100 by a disulfide bond. The apo(a) coding gene (LPA gene, 6q26-27) [72] has a variable number of tandem repeats, constituted by the plasminogen-like kringle IV-type 2 coding domain (KIV-kringle) and the apo(a) protein is structurally homologous to plasminogen [73] (Figure 1).

The LPA gene polymorphism is largely responsible for the inter-individual variability of apo(a) isoforms size (range 300-800 kDa) that characterizes human populations, and for at least 50% of Lp(a) concentrations variability in Caucasian population [74]. Several single nucleotide polymorphisms have been identified in the LPA gene 5'-flanking region that have a role in modulating the promoter activity [75]. There is an inverse relationship between Lp(a) concentration and apo(a) size, although this relation is not linear and differs among populations [76].

Many studies have been conducted on the pathophysiological role of Lp(a) in circulation. Although the findings are not exhaustive, it is well known that elevated plasma concentrations of Lp(a) (above 30mg/dl) and small dimensions of apo(a) are associated with increased risk of cardiovascular and cerebrovascular diseases [74,77-80]. The size polymorphism of apo(a) may be of importance in conveying the Lp(a)-related risk also for vascular dementia and AD [81].

The pathogenicity of Lp(a) is due to different mechanisms. Due to the high similarity of apo(a) with the fibrinolytic proenzyme plasminogen, Lp(a) competes with it for binding to lysine residues of cell membrane proteins or fibrin surfaces, resulting in decreased plasmin formation and inhibiting the breakdown of thrombi formed in the vasculature. *In vitro* data showed that fibrin and cells have higher affinity for small apo(a) isoforms than for large ones and supported a major role of small apo(a) isoforms in atherothrombotic risk [82-86]. Further,

Lp(a) can interacts with homocysteine, another independent risk factor for atherothrombosis: the additive effect of these molecules increases their pathogenic role [87]. Apo(a) also interferes with plasmin(ogen)–induced cell detachment and apoptosis of adherent cells, with an additional pathogenic potential [88]. Therefore, interaction of Lp(a) with monocyte-macrophages, for which it is a potent chemoattractant [89], may stimulate cytokines production [90,91] and contribute to the inflammatory processes inducing atheroma formation. On the other hand, according to the previous hypothesis of Brown and Goldstein [92] and the evidence of Yano et al. [93], our study on patients undergoing abdominal surgery indicated a possible role of Lp(a) in wound healing, as the cholesterol-rich particle would concentrate at sites of tissue injury [94]. Thus, the Lp(a) physiology and pathogenicity seems to generate more questions than answers [95].

Lp(a) is a ligand for the members of LDL-receptor family. Megalin/gp330, which is expressed by several cells like ependymal cells and the choroids plexus in brain, acts as a receptor of Lp(a) *in vitro* [96]. The LDL receptor related protein present on different cells, as well as the activated glial cells [97], is also able to internalize Lp(a) particles in a size-dependent manner [98]. Although the affinity of Lp(a) for these receptors is low, and a specific Lp(a) receptor is still unknown, there is evidence suggesting that *in vivo* Lp(a) may interact with several types of cells, including nerve cells, possibly eliciting their response.

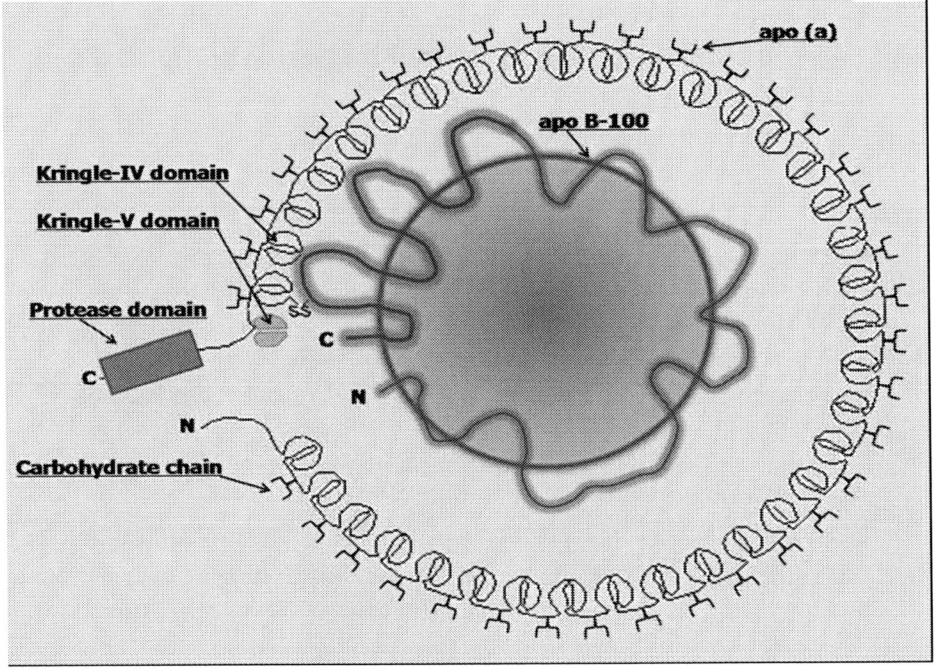

Figure 1. Model of Lp(a) particle. The LDL core of neutral lipids is surrounded by one molecule of apo B-100 which is attached to one molecule of highly glycosilated apo(a) by a single disulfide bond between the KIV-9 repeat in apo(a) and the C-terminus of apo B-100. In apo(a), KI to KIII-kringle homologous to plasminogen are not present; KIV-type 1, type 3 to 10, and KV domains are present only once; KIV-type 2 domain has a variable number; protease domain is inactive.

Lp(a) and CNS: A Study on Patients Affected by Neurological Diseases with Blood-CSF Barrier Dysfunction

No data were available about the presence of Lp(a) in the CSF until we were able to demonstrate that entire Lp(a) can cross a dysfunctional blood-CSF barrier and be found in CSF of patients with neurological diseases [11].

Paired CSF/serum samples were collected from 77 patients and routine assays were performed. The ratio of CSF to serum albumin was also calculated as the marker of blood-CSF barrier dysfunction [99].

On the basis of the diagnoses, the patients were grouped according to the state of blood-CSF barrier as follows: patients with inflammatory barrier dysfunction (IBD) caused by CNS infection (10 cases of encephalitis and 10 of meningitis), patients with non-inflammatory barrier dysfunction (NIBD) (19 affected by the Guillain Barré syndrome, 6 by chronic inflammatory demyielinating polyradiculoneuropathy, 6 by spinal stenosis, and 3 by amyotrophic lateral sclerosis) and patients with an inflammatory CNS disorder (23 patients with multiple sclerosis) but without CSF signs of barrier dysfunction (WBD).

Apo(a) was immunodetected in the CSF samples of IBD (30%) and NIBD patients (42%), but not in WBD patients, with no significant differences between the two positive groups ($P = 0.399$) (Figure 2A and 2B). Furthermore, comparison of the samples analyzed in reduced and in native conditions clearly indicated that the apo(a) detected in CSF samples was linked to apo B-100, as it was in the serum samples (Figure 2C). This finding suggests that a barrier dysfunction can permit the transmigration of the entire Lp(a) from serum into the CSF.

A wide size range of apo(a) isoforms were found in the CSF, from 18 to 35 KIV-kringles; thus, even Lp(a) particles with larger apo(a) isoform resulted able to cross the blood-CSF barrier. However, the smaller apo(a) isoforms were the most frequent in CSF. Since small apo(a) isoforms are associated with high Lp(a) concentrations in plasma, and are an independent risk factor for cardiovascular diseases, Lp(a) may have similar functional heterogeneity in the CNS.

By ELISA Lp(a) was measured in CSF samples and the results were concordant with qualitative ECL. Apo(a) was detected in the CSF from both IBD (0.11 mg/L, range 0.09–0.9) and NIBD patients (0.16 mg/L, range 0.09–0.04) and not in CSF from WBD patients (0.01 mg/L, range 0.0–0.08) with significant differences ($P = 0.002$), as shown in Figure 3.

These results suggested that the passage of Lp(a) into CSF is not influenced by the pathophysiologic mechanisms (inflammation or not inflammation) determining the blood-CSF barrier dysfunction. Instead, the amount of Lp(a) found in CSF was correlated to the degree of barrier dysfunction and to Lp(a) serum concentration.

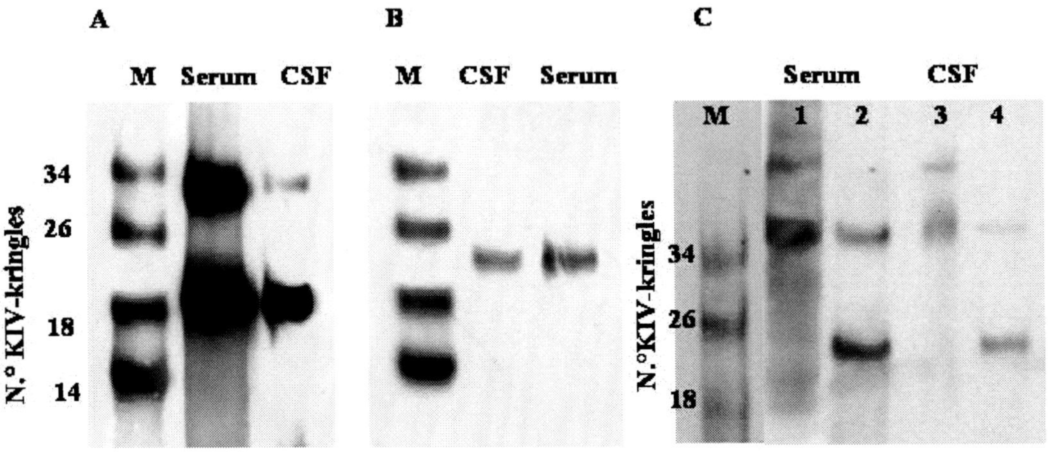

Figure 2. Apo(a) phenotyping in paired serum and CSF samples. Western blot immunodetection of (A) a sample composed by 33/19 KIV-kringles isoforms and (B) a sample composed by 25/25 KIV-kringles isoforms. Samples and marker were reduced with 2-mercaptoethanol before loading. M, mixture of recombinant apo(a) as marker. (C) Immunoblot analysis of serum and CSF samples in native and reducing conditions: lane 1, serum sample run in native conditions (loading buffer without 2-mercaptoethanol); lane 2, serum sample run after reduction with 0.5% 2-mercaptoethanol; lane 3, CSF sample run in native conditions; lane 4, CSF sample run under reducing conditions; M, a mixture of recombinant apo(a) as marker run under reducing conditions. Modified from Pepe et al. [11]. Used with permission.

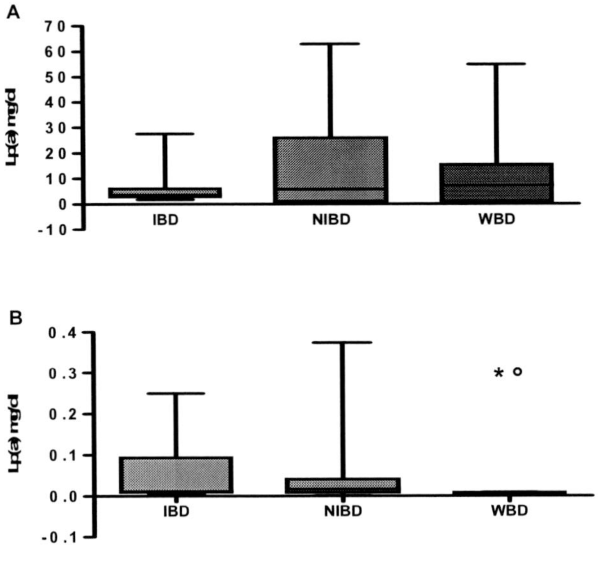

Figure 3. Lp(a) concentrations determined by ELISA. Box and whiskers representation. (A), Lp(a) concentrations in serum samples in the 3 study groups, Kruskall Wallis test; P = 0.846. (B), Lp(a) concentrations in CSF samples in the 3 study groups; Kruskall Wallis test: P = 0.002. Dunn's multiple comparison post-test; * P < 0.050 for WBD vs IBD; ° P < 0.050 for WBD vs NIBD. Reproduced from Pepe et al. [11]. Used with permission.

CONCLUSIONS

Despite the existence of the blood-brain barrier, Lps are present not only in the plasma but also in the CSF: their protein components in part filtered through the barrier from the vascular compartment, in part may originate from the nervous cells. The presence of Lps in human CSF ensures cholesterol homeostasis in CNS, however Lps with their apos are far more than lipid transporters. In particular, apo E in brain performs other neurobiological roles involved in neurotransmission, neuron growth and immune response, thus acting as a critical and multifunctional signaling molecule. The pleiotropic effects of the apo E isoforms implies that the quantitative alteration of apo E levels, or the qualitative change in apo E4 isoform is crucial for the correct functions of the brain, thus contributing to pathologies, the most frequent of them being AD.

The clear association of apo E4 with pathological processes in CNS stimulated the increased interest on the study of the role of this apo in the risk for the disease and on the research of its therapeutic potentiality. Novel therapeutic strategies have been recently designed in order to modify the pathogenic apo E4 isoform to the benefic apo E3 isoform, or use part of the molecule to improve clinical outcomes of brain injuries.

Lp(a) is another lipoparticle well known for its properties in the vascular system and with clear functions as independent risk factor for atherotrombosis. However, some evidence indicates its possible role in wound healing.

The recent discovery that, in neurological disorders characterized by the blood-CSF dysfunction, Lp(a) can be present in the CSF, which is an unusual environment for this molecule, raises new questions on its possible role in CNS where Lp(a) may extend some of its effects. It may interfere with the plasmin(ogen) system, induce cytokines production, or have other effects with possible consequences on the neuronal survival and involvement in the neurological diseases progression.

Further studies are ongoing in our laboratories to clarify the role of Lp(a) in the CNS.

ACKNOWLEDGEMENTS

The authors thank Mr. V. Cataldo for his skillful assistance in preparing the artwork.

REFERENCES

[1] Swahn, B; Bronnestam, R; Dencker SJ. On the origin of the lipoproteins in the cerebrospinal fluid. *Neurology*. 1961 11, 437-440.

[2] Roheim, PS; Carey, M; Forte, T; Vega GL. Apolipoproteins in human cerebrospinal fluid. *Proc. Natl. Acad Sci. USA*. 1979 76, 4646-4649.

[3] Pitas, RE; Boyles, JK; Lee, SH; Hui, D; Weisgraber, KH. Lipoproteins and their receptors in the central nervous system. Characterization of the lipoproteins in

cerebrospinal fluid and identification of apolipoprotein B, E(LDL) receptors in the brain. *J. Biol. Chem.* 1987 262,14352-14360.

[4] Nakai, M; Kawamata, T; Taniguchi, K.; Maeda, K; Tanaka, C. Expression of apolipoprotein E mRNA in rat microglia. *Neurol. Sci Lett.* 1996 211, 41-44.

[5] Elshourbagy, NA; Liao, WS; Mahley, RW; Taylor, M. Apolipoprotein E mRNA is abundant in the brain and adrenals, as well as in the liver, and is present in other peripheral tissues of rats and marmosets. *Proc. Natl. Acad. Sci. USA.* 1985 82, 203-207.

[6] Boyles, JK; Pitas, RE; Wilson, E; Mahley, RW; Taylor, JM. Apolipoprotein E associated with astrocytic glia of the central nervous system and with non myelinating glia of the peripheral nervous system. *J. Clin. Invest.* 1985 76, 1501-1513.

[7] Koch, S; Beisiegel, U. Lipoproteins in the brain: a new frontier? In: Betteridge, DJ., Dunitz, M. editors, Lipids and vascular disease. London. 2000, 51-64.

[8] Elshourbagy, NA; Boguski, MS; Liao, WS; Jefferson, LS; Gordon, JI; Taylor, JM. Expression of rat apolipoprotein A-IV and A-I genes: mRNA induction during development and in response to glucocorticoids and insulin. *Proc. Nat. Acad. Sci. USA.* 1985 82, 8242-8246.

[9] Borghini, I; Barja, F; Pometta, D; James, RW. Characterization of subpopulations of lipoprotein particles isolated from human cerebrospinal fluid. *Biochim. Biophys. Acta* 1995 1255, 192-200.

[10] Koch, S; Donarski, N; Goetze, K; Kreckel, M; Stuerenburg, H-j; Beisiegel, U. Characterization of four lipoprotein classes in human cerebrospinal fluid. *J. Lipid Res.* 2001 42, 1143-1150.

[11] Pepe, G; Chimienti, G; Liuzzi, GM; Lamanuzzi, BL; Nardulli, M; Lolli, F; Anglés-Cano, E; Matà, S. Lipoprotein(a) in the cerebrospinal fluid of neurological patients with blood-cerebrospinal fluid barrier dysfunction. *Clin.Chem.* 2006 52, 2043-2048.

[12] Felgenhauer, D. Protein size and cerebrospinal fluid composition. *Klin. Wochenschr.* 1974 52, 1158-1164.

[13] Patel, SC; Asotra, K; Patel, YC; McConathy, WJ; Patel, RC; Suresh, S. Astrocytes synthesize and secrete the lipophilic ligand carrier apolipoprotein D. *Neuroreport.* 1995 6, 653-7.

[14] Harr, SD; Uint, L; Hollister, R, Hyman, BT; Mendez, AJ. Brain expression of apolipoproteins E, J, and A-I in Alzheimer's disease. *J. Neurochem.*1996 66, 2429-2435.

[15] LaDu, MJ; Gilligan, SM; Lukens, JR; Cabana, VG; Reardon, CA; Van Eldik, LJ; Holtzman, DM. Nascent astrocyte particles differ from lipoproteins in CSF. J. Neurochem. 1998 70, 2070-2081.

[16] Mockel, B; Zinke, H; Flach, R; Weiss, B; Weiler-Guttler, H; Gasses, HG. Expression of apolipoprotein AI in porcine brain endothelium in vitro. *J. Neurochem.* 1994 62,788-798.

[17] Weiler-Guttler, H; Sommerfeldt, M; Papandrikopoulou, A; Mischek, U; Bonitz, D; Fery, A; Gruppe, M; Scheerer, J; Gassen, HG. Synthesis of apolipoprotein AI in pig brain microvascular endothelial cells. *J. Neurochem.* 1990 54, 444-450.

[18] Basset, CN; Montine, KS; Neely, MD; Swift, LL; Montine, TJ. Cerebrospinal fluid lipoproteins in Alzheimer's disease. *Micros. Res. Tech.* 2000 50, 282-286.

[19] Vance, JE; Hayashi, H; Karten, B. Cholesterol homeostasis in neurons and glial cells. *Semin Cell Dev Biol.* 2005 16,193-212.

[20] Mahley, RW. Apolipoprotein E: cholesterol transport protein with expanding role in cell biology. *Science* 1988 240, 622-630.

[21] Gee, JR.; Keller, JN. Astrocytes: regulation of brain homeostasis via apolipoprotein E. *Int. J. Biochem Cell Biol.* 2005 37, 1145-1150.

[22] Swertfeger, DK; Hui, DY. Apolipoprotein E: a cholesterol transport protein with lipid transport-independent cell signalling properties. *Front Biosci.* 2001 6, D526-35.

[23] Mahley, RW. Apolipoprotein E: far more than a lipid transport protein. *Annu. Rev. Genomics Hum. Genet.* 2000 1, 507-37.

[24] Laskowitz, DT; Lee, DM; Schmechel, D; Staats, HF. Altered immune responses in apolipoprotein E-deficient mice. *J Lipid Res.* 2000 41, 613-20.

[25] Laskowitz DT., Fillit H., Yeung N., Toku K., Vitek MP. Apolipoprotein E-derived peptides reduce CNS inflammation: implications for therapy of neurological disease. Acta Neurol. Scand. Suppl. 2006;185:15-20.

[26] Lynch, JR; Tang, W; Wang, H, Vitek, MP; Bennett, ER; Sullivan, PM; Warner, DS; Laskowitz, DT. APO E genotype and an Apo E-mimetic peptide modify the systemic and central nervous system inflammatory response. *J Biol Chem.* 2003 278, 48529-33.

[27] Ignatius, MJ; Gebicke-Harter, PJ; Skene, JH, Schilling, JW; Weisgraber, KH; Mahley, RW; Shooter, EM. Expression of apolipoprotein E during nerve degeneration and regeneration. *Proc. Natl. Acad. Sci. USA.* 1986 83,1125-1129.

[28] Snipes, GJ; McGuire, CB; Norden, JJ; Freeman, JA. Nerve injury stimulates the secretion of apolipoprotein E by non-neuronal cells. *Proc. Natl. Acad. Sci. USA.* 1986 83, 1130-1134.

[29] Boyles, JK; Zoellner, CD; Anderson, LJ; Kosik, LM; Pitas, RE; Weisgraber, KH; Hui,DY;. Mahley, RW; Gebicke-Haerter, PJ; Ignatius, MJ; Shooter, EM. A role for Apolipoprotein E, Apolipoprotein A-I, and Low Density Lipoprotein receptors in cholesterol transport during regeneration and remyelination of the rat sciatic nerve. *J. Clin. Inv.* 1989 83, 1015-1031.

[30] Graham, DI; Horsburgh, K; Nicoll, JA; Teasdale, GM. Apolipoprotein E and the response of the brain to injury. *Acta Neurochir Suppl (Wien)* 1999 73, 89-92.

[31] White, F; Nicoll, JA; Horsburgh, K. Alterations in Apo E and ApoJ in relation to degeneration and regeneration in a mouse model of entorhinal cortex lesion. *Exp Neurol* 2001 169, 307-318.

[32] Siest, G; Pillot, T; Régis-Bailly, A; Leininger-Muller, B; Steinmetz, J; Galteau, MM; Visvikis, S Apolipoprotein E: an important gene and protein to follow in laboratory medicine. *Clinical Chemistry* 1995 41, 1068–1086.

[33] Mahley, RW; Huang, Y. Apolipoprotein (apo)E4 and Alzheimer's disease: unique conformational and biophysical properties of apo E4 can modulate neuropathology. *Acta Neurol. Scand.* 2006 114, 8-14.

[34] Utermann, G. Apolipoprotein E polymorphism in health and disease. *Am Heart J.* 1987 113,433-440.

[35] Alberts, MJ; Graffagnino, C; McClenny, C; DeLong, D; Strittmatter, W; Saunders, AM; Roses, AD. Apo E genotype and survival from intracerebral haemorrhage. *Lancet* 1995 346, 575-578.

[36] Teasdale, GM; Nicoll, JA; Murray, G; Fiddes, M. Association of apolipoprotein E polymorphism with outcome after head injury. *Lancet* 1997 350,1069-1071.

[37] McCarron, MO; Muir, KW; Nicoll, JA; Stewart, J; Currie, Y; Brown, K; Bone, I. Prospective study of apolipoprotein E genotype and functional outcome following ischemic stroke. *Arch Neurol* 2000 57,1480-1484.

[38] Kay, AD; Day, SP; Kerr, M; Nicoll, JA; Packard, CJ; Caslake, MJ. Remodelling of cerebrospinal fluid lipoprotein particles after human traumatic brain injury. *J. Neurotrauma*. 2003 20,717-723.

[39] Kay, AD; Day, SP; Kerr, M; Nicoll, JA; Packard, CJ; Caslake, MJ. Remodelling of cerebrospinal fluid lipoprotein after subarachnoid hemorrhage. *Atheroscl.* 2003 170, 141-146.

[40] Corder, EH; Saunders, AM; Risch, NJ; Strittmatter, WH; Schmechel, DE; Gaskell, PJ; Rimmler, JB; Locke, PA; Conneally, PM; Schmader, KE. Protective effect of apolipoprotein E type 2 allele for late onset Alzheimer's disease. *Nat. Genet.* 1994 7,180-184.

[41] Lippa, CF; Smith, TW; Saunders, AM, Hulette, C, Pulaski-Salo, D, Roses, AD. Apolipoprotein E-epsilon 2 and Alzheimer's disease: genotype influences pathologic phenotype. *Neurology.* 1997 48, 515-519.

[42] Corder, EH; Saunders, AM; Strittmatter, WJ; Schmechel, DE; Gaskell, PC; Small, GW; Roses, AD; Haines, JL; Pericak-Vance, MA. Gene dose of apolipoprotein E type 4 allele and the risk of Alzheimer's disease in late onset families. *Science.* 1993 26, 921-3.

[43] Poirier, J; Davignon, J; Bouthillier, D, Kogan, S; Bertrand, J; Gauthier, S. Apolipoprotein E polymorphism and Alzheimer's disease. *Lancet* 1993 342, 697–699.

[44] Strittmatter, WJ; Roses, AD. Apolipoprotein E and Alzheimer's diseases. *Proc. Natl. Acad. Sci. USA* 1995 92, 4725-4727.

[45] Poirier, J. Apolipoprotein E, cholesterol transport and synthesis in sporadic Alzheimer's disease. *Neurol Aging.* 2005 26, 355-361.

[46] Roses, AD. On the discovery of the genetic association of Apolipoprotein E genotypes and common late-onset Alzheimer disease. *J. Alzheimer's Dis.* 2006 9, 361-6.

[47] Arendt, T; Schindler, C; Bruckner, MK; Eschrich, K; Bigl, V; Zedlick, D, Marcova, L. Plastic neuronal remodeling is impaired in patients with Alzheimer's disease carrying apolipoprotein epsilon 4 allele. *J Neurosci* 1997 17, 516–29.

[48] Beffert, U; Cohn, JS; Petit-Turcotte, C; Tremblay, M; Aumont, N; Ramassamy, C, Davignon, J ; Poirier, J. Apolipoprotein E and beta amyloid levels in the hippocampus and frontal cortex of Alzheimer's disease subjects are disease-related and apolipoprotein E genotype dependant. *Brain Res.* 1999 843, 87–94.

[49] Poirier, J. Apolipoprotein E: A pharmacogenetic target for the treatment of Alzheimer's disease. *Mol Diagnosis* 1999 4, 335-341.

[50] Mahley, RW; Weisgraber, KH; Huang, Y. Apolipoprotein E4: a causative factor and therapeutic target in neuropathology, including Alzheimer's disease. *Proc. Natl Acad. Sci USA* 2006 103, 5644-5651.

[51] Sanan, DA; Weisgraber, KH; Russell, SJ; Mahley, RW; Huang, D; Saunders, A; Schmechel, D; Wisniewski, T; Frangione, B; Roses, AD. Apolipoprotein E associates with beta amyloid peptide of Alzheimer's disease to form novel monofibrils. Isoform apo E4 associates more efficiently than apo E3. *J.Clin.Invest.*1994 94, 860-869.

[52] Cacabelos, R. Molecular pathology and pharmacogenomics in Alzheimer's disease: polygenic-related effects of multifactorial treatments on cognition, anxiety and depression. *Methods Find Exp. Clin. Pharmacol.* 2007 29, 1-91.

[53] Danik, M; Champagne, D; Petit-Turcotte, C; Beffert, U; Poirier, J. Brain lipoprotein metabolism and its relation to neurodegenerative disease. *Crit. Rev. Neurobiol.* 1999 13, 357-407.

[54] Mahley RW, Nathan BP, Bellosta S, Pitas RE. Apolipoprotein E: impact of cytoskeletal stability in neurons and the relationship to Alzheimer's disease. *Curr Opin Lipidol.* 1995 6, 86-91.

[55] Lauderback, CM; Kanski, J; Hackett, JM; Maeda, N; Kindy, MS; Butterfield, DA. Apolipoprotein E modulates Alzheimer's Abeta(1-42)-induced oxidative damage to synaptosomes in an allele-specific manner. *Brain Res.* 2002 924, 90-7.

[56] Miyata, M; Smith, JD. Apolipoprotein E allele-specific antioxidant activity and effects on cytotoxicity by oxidative insults and beta-amyloid peptides. *Nat Genet.* 1996 14, 55-61.

[57] Roses, AD. On the metabolism of apolipoprotein E and the Alzheimer diseases. *Exp Neurol.* 1995 132, 149-56.

[58] Montine, TJ; Montine, KS; Swift, LL. Central nervous system lipoproteins in Alzheimer's diseases. *Am. J. Pathol.* 1997 151, 1571-1575.

[59] Lambert, JC; Pasquier, F; Cottel, D; Frigard, B; Amouyel, P; Chartier-Harlin, MC. A new polymorphism in the APO E promoter associated with risk of developing Alzheimer's disease. *Hum. Mol. Genet.* 1998 7, 533–540.

[60] Lambert, JC; Brousseau, T; Defisse, V; Evans, A; Arveiler, D; Ruidavets, JB; Haas, B; Cambou, JP; Luc, G; Ducimetière, P.; Cambien, F; Chartier-Harlin, MC; Amouyel, P. Independent association of an APO E gene promoter polymorphism with increased risk of myocardial infarction and decreased APO E plasma concentrations—the ECTIM Study. *Hum Mol Genetics,* 2000 9, 1, 57-61.

[61] Poirier, J. Apolipoprotein E in animal models of CNS injury and in Alzheimer's disease. *TINS* 1994 17,525-530.

[62] Hafezi-Moghadam, A; Thomas, KL; Wagner, DD. Apo E deficiency leads to a progressive age-dependent blood-brain barrier leakage. *Am. J. Physiol. Cell Physiol.* 2007 292,1256-1262.

[63] Horkko, S; Binder, CJ; Shaw, PX; Chang, MK; Silverman, G; Palinski, W; Witztum, JL; Immunological responses to oxidized LDL. *Free Rad.Biol. Med.* 2000 28,1771-1779.

[64] Shie, FS; Neely, MD; Maezawa, I.; Wu, H; Olson, SJ; Jutgens, G; Montine, KS; Montine, TJ; Oxidized Low Density Lipoprotein is present in astrocytes surrounding

cerebral infarcts and stimulates astrocyte interleukin-6 secretion. *Am. J. Pathol.* 2004 164,1173-1181.

[65] Bassett, CN; Neely, MD; Sidell, KR; Swift, LL; Montine, TJ. CSF lipoproteins are more vulnerable to oxidation in Alzheimer's disease and are neurotoxic when oxidized ex vivo. *Lipids* 1999 34,1273-1280.

[66] Huang, X; Chen, PC; Poole, C. *APO E*-2 allele associated with higher prevalence of sporadic Parkinson disease. *Neurology* 2004 62, 2198–2202.

[67] Jasinska-Myga, B; Opala, G; Goetz, CG; Tustanowski, J; Ochudlo, S; Gorzkowska, A; Tyrpa, J. Apolipoprotein E gene polymorphism, total plasma cholesterol level, and Parkinson disease dementia. *Arch Neurol.* 2007 64, 261-5.

[68] Huang, X; Chen, P; Kaufer, DI; Tröster, AI; Poole, C. Apolipoprotein E and dementia in Parkinson disease: a meta-analysis. *Arch Neurol.* 2006 63,189-93.

[69] Pinholta, M; Frederiksen, JL; Christiansen, M. The association between apolipoprotein E and multiple sclerosis. *Eur. J. Neurol.* 2006 13, 573–580.

[70] Burwick, RM; Ramsay, PP; Haines, JL; Hauser, SL; Oksenberg, JR; Pericak-Vance, MA; Schmidt, S; Compston, A; Sawcer, S; Cittadella, R; Savettieri, G; Quattrone, A; Polman,CH; Uitdehaag, BM; Zwemmer, JN; Hawkins, CP; Ollier, WE; Weatherby, S; Enzinger, C; Fazekas, F; Schmidt, H; Schmidt, R; Hillert, J; Masterman, T; Hogh, P; Niino, M; Kikuchi, S; Maciel, P; Santos, M; Rio, ME; Kwiecinski, H; Zakrzewska-Pniewska, B; Evangelou, N; Palace, J; Barcellos, LF. *APO E* epsilon variation in multiple sclerosis susceptibility and disease severity: Some answers. *Neurology* 2006 66,1373-1383.

[71] Fazekas, F.; Enzinger, C; Ropele, S; Schmidt, H; Strasser-Fuchs, S. The impact of our genes: consequences of the apolipoprotein E polymorphysm in Alzheimer disease and multiple sclerosis. *J. Neurol.Sci.* 2006 245,35-39.

[72] Frank, SL; Klisak, I; Sparkes, RS; Mohandas, T; Tomlinson, JE; McLean, JW; Lawn, RM; Lusis, AJ. The apolipoprotein(a) gene resides on human chromosome 6q26-27, in close proximity to the homologous gene for plasminogen. *Hum. Genet.* 1988 79, 352–356.

[73] McLean, JW; Tomlinson, JE; Kuang, WJ; Eaton, DL; Chen, EY; Fless, GM; Scanu, AM; Lawn, RM. cDNA sequence of human apolipoprotein(a) is homologous to plasminogen. *Nature* 1987 300,132-7.

[74] Utermann, G. Lipoprotein(a). In: Scriver CR., Beaudet AL., Sly WS., Stambury JB., Wyngaarden JB., Fredrickson DS. Editors. The metabolic and molecular bases of inherited diseases. New York: McGrow-Hill, Inc.; 1995;1887-912.

[75] Suzuki,K; Kuriyama, M; Saito, T; Ichinose, A. Plasma lipoprotein(a) levels and expression of the apolipoprotein(a) gene are dependent on the nucleotide polymorphisms in its 5'-flanking region. *J. Clin. Invest.* 1997 99, 1361–1366.

[76] Kraft, HG; Lingenhel, A; Pang, RW; Delport, R; Trommsdorff, M; Vermaak, H; Janus, ED; Utermann, G. Frequency distribution of apolipoprotein(a) kringle IV repeat alleles and their effects on lipoprotein(a) levels in Caucasian, Asian, and African populations: the distribution of null alleles is non-random. *Eur. J. Hum. Genet.* 1996 4, 74-87.

[77] de la Pena-Diaz, A; Izaguirre-Avila, R; Anglés-Cano, E. Lipoprotein Lp(a) and atherothrombotic disease. *Arch. Med. Res.* 2000 31, 353-9.

[78] Chimienti, G; Lamanuzzi, BL; Nardulli, M; Colacicco, AM; Capurso, A; La Gioia, R; Scrutinio, D; Pepe, G. Apo(a) variants and Lipoprotein(a) in men with or without myocardial infarction. *Exp. Mo.l Pathol.* 2002 73, 28-34.

[79] Morrisett, JD. The role of lipoprotein(a) in atherosclerosis. *Curr. Atheroscler. Rep.* 2000 2, 243-250.

[80] Kamstrup, PR; Benn, M; Tybjærg-Hansen, A; Nordestgaard, BG. Extreme Lipoprotein(a) Levels and Risk of Myocardial Infarction in the General Population. The Copenhagen City Heart Study. *Circulation* 2008 117,176-184.

[81] Emanuele, E; Peros, E; Tomaino, C; Feudatari, E; Bernardi, L; Binetti, G; Maletta, R; Micieli, G; Bruni, AC; Geroldi, D. Relation of apolipoprotein(a) size to Alzheimer's disease and vascular dementia. *Dement. Geriatr. Cogn. Disord.* 2004 18, 189-196.

[82] Kang, C; Durlach, V; Soulat, T; Fournier, C; Anglés-Cano, E. Lipoprotein(a) isoforms display differences in affinity for plasminogen-like binding to human mononuclear cells. *Arterioscler. Thromb. Vasc. Biol.* 1997 17, 2036-43.

[83] Lamanuzzi, BL; Mtairag, EM, Pepe, G; Anglés-Cano, E. Neutrophils stimulated by apolipoprotein(a) generate fragments that are stronger inhibitors of plasmin formation than apo(a). *Thromb. Haemost.* 2004 92, 1066-75.

[84] Marcovina, SM; Koschinsky, ML. Evaluation of lipoprotein(a) as a prothrombotic factor: progress from bench to bedside. *Curr. Opin. Lipidol.* 2003 14, 361-366.

[85] Soulat, T; Loyau, S ; Baudouin, V ; Maisonneuve, L ; Hurtaud-Roux, MF ; Schlegel, N ; Loirat, C ; Anglés-Cano, E. Effect of individual plasma lipoprotein(a) variations in vivo on its competition with plasminogen for fibrin and cell binding: An in vitro study using plasma from children with idiopathic nephrotic syndrome. *Arterioscler. Thromb.Vasc. Biol.* 2000 20, 575-584.

[86] Emanuele, E; Peros, E; Minoretti, P; D'Angelo, A; Montagna, L; Falcone, C; Geroldi, D. Significance of apolipoprotein(a) phenotypes in acute coronary syndromes: relation with clinical presentation. *Clin Chim Acta* 2004 350, 159-65.

[87] Nardulli, M; Durlach, V; Pepe, G; Anglés-Cano, E. Mechanism for the homocysteine-enhanced antifibrinolytic potential of lipoprotein(a) in human plasma. *Thromb. Haem.* 2000 94, 75-81.

[88] Ho-Tin-Noé, B; Meilhac, O; Rossignol, P; Lijnen, R; Anglés-Cano, E. Dual effect of apolipoprotein(a) on plasmin(ogen)-induced apoptosis through modulation of cell detachment of adherent cells. *Thromb. Haemost.* 2006 95, 2-9.

[89] Poon, M; Zhang, X; Dunsky, KG; Taubman, MB; Harpel, PC. Apolipoprotein(a) induces monocyte chemotactic activity in human vascular endothelial cells. *Circulation* 1997 96, 2514-2519.

[90] Klezovitch, O; Edelstein, C; Scanu, AM. Stimulation of interleukin-8 production in human THP-1 macrophages by apolipoprotein(a). *J. Biol. Chem.* 2001 276, 46864-46869.

[91] Buechler, C; Ullrich, H; Aslanidis, C; Bared, SM; Lingenhel, A; Ritter, M; Schmitz, G. Lipoprotein(a) downregulates lysosomal acid lipase and induces interleukin-6 in human blood monocytes. *Biochim. Biophys. Acta* 2003 1642, 25-31.

[92] Brown, MS, Goldstein, JL. Plasma lipoproteins: teaching old dogmas new tricks. *Nature* 1987 330, 113-114.

[93] Yano, Y; Shimokawa, K; Okada, Y; Noma, A Immunolocalization of lipoprotein(a) in wounded tissues. *J Histochem Cytochem.* 1997 45, 559-568.

[94] Chimienti, G; Aquilino, F; Rotelli, MT; Russo, F; Lupo, L; Pepe, G. Lipoprotein(a), lipids and proinflammatory cytokines in patients undergoing major abdominal surgery. *Br J Surg.* 2006 93, 347-353.

[95] Koschinsky, ML. Novel insights into Lp(a) physiology and pathogenicity: more questions than answers *Cardiovasc Hematol Disord Drug Targets.* 2006 6:267-278.

[96] Niemeier, A; Willnow, T; Dieplinger, H; Jacobsen, C; Meyer, N; Hilpert, J; Beisiegel, U. Identification of megalin/gp330 as a receptor for lipoprotein (a) in vitro. *Arterioscler. Thromb. Vasc. Biol.* 1999 19, 552–61.

[97] Bauer, J.; Strauss, S; Schreiter-Gasser, U; Ganter, U; Schlegel, P; Witt, I; Yolk, B; Berger, M. Interleukin IL-6 and alfa-macroglobulin indicate an acute phase state in Alzheimer's disease cortices. *FEBS Lett.* 1991 285, 111-114.

[98] Marz, W; Beckmann, A; Scharnagl, H; Siekmeier, R; Mondorf, U; Held, I; Schneider, W; Preissner, KT; Curtiss, LK; Gross, W; Hüttinger, M. Heterogeneous lipoprotein(a) size isoforms differ by their interaction with the low density lipoprotein receptor and the low density lipoprotein receptor-related protein/2-macroglobulin receptor. *FEBS Lett.* 1993 325, 271–275.

[99] Tibbling, G; Link, H; Ohman, S. Principles of albumin and IgG analyses in neurological disorders: I. Establishment of reference value. *Scand. J. Clin. Lab. Inves.* 1977 37, 385–390.

Reviewed by Dr. Diego Geroldi, Department of Internal Medicine and Medical Therapeutics, Section of Internal Medicine, Vascular and Metabolic Diseases, IRCCS Policlinico San Matteo, P.le Golgi, 2, 27100 Pavia, Italy. e-mail: d.geroldi@smatteo.pv.it.

INDEX

A

B

C

D

E

F

G

H

I

J

K

L

M

N

O

P

Q

R

S

T

U

V

W

Y

Z